Test Item File
to accompany

Abnormal Psychology

Susan Nolen-Hoeksema
University of Michigan

Prepared by
Anita Rosenfield
Chaffey Community College

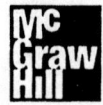

Boston, Massachusetts   Burr Ridge, Illinois   Dubuque, Iowa
Madison, Wisconsin   New York, New York   San Francisco, California   St. Louis, Missouri

McGraw-Hill

A Division of The McGraw-Hill Companies

Test Item File to accompany
ABNORMAL PSYCHOLOGY

Copyright ©1998 by The McGraw-Hill Companies, Inc. All rights reserved.
Printed in the United States of America.

The contents of, or parts thereof, may be reproduced for use with
ABNORMAL PSYCHOLOGY by Susan Nolen-Hoeksema,
provided such reproductions bear copyright notice and may be reproduced in
any form for any other purpose without permission of the publisher.

Acid-free paper
This book is printed on acid-free paper.

1 2 3 4 5 6 7 8 9 0 QPD/QPD 9 0 9 8 7

ISBN 0-697-25270-1

www.mhhe.com

Contents

Preface ... iv

Acknowledgments ... v

Learning Objectives ... vi

Part 1 Understanding and Treating Abnormality
1. Looking at Abnormality ... 1
2. Assessing and Diagnosing Abnormality ... 22
3. Approaching and Treating Abnormality ... 47

Part 2 Disorders of Anxiety, Mood, Psychosis, and Personality
4. Anxiety Disorders ... 73
5. Mood Disorders ... 98
6. The Schizophrenias ... 123
7. Dissociative and Somatoform Disorders ... 148
8. Personality Disorders ... 172

Part 3 Developmental and Health-Related Disorders
9. Childhood Disorders ... 198
10. Eating Disorders ... 221
11. Sexual Disorders ... 245
12. Substance Use Disorders ... 270
13. Personality, Behavior, and the Body ... 295
14. The Cognitive Disorders: Dementia, Delirium, and Amnesia ... 319

Part 4 The Methods, Ethics, and Policy of Abnormal Psychology
15. The Research Endeavor ... 342
16. Society and Mental Health ... 366

Preface

The classroom instructor is sufficiently overloaded with so many out-of-classroom demands, such as creating lesson plans, developing assignments, and grading papers, that adding the additional task of writing exam questions can become burdensome. It is to help lighten this load that test banks are created, thereby allowing faculty to direct their energies toward the more student-oriented activities. However, as a classroom instructor myself, I see tests as another means of educating students, rather than merely as an assessment of what they have learned; thus, the questions in this Test Item File have been written with both goals in mind.

It is often said that "good" test questions make the student think and require students to choose among several potentially tempting options. However, I try to bear in mind Lashley's rats and attempt to avoid creating in my students the "experimental neurosis" caused by not being able to distinguish between much-too-similar stimuli. Also, lest students become totally discouraged and just give up, I believe they need to see some questions that allow them to take a breather and say to themselves, "Whew! I DO know something!" Consequently, scattered in among the more difficult and demanding questions are some that may seem obvious--just as I wish to lighten the load of the faculty, I want to do the same for students. It is, of course, the instructor's choice to pick the questions that best fit that instructor's particular teaching style and goals.

The test bank consists of approximately 95 multiple choice questions and 5 or 6 essay questions per chapter. After each essay question, you will find the basic elements that would comprise a correct answer. Each multiple choice question is followed by the correct answer, a specific learning objective, whether it is factual, conceptual, or applied, and the page(s) where the information is found:

    Answer: a   LO: 1; conceptual   page: 273

The learning objectives are contained on the pages that follow, as well as in the Student Study Guide and the Instructor Course Planner. Note that a few questions were included from material contained in the text that did not fit into a stated learning objective; thus, no "LO" is indicated. With respect to whether the question is factual, conceptual, or applied, note that some are both factual and conceptual, and this is often a judgment call by the person teaching the course.

Personally, I rarely ask my students to remember numbers or dates, perhaps because they are difficult for me to remember. However, I am aware that this may be a personal issue for me, and so there are some questions that ask for numbers, percents, or dates. The applied questions range from relatively simple one- or two-line stems to much more complex scenarios. These offer the student an opportunity to consider what has been learned and to apply that information in a more practical way. Not all instructors will respond to each question in the same manner; thus, a variety of questions are provided so instructors may choose according to their own preferences. Also, you will occasionally note that the "same" question is asked more than once (although using different wording. Again, this is to allow you to choose the form of the question you prefer.

I hope you find this test bank useful and that it does, indeed, help lighten your out-of-classroom load so that you may enjoy your time in the classroom with your students as much as I enjoy my classroom time with my students.

Acknowledgments

There are many people who have helped me get this test item file (TIF) from its initial conception to its final completion. I would like to thank all of them for their help in that process. The first were Brown & Benchmark folk. My former sales representative, Lorraine Zelinski, was always on top of everything in terms of getting me the texts and ancillaries I needed for all of my classes, and she was the person who first connected me with Ted Underhill, Senior Editor at Brown & Benchmark, with whom I worked for several years as a reviewer. It was Ted who asked if I would like to write the Instructor Course Planner that will accompany this package, and that has been an absolutely exciting project for me. A week later, Kevin Campbell invited me to write this test item file, and Ted agreed that it would be appropriate for me to do both. So, to Lorraine, Ted, and Kevin, thank you for involving me in this project.

Two reviewers have been extremely helpful in critiquing the questions contained in this TIF. Both Beth Rienzi of California State University, Bakersfield and Lorry J. Cology of Owens Community College in Ohio, have devoted many hours of their time, plus their expertise, to help make this a useful and accurate test bank. In addition to checking for accuracy, Professor Cology has offered me a great deal of instruction on the proper form for multiple choice questions. Professor Rienzi, who also kept me accurate on all of the questions, offered a great deal of support and excellent ideas and suggestions particularly for structuring the essay questions. I am truly appreciative of the assistance both have provided and acknowledge their important contributions to this project. However, if any errors currently exist (hopefully not), I take full responsibility, since (pursuant to their extremely helpful suggestions) I made several changes after reviewing their comments.

Meera Dash, Senior Developmental Editor at McGraw-Hill, has also had a major impact on this TIF, providing input on form and requirements and answering many of my often unending questions. I appreciate her assistance and support.

Most of all, I would like to thank Susan Kunchandy, Editorial Coordinator at McGraw-Hill. Susan has answered ALL of my questions, and she has been patient, supportive, and a wonderful motivator. She has assisted me all the way through this project and has provided all of the assistance I have requested. Susan has helped me keep my perspective and my enthusiasm, and without her, this project would not be in your hands today. THANK YOU, SUSAN!

                                            Anita Rosenfield, Ph.D.

Learning Objectives

Chapter 1 Looking at Abnormality

1. Discuss the factors that influence whether a behavior is regarded as normal or abnormal.
2. Summarize five proposed ways to define abnormality, and discuss the merits and problems that each theory faces.
3. Describe the aspects of maladaptive or dysfunctional behavior.
4. Distinguish among supernatural, natural, and psychological theories of abnormality, and discuss how each type of theory has led to different ways of treating mentally ill people throughout history.
5. Summarize how the Ancient Chinese, Egyptians, Greeks, and Hebrews thought about abnormality and how each respective culture treated the mentally ill differently as a result.
6. Summarize the evidence for and against the idea that many people accused of witchcraft during the Middle Ages actually suffered from a mental illness.
7. Discuss the historical shift from the early mental asylums in Europe and America to the humanitarian and mental hygiene movements.
8. Discuss the different professions within Abnormal Psychology and the typical tasks of each type of professional.

Chapter 2 Assessing and Diagnosing Abnormality

1. Discuss the types of information that should be obtained during an assessment and why they are important. Also, describe the types of information required to devise an effective treatment plan.
2. Describe and give examples of each of the various tools (including biological, neuropsychological, intelligence, clinical interviews, symptom questionnaires, personality inventories, observation, and projective) used by clinicians to gather information during an assessment.
3. Discuss the advantages and disadvantages of each assessment tool.
4. Understand the differences in symptoms that clients from cultures other than an assessor's own can present.
5. Define and distinguish among the various psychometric properties (i.e., validity and reliability) that set the standard by which various assessment tools are evaluated.
6. Discuss the problems in assessment and how they might be overcome or diminished.
7. Discuss the modern method for diagnosing mental disorders, the DSM-IV, and discuss its five axes.
8. Discuss the changes in the DSM from its earliest version to its most recent version and the factors that have influenced the changes.
9. Discuss the dangers inherent in diagnosing a person with a mental disorder.

Chapter 3　　Approaching and Treating Abnormality

1. Distinguish between a biological approach and a psychosocial approach to abnormality, and discuss how each approach leads to different conceptions of the causes of abnormality and the most appropriate treatments for abnormality. Also, discuss how these two approaches are not mutually exclusive, and summarize how advocates of both approaches might work together to treat a single patient.
2. Discuss the three biological causes of abnormality, and describe the relationship between structural brain abnormalities and psychological impairment. Summarize the processes involved in communication between neurons and what aspects of this process may break down, resulting in psychological distress. Summarize how researchers investigate genetic contributions to psychopathology and the current polygenic model.
3. Describe the basic foundation of psychodynamic theory, and know each defense mechanism. Discuss how Erikson and the object relations school differ from the traditional perspective.
4. Summarize classical and operant conditioning, and give examples of each.
5. Discuss Bandura's social learning theory, and relate it to both the "pure" behavioral theories and to the cognitive theories.
6. Know and be able to distinguish among causal attributions, control beliefs, self-efficacy, dysfunctional assumptions, and automatic thoughts.
7. Discuss the elements of both humanistic and existential theories, and how they differ.
8. Know the major types of drug treatments and the symptoms they can alleviate, as well as the side effects they can cause.
9. Know the basic processes in psychodynamic, behavioral, humanistic-existential, and cognitive therapies. Describe how each therapy is predicated upon beliefs about the causes of abnormality discussed earlier in the chapter. Discuss which of these therapies have been shown to be effective. Describe how the therapist and client relate differently to one another in each therapy.
10. Distinguish between conjoint and structural family therapy.
11. Know the most effective treatments for children, the problems often encountered when treating them, and the status of drug treatments for them.
12. Discuss what the evidence has shown about matching therapist and client on race, ethnicity, and/or gender. Discuss the common components of successful therapies, and what clinicians should consider when treating clients from different cultural backgrounds.

Chapter 4　　Anxiety Disorders

1. Identify and give examples of four types of symptoms that constitute anxiety.
2. Explain the distinction between adaptive (fight-or-flight) anxiety and maladaptive anxiety.
3. Discuss the key symptoms of panic disorder, panic with agoraphobia, phobias, post-traumatic stress disorder, generalized anxiety disorder, and obsessive-compulsive disorder.
4. Discuss what it is that people who have panic with agoraphobia fear, and explain how their condition may develop in people who already have panic disorder.
5. Discuss the biological theories of panic disorder and panic with agoraphobia, as well as the evidence for them, including the safety signal hypothesis and the roles of classical and operant conditioning, cognition, and control beliefs. Also, discuss how the psychological and biological theories may be integrated into a vulnerability-stress model.

7. Discuss and contrast the biological therapies for panic disorder and panic with agoraphobia, including their effectiveness, the mechanisms by which they operate, and any negative effects that they can induce.
8. List and describe the elements of cognitive-behavioral therapies for panic disorder and panic with agoraphobia, and discuss the effectiveness of those treatments and how they compare to other treatments in terms of their effectiveness.
9. List the four most common types of specific phobias, and discuss how people with them differ from people who have mild fears of similar objects or events but who are not phobic.
10. Describe social phobia, and discuss how it might develop.
11. Discuss the psychodynamic, behavioral (including the roles of classical and operant conditioning, observational learning, and prepared classical conditioning), and biological theories of phobias, as well as the evidence for each theory.
12. Discuss the behavioral therapies for phobias (including the roles of systematic desensitization, modeling, and flooding), cognitive techniques in therapy for phobias, how people with blood-injection-injury phobias and social phobias should be treated differently from people with other types of phobias and the drug therapies for phobias. Be able to discuss how these therapies work and their effectiveness.
13. Discuss the symptoms of post-traumatic stress disorder (PTSD) and how they are manifested differently in children. Discuss the types of events that lead to PTSD and what aspects of the events themselves or the people who experience them can make PTSD more likely to develop.
14. Discuss the basic assumptions that traumatic events can shatter and the factors that predict and can account for why there are wide individual differences in reactions to traumatic events.
15. Discuss the psychosocial treatments for PTSD and how and why different types of people may need different types of therapeutic approaches to treating their conditions. Discuss also how drug therapies are used to treat PTSD and how they may be combined with psychosocial treatments.
16. Discuss how generalized anxiety disorder (GAD) differs from other anxiety disorders.
17. Describe how the conscious cognitions of people with GAD are debilitating and hinder recovery from GAD. Discuss the idea that people with GAD are vigilant for impending threats at even an unconscious level and the evidence for this idea. Discuss the most effective treatment(s) for GAD.
18. List the anxiety disorders that women are more likely than men to experience. Discuss the biological and psychosocial explanations for these gender differences.
19. Discuss how anxiety may be manifested differently among people of different cultures and how clinicians should treat them (and not treat them) in light of these differences.
20. Discuss how the prevalence of certain anxiety disorders differs among people of lower socioeconomic and educational status and what factors may lead certain groups of people to avoid developing anxiety disorders.
21. Discuss what the most common types of obsessions are, how they are distinguished from psychotic thoughts, and how they lead to compulsions.
22. Discuss the biological, psychodynamic, and cognitive theories of obsessive-compulsive disorder (OCD), as well as the evidence for them. Also, be able to discuss the treatments derived from these theories, how each treatment operates, and how effective it is for treating OCD.

Chapter 5   Mood Disorders

1. Distinguish between unipolar and bipolar depression, and know the diagnostic criteria for the disorders that fall under each category: major depression (and its associated subtypes), dysthymic disorder, double depression, Bipolar I Disorder (and its associated subtypes), Bipolar II Disorder, cyclothymic disorder, and rapid cycling bipolar disorder.
2. Explain how depression affects the whole person, i.e., cognitively, emotionally, behaviorally, and physiologically.
3. Discuss how rates of unipolar depression vary as a function of age, gender, and culture, as well as the proposed explanations for these differences.
4. Discuss the similarities and differences between unipolar depression and bipolar disorder.
5. Discuss how the manifestation of bipolar disorder may differ across cultures.
6. Summarize the evidence for the idea that bipolar disorder is linked to creativity.
7. Summarize the evidence for and against the idea that genetics partially determine who will develop a mood disorder.
8. Discuss the monoamine theory of depression, the methodological difficulties of measuring neurotransmitter levels, and the resulting limits on our knowledge of the role of neurotransmitters in depression.
9. Discuss the neuroendocrine and neurophysiological abnormalities in depression.
10. Discuss the positive and negative aspects of lithium treatment for bipolar disorder and other therapies available for this disorder.
11. Discuss how tricyclic antidepressants, monoamine oxidase inhibitors, and selective serotonin reuptake inhibitors work, their side effects, and their effectiveness at treating depression.
12. Discuss the type of patient most likely to receive electroconvulsive therapy, what the therapy entails, and how it might work.
13. Explain how light therapy for seasonal affective disorder (SAD) might work.
14. Discuss the link between stress and depression and how the behavioral and learned helplessness theories explain this link.
15. Explain the cognitive distortion theory and depressive realism, and discuss the controversy that emerges from integrating these two views.
16. Explain the reformulated learned helplessness theory, and summarize the evidence for it.
17. Discuss Freud's theory of depression, and know the aspects of it that are supported by evidence and those that are not.
18. Discuss the foci of cognitive-behavioral and interpersonal therapy and how these two therapies are similar and different.
19. Know the specific steps taken by a cognitive-behavioral and interpersonal therapist to treat depression.
20. With respect to effectiveness of treatment for depression, know how the psychosocial therapies compare to drug therapy and use of placebos.
21. Discuss the biological theories of gender differences in depression.
22. Discuss how personality and social factors may explain women's higher rates of depression.
23. Discuss the gender and cultural differences in suicide, as well as the psychological, social, and biological risk factors for suicide.
24. Summarize the arguments for and against the idea that people have a fundamental right to die.

Chapter 6   The Schizophrenias

1. Discuss what the term *schizophrenia* means, compared to the inaccurate usage of the term in popular discourse.
2. Define and describe delusions and hallucinations as well as the different types of delusions and hallucinations, and how they vary and do not vary across cultures.
3. Describe the disorganized thought and speech in schizophrenia and a proposed reason for these symptoms.
4. Distinguish among Type I and Type II symptoms, as well as prodromal and residual symptoms.
5. Know the key symptoms and prognosis for each of the five types of schizophrenia: paranoid, disorganized, catatonic, undifferentiated, and residual.
6. Know the evidence for a genetic transmission of schizophrenia and which people are most at risk for developing schizophrenia.
7. Know the brain areas implicated in schizophrenia, as well as their functions, and be able to discuss how they are different in the brains of people with schizophrenia compared to people without schizophrenia, both biologically and psychologically.
8. Know the progression of hypotheses that implicate the neurotransmitter dopamine as a key agent in the development and treatment of schizophrenia, and how different drugs can affect dopamine.
9. Know the psychosocial factors associated with schizophrenia, the evidence for them, and their limits.
10. Know the drug therapies most commonly prescribed for schizophrenia, their side effects, and which symptoms they treat most effectively, and which they do not. Also, be able to describe the mechanisms by which they operate on schizophrenia.
11. Discuss the behavioral, cognitive, and social interventions designed for people with schizophrenia, including family therapy and the folk and religious treatments. Give examples of interventions that evidence has found to be beneficial for schizophrenic people.
12. Know the prevalence of schizophrenia across cultures, as well as how culture and gender can influence the prognosis for people with schizophrenia.

Chapter 7   Dissociative and Somatoform Disorders

1. Discuss how early theorists, such as Janet and Freud, viewed dissociation, how Hilgard's experiments provided insight into the "hidden observer" phenomenon, and how these views have shaped our modern understanding of dissociative disorders.
2. Identify the symptoms of dissociative identity disorder (DID), discuss the characteristics that each personality may exhibit and the three types of alternate personalities, as well as the functions performed by each.
3. Discuss the comorbidity of DID with other disorders, the differences between it and schizophrenia, and its differences across culture and gender, as well as the reasons for these differences.
4. Summarize the debate and evidence surrounding the possible creation of DID by therapists and the claim that American clinicians are too quick to diagnose DID, as well as the responses to these claims.
5. Discuss the theories of how DID develops, and summarize the different approaches to treating it.
6. Define dissociative fugue, and explain how it is similar to and different from DID and other dissociative disorders.

7. Discuss the conditions that may precede a dissociative fugue.
8. Distinguish among anterograde, retrograde, organic, and psychogenic amnesia, and know the types of information that tend to be lost and retained in each type.
9. Summarize the causes of organic amnesia and psychogenic amnesia, and explain how this information may apply to claims made by accused murderers that they have amnesia for the period during which they were accused of homicide.
10. Define depersonalization disorder.
11. Distinguish among somatoform disorders, psychosomatic disorders, malingering, and factitious disorders.
12. Define conversion disorder and *la belle indifference*, and discuss how early physicians and psychodynamic theorists view it.
13. Discuss the types of events frequently experienced by people with conversion disorder and the other disorders that often accompany it.
14. Describe the psychodynamic and behavioral treatments for conversion disorder and the reasons why people with this disorder are often difficult to treat.
15. Distinguish between somatization disorder, pain disorder, conversion disorder, and hypochondriasis.
16. Discuss the cultural and cohort variations in the rates of somatization disorder, as well as the disorders that often accompany it and those that are similar to it, making it difficult to diagnose.
17. Discuss the family history evidence for somatization disorder and three explanations for it. Discuss the cognitive theory of somatization.
18. Summarize how clinicians conduct psychotherapy for people with somatization disorder.
19. Define hypochondriasis, and discuss its similarities with somatization disorder.
20. Define body dysmorphic disorder, and identify the behaviors that people with this disorder engage in to compensate for their "defective" body part(s).
21. Summarize the debate surrounding the claim that body dysmorphic disorder may not be a disorder in its own right and the arguments given by proponents on both sides of this debate.
22. Discuss the treatments available for body dysmorphic disorder.

Chapter 8   Personality Disorders

1. Identify the differences between personality disorders and acute disorders.
2. Identify the three clusters of personality disorders, the disorders in each cluster, and the ways in which the disorders in each cluster are related.
3. Discuss the controversies that surround the personality disorders, including diagnostic issues and claims that they contain inherent gender-based and cultural biases.
4. Identify the similarities and differences between schizophrenia and the odd-eccentric personality disorders.
5. Describe the key symptoms and characteristics of paranoid personality disorder (including gender differences and associated symptoms or disorders), as well as the genetic, psychodynamic, and cognitive theories that attempt to explain this disorder.
6. Discuss the ways in which paranoid personality disorder is treated.
7. Describe the key symptoms and characteristics of schizoid personality disorder (including gender differences and associated symptoms or disorders), as well as the genetic, psychodynamic, and cognitive theories that attempt to explain this disorder.
8. Discuss the ways in which schizoid personality disorder is treated.

9. Describe the key symptoms and characteristics of schizotypal personality disorder (including gender differences and associated symptoms or disorders), as well as the evidence for a genetic transmission of this disorder, and its biopsychological similarities to schizophrenia.
10. Discuss the ways in which schizoid personality disorder is treated.
11. Describe the key symptoms and characteristics of antisocial personality disorder (including gender differences and associated symptoms or disorders), as well as the genetic, biological, and cognitive theories that attempt to explain this disorder.
12. Discuss the few treatments available for antisocial personality disorder, and explain why treatment of this disorder is especially difficult.
13. Describe the key symptoms and characteristics of borderline personality disorder (including gender differences and associated symptoms or disorders), as well as the genetic, biological, and cognitive theories that attempt to explain this disorder.
14. Discuss the ways in which borderline personality disorder is treated and the special considerations that therapists who work with these clients should keep in mind.
15. Describe the key symptoms and characteristics of histrionic personality disorder (including gender differences and associated symptoms or disorders), as well as the genetic, biological, and cognitive theories that attempt to explain this disorder.
16. Discuss the ways in which histrionic personality disorder is treated.
17. Describe the key symptoms and characteristics of narcissistic personality disorder (including gender differences and associated symptoms or disorders), as well as the psychodynamic, social learning, and cognitive theories that attempt to explain this disorder.
18. Discuss the ways in which narcissistic personality disorder is treated.
19. Describe the key symptoms and characteristics of avoidant personality disorder (including gender differences and associated symptoms or disorders), as well as the psychodynamic and cognitive theories that attempt to explain this disorder.
20. Identify the differences among avoidant personality disorder, social phobia, and schizoid personality disorder.
21. Discuss the ways in which avoidant personality disorder is treated.
22. Describe the key symptoms and characteristics of dependent personality disorder (including gender differences and associated symptoms or disorders), as well as the psychodynamic theory that attempts to explain this disorder.
23. Discuss the ways in which dependent personality disorder is treated.
24. Describe the key symptoms and characteristics of obsessive-compulsive personality disorder (including gender differences and associated symptoms or disorders), as well as the psychodynamic and social learning theories that attempt to explain this disorder.
25. Identify the similarities and differences between obsessive-compulsive disorder and obsessive-compulsive personality disorder.
26. Discuss the ways in which obsessive-compulsive personality disorder is treated.
27. Be able to describe the types of parenting practices, and their effects on the child, that have been hypothesized to lead to each of the disorders presented in this chapter.

Chapter 9   Childhood Disorders

1. Discuss how biological and psychosocial factors can interact to influence the development and course of the childhood disorders.
2. List the symptoms of attention deficit/hyperactivity disorder (ADHD), describe how it affects a child's social and intellectual functioning, and discuss how it affects children as they enter adolescence and adulthood.

3. Discuss the genetic and neurological contributors to ADHD and the factors that put children at risk for developing abnormalities that contribute to ADHD.
4. Describe the drug and psychosocial therapies for ADHD.
5. Discuss the similarities and differences among conduct disorder, oppositional defiant disorder, and ADHD.
6. Discuss the symptoms and course of conduct disorder and oppositional defiant disorder.
7. Describe the genetic, neurological, hormonal, and temperamental contributors to conduct disorder and oppositional defiant disorder.
8. Discuss the parenting practices, social correlates, and cognitive factors that are associated with conduct disorder.
9. Describe how psychosocial therapy for conduct disorder brings about behavioral change, and describe the steps this therapy entails.
10. List the drugs used to control aggressive behavior in children with conduct disorder.
11. Discuss the symptoms of separation anxiety disorder and how they are similar to panic attacks.
12. Discuss the genetic factors and parenting practices that may lead to separation anxiety disorder.
13. Describe the elements of effective therapy for separation anxiety disorder.
14. Discuss the diagnostic criteria for enuresis and encopresis; the genetic, psychodynamic, and behavioral theories of enuresis; and the most effective treatment for enuresis.
15. Know the types of developmental disorders that affect only specific skills.
16. Discuss what is required for a diagnosis of mental retardation, the difference between organic and cultural-familial mental retardation, and how the symptoms of the disorder vary in severity from mild to moderate to severe to profound.
17. Summarize the evidence for a genetic contribution to mental retardation.
18. Discuss and distinguish among the numerous diseases, maternal behaviors, and aspects of pregnancy and birth that can lead to mental retardation.
19. Discuss the sociocultural factors that may contribute to mental retardation.
20. Describe the qualities of an effective intervention for mental retardation.
21. Summarize the arguments for and against the inclusion of mentally retarded children in normal classrooms and the evidence pertaining to the outcomes of doing so.
22. Describe the deficits in social interaction, communication, and activities and interests of autistic children.
23. Describe the differential course of autism.
24. Discuss the genetic and biological causes of autism.
25. Discuss the four drugs used to treat the symptoms of autism and the behavioral methods used to treat autistic children.
26. Discuss the gender differences in the rates of childhood disorders, how these rates change with the onset of puberty, and the proposed explanations for these differences.

Chapter 10   Eating Disorders

1. Discuss the societal pressures on people (especially women) to maintain a slim appearance, and discuss the behaviors people engage in to meet these expectations.
2. Discuss the four key symptoms of anorexia nervosa, and distinguish between the restricting and binge-purge type.
3. Discuss the prevalence of anorexia and its associated health risks.
4. Discuss the contributions of Sir William Gull and Charles Lesegue to our understanding of anorexia.

5. Discuss the three key symptoms of bulimia nervosa, and distinguish between the purging and nonpurging type.
6. Discuss the prevalence of bulimia and its associated health risks.
7. Identify the differences between anorexia and bulimia.
8. Discuss binge-eating disorder and how it differs from anorexia and bulimia.
9. Discuss the physiological and emotional effects of dieting and how dieting may lead to both anorexia and bulimia.
10. Discuss why athletes have higher rates of eating disorders.
11. Discuss the gender similarities and differences in the eating disorders.
12. Discuss the cross-cultural, cross-ethnic, and cross-national differences in the eating disorders.
13. Summarize the theories of Hilda Bruch and Salvador Minuchin, and discuss the evidence that supports their theories.
14. Discuss the proposed explanations for why girls are at an increased risk for eating disorders compared to boys.
15. Discuss the argument that eating disorders result from sexual abuse, and summarize what the evidence suggests about this idea.
16. Discuss the evidence that genetic factors contribute to the development of eating disorders.
17. Discuss the link between eating disorders and mood disorders.
18. Discuss the biological abnormalities in anorexia and bulimia.
19. Discuss the difficulties faced by therapists who treat anorexic clients, and explain the ingredients of therapy for anorexia.
20. Discuss interpersonal, supportive-expressive, cognitive-behavioral, and behavioral therapies for bulimia, and describe their respective efficacy.
21. Describe how efficacious or inefficacious tricyclic antidepressants, MAO inhibitors, and selective serotonin reuptake inhibitors are for treating anorexia and bulimia.
22. Describe how a combination of biological, psychological, and social factors may interact to produce eating disorders.

Chapter 11   Sexual Disorders

1. Identify and describe the five stages of the sexual response cycle and the gender differences evident in it.
2. Distinguish among generalized hypoactive sexual desire, situational hypoactive sexual desire, and sexual aversion disorder, and identify when these conditions are not diagnosed.
3. Describe female sexual arousal disorder and male erectile disorder.
4. Describe female orgasmic disorder (anorgasmia), male orgasmic disorder, and premature ejaculation.
5. Describe dyspareunia and vaginismus.
6. Discuss the biological causes of sexual dysfunctions, including specific medical conditions and drugs and how biologically-caused dysfunctions differ from those caused by psychological factors.
7. Discuss the relationship problems, traumas, and attitudes that can cause sexual dysfunctions.
8. Discuss how cultures differ in their beliefs about sexual practices, sexual dysfunctions, and the prevalence of sexual dysfunctions.
9. Discuss the drug and biological procedures used to treat sexual dysfunctions.

10. Discuss the components of sex therapy with particular respect to sensate focus therapy, the stop-start technique, and the squeeze technique. Describe how couples therapy and individual psychotherapy can be used in addition to or instead of sex therapy and when each type of therapy is most appropriate.
11. Discuss how clinicians should confront clients whose values about sex differ from their own.
12. Discuss the differences between paraphilias and normal sexual fantasies.
13. Describe fetishism, sexual sadism, sexual masochism, voyeurism, exhibitionism, and frotteurism.
14. Discuss the causes, characteristics, and available treatments for pedophilia.
15. Distinguish among gender identity, gender role, and sexual orientation.
16. Discuss the characteristics and treatments for gender identity disorder.
17. Distinguish between transsexualism and transvestitism.

Chapter 12   Substance Use Disorders

1. Distinguish among different ways in which people use substances, and identify those uses that lead to substance-related disorders.
2. Discuss the prevalence, patterns, and trends of substance use over the past several decades.
3. Distinguish among and define substance intoxication, withdrawal, abuse, and dependence and the factors associated with different manifestations of intoxication, withdrawal, and dependence.
4. Describe the physiological, cognitive, affective, and behavioral effects of alcohol, benzodiazepines, barbiturates, inhalants, cocaine, amphetamines, opioids, hallucinogens, PCP, cannabis, and nicotine; how these effects differ when larger doses are ingested; and the effects of extreme doses.
5. Distinguish between legal and psychological alcohol intoxication.
6. Discuss the negative effects of the substances described in this chapter on physical and mental health.
7. Describe the three stages of alcohol withdrawal.
8. Discuss the patterns of use of alcohol, benzodiazepines, barbiturates, and cocaine that lead to dependence on these substances.
9. Define and describe Wernicke's encephalopathy, Korsakoff's psychosis, alcohol-induced dementia, and fetal alcohol syndrome.
10. Discuss how the rates of alcohol use and problems vary across cultures.
11. Discuss the gender and age differences in alcohol use and abuse, and the proposed explanations for these differences.
12. Discuss the most frequent causes of death and the negative health conditions associated with each of the substances in this chapter.
13. Discuss the effects of a pregnant woman's use of alcohol, cocaine, and nicotine on her developing fetus and newborn child.
14. Distinguish between the disease model of alcoholism and the controlled drinking perspective.
15. Summarize the contributions of the mesolimbic dopamine system and opponent processes to substance use behavior.
16. Discuss the role of genetics in alcoholism, and describe what might be inherited in the children of alcoholics.
17. Summarize the arguments and evidence for and against the idea that alcoholism is a form of depression.

18. Discuss the social and cognitive factors that lead to substance use.
19. Describe how methadone, naltrexone, naloxone, disulfiram, and antidepressants may be used to treat people with particular substance-related disorders.
20. Describe Alcoholics Anonymous and its treatment philosophy.
21. Discuss the behavioral treatments for alcoholism: aversive classical conditioning, cover sensitization therapy, and cue exposure and response prevention.
22. Describe the elements of cognitive therapies for alcoholism, and describe the elements of relapse prevention programs.
23. Discuss how men and women differ in their patterns of substance use, and discuss the proposed explanations for these differences.
24. Give examples of how different countries view substance abuse and how they enact laws based upon these views.

Chapter 13   Personality, Behavior, and the Body

1. Discuss the three predominant models of mind-body interaction in health psychology and the evidence that favors each one.
2. Discuss the characteristics of events that lead people to perceive them as stressful, and explain why events that do not share these characteristics are not perceived as stressful.
3. Explain the safety signal hypothesis and the phenomena it seeks to explain.
4. Explain why positive events can be stressful.
5. Describe the fight-or-flight response and the ways in which it is adaptive, as well as the ways in which it is maladaptive.
6. Discuss the physiological changes activated during the fight-or-flight response.
7. Discuss coronary heart disease, its physiological causes, psychological risk factors, and associated conditions.
8. Discuss hypertension, its physiological causes, psychological risk factors, and associated conditions.
9. Discuss how psychological factors can influence immunocompetence and the evidence that psychological factors influence the development and course of physical illness.
10. Discuss the negative physiological and psychological effects of sleep deprivation.
11. Explain how dispositional pessimism may contribute to physical illness and the specific evidence that supports this view.
12. Distinguish between Type A and Type B personalities, and discuss the evidence that Type A personality is associated with early mortality and coronary heart disease.
13. Explain the specific aspects of Type A personality that are most detrimental to health.
14. Explain why men are more likely than women to develop Type A personalities.
15. Define repressive coping style, and summarize the evidence for its negative effect on physical health.
16. Define John Henryism, and explain how it might partly explain higher rates of hypertension in African-American men.
17. Summarize the evidence for the idea that seeking social support has a positive impact upon physical health.
18. Describe the elements of guided mastery techniques, cognitive therapy, biofeedback, and time management training.
19. Explain how the psychosocial interventions previously listed assist with promoting health-related behavior, the specific health conditions for which each intervention is most appropriate, and the evidence that supports these links.

Chapter 14 The Cognitive Disorders: Dementia, Delirium, and Amnesia

1. Explain why the cognitive disorders are no longer known as "organic brain disorders."
2. Identify when a set of symptoms should be diagnosed as a cognitive disorder and when it should not be.
3. List five types of cognitive impairment in the cognitive disorders.
4. List and describe five types of cognitive impairment in dementia.
5. Describe the effects of dementia on a patient's psychological and social functioning.
6. Discuss the prevalence of dementia.
7. Discuss the prevalence of Alzheimer's disease.
8. Discuss the effects of having a loved one with Alzheimer's on caregivers.
9. Identify and describe the brain changes that occur in Alzheimer's disease and the conditions thought to cause them.
10. Discuss the evidence for a genetic contribution to Alzheimer's.
11. Discuss vascular dementia and identify its causes.
12. Distinguish between penetrating injuries and closed head injuries, and identify the most common types that lead to dementia.
13. Identify five medical conditions that can lead to dementia.
14. Discuss the symptoms of Parkinson's disease, HIV, and Huntington's disease.
15. Discuss the available treatments for dementia.
16. Identify the symptoms of delirium, their typical progression, and the conditions that make a diagnosis likely.
17. Discuss the causes of delirium and risk factors for delirium.
18. Discuss the ways in which delirium can be treated.
19. Distinguish between anterograde and retrograde amnesia.
20. Identify the causes of amnestic disorders.
21. Discuss four ways to treat someone with an amnestic disorder.
22. Identify the gender and cultural differences in the cognitive disorders.
23. Explain how psychological and social factors can influence the cognitive disorders.

Chapter 15 The Research Endeavor

1. Explain the difficulties inherent in psychological research and one way in which these difficulties may be overcome.
2. Define and distinguish between a hypothesis and a null hypothesis.
3. Define and distinguish between independent and dependent variables.
4. Explain the concept of operationalization.
5. Describe the elements of cross-sectional, longitudinal, prospective longitudinal, correlational, human laboratory, therapy outcome, animal studies, and single case studies, as well as the strengths and weaknesses of each type of study.
6. Explain why it is important to have a representative sample.
7. Explain why it can be important to match subjects on certain variables when comparing two groups.
8. Discuss what "significant differences" are between groups and how significance is determined.
9. Define and distinguish among control groups, placebo control groups, wait list control groups, and experimental groups, and explain the circumstances in which each would be appropriate and why (with regard to therapy outcome studies).

10. Discuss the ethical problems raised by human laboratory, therapy outcome, and animal studies and ways in which researchers attempt to avoid these problems.
11. Discuss what third variables are and how they may be minimized or eliminated.
12. Discuss the challenges inherent in cross-cultural research.

Chapter 16   Society and Mental Health

1. Discuss the limitations in the ability of psychological research to inform legal decisions.
2. Discuss how competency to stand trial is determined.
3. Discuss the characteristics of people most likely to be referred for competency evaluations and the characteristics of people most likely to be found incompetent to stand trial.
4. Discuss the frequency with which the insanity defense is used and the typical judgments that result when it is used.
5. Summarize how insanity pleas are evaluated according to the M'Naghten Rule, irresistible impulse rule, Durham Rule, ALI Rule, and the American Psychiatric Association's definition of insanity.
6. Discuss the pros and cons of each rule previously listed, and describe how each rule either broadened or constricted the legal definition of insanity.
7. Discuss the significance of *Barrett v. United States* (1977).
8. Discuss the use of the verdict guilty but mentally ill (GBMI).
9. Discuss the professional concerns that some mental health professionals have about the insanity defense.
10. Discuss the need for treatment as a justification for civil commitment.
11. Discuss the modern criteria used to enable civil commitment and the variations in how states treat the legal issue of civil commitment.
12. Discuss the significance of *Donaldson v. O'Connor* (1975).
13. Discuss the problems with predictions of dangerousness to others and the factors that predict violence over the short term.
14. Discuss the rights of patients to treatment and to refuse treatment, and describe the variations among states as to the recognition of these rights.
15. Discuss the circumstances in which patients' rights can be violated.
16. Summarize the goals of the deinstitutionalization movement, as well as its accomplishments and failures.
17. Identify the culture and gender issues surrounding competency evaluations, the insanity defense, and psychologists' predictions of dangerousness to others.
18. Identify and describe the clinician's duties to the client and society.
19. Discuss when confidentiality may and may not be broken.
20. Discuss the significance of *Tarasoff v. Regents of the University of California* (1974).
21. Summarize the recent trends in family law in general.
22. Summarize the recent trends in child custody law.
23. Identify the guidelines that clinicians should follow when conducting independent assessments in child custody disputes.
24. Discuss the roles that psychologists assume in child maltreatment cases, and discuss the pros and cons of having psychologists involved in these matters.
25. Identify and describe the controversy in the repressed/recovered/false memory debate, the viewpoints held, and the evidence that supports or weakens each viewpoint.

Chapter 1 Looking at Abnormality

1. As stated in the text, throughout history deciding if a person's behavior is abnormal has depended on all of the following *except*:
   a. cultural norms.
   b. gender.
   c. ethnicity.
   d. innate abilities.
   Answer: d LO: 1; factual page: 2

2. An official guidebook used for diagnosing psychological disorders is:
   a. *The Diagnostic and Statistical Manual of Mental Disorders (DSM)*.
   b. *The Guidebook for Diagnosing Psychological Disorders (GDPD)*.
   c. *The Guidebook of the Psychiatric and Psychological Associations of America (GPPAA)*.
   d. *The Official Diagnostic Guidebook for Psychological Disorders (ODGPD)*.
   Answer: a LO: 1; factual page: 2

3. Whether a behavior is labeled as "normal" or "abnormal" is greatly influenced by:
   a. reality.
   b. context.
   c. physical geography.
   d. individual perceptions.
   Answer: b LO: 1; factual page: 6

4. Two factors noted in the text that determine the context of a behavior are:
   a. cultural norms and gender.
   b. geography and weather.
   c. personal traits and society.
   d. religion and perception.
   Answer: a LO: 1; factual page: 6

5. Sarah face is painted bright colors and she is wearing strange looking clothes. It is evening as she wanders the streets with a large sack, knocking on people's doors and asking for candy. Which of the following must be considered in determining whether her behavior is abnormal?
   a. weather
   b. context
   c. financial status
   d. gender
   Answer: b LO: 1; applied page: 6

Chapter 1

6. Which of the following *is not* a criterion stated in the text for determining abnormality?
    a. cultural relativism
    b. subjective discomfort
    c. mental disease
    d. objective reality
    Answer: d   LO: 2; factual   pages: 6-10

7. According to the cultural relativism perspective of abnormality:
    a. although it may be difficult, we can agree on a universal definition of abnormality.
    b. there is one agreed upon, universal definition of abnormality.
    c. there are a few relatively universal definitions of abnormality agreed on by most cultures.
    d. different cultures have different definitions of abnormality.
    Answer: d   LO: 2; factual   page: 7

8. The notion that "there is no one, universal definition of abnormality, but different definitions" for different groups expresses which perspective of abnormality?
    a. statistical deviance
    b. subjective discomfort
    c. cultural relativism
    d. mental disease
    Answer: c   LO: 2; factual   page: 7

9. Opponents of the cultural relativism perspective of abnormality note that:
    a. not all people in a given culture will agree on a definition of what is or is not abnormal.
    b. there are some behaviors or experiences that almost all cultures consider abnormal or undesirable.
    c. all behavior is judged by personal perspectives, and therefore, we cannot assume a societal norm.
    d. every society has unpopular groups, but they don't generally label their behaviors as abnormal.
    Answer: b   LO: 2; factual   page: 7

10. A concern that societies may label persons or groups as abnormal in order to justify controlling or silencing them is expressed by:
    a. proponents of the cultural relativism perspective of abnormality.
    b. opponents of the cultural relativism perspective of abnormality.
    c. proponents of the subjective discomfort perspective of abnormality.
    d. opponents of the subjective discomfort perspective of abnormality.
    Answer: b   LO: 2; factual   page: 7

11. The term *drapetomania* refers to:
    a. an extremely excitable person.
    b. a person who cycles between high and low moods.
    c. a sickness that causes slaves to desire freedom.
    d. a mental disorder sometimes found in interior decorators.
    Answer: c   LO: 2; factual   page: 7

12. By attributing a medical term (*dysaesthesia Aethiopis*) to a slave's refusal to work, Dr. Samuel Cartwright justified:
    a. whipping slaves and putting them to hard work in order to cure them.
    b. taking care of an ill slave until the slave was again able to return to work.
    c. hanging the slave, since Dr. Cartwright determined the disease was incurable.
    d. enacting legislation to end slavery because it caused mental and physical distress.
    Answer: a   LO: 2; conceptual   page: 7

13. The criterion that might be used to designate Albert Einstein as abnormal because of his intellectual genius is:
    a. cultural relativism.
    b. statistical deviance.
    c. subjective discomfort.
    d. dysfunctional behavior.
    Answer: b   LO: 2; conceptual   page: 8

14. One objection of therapists to the subjective discomfort criterion of mental illness is that:
    a. what disturbs one person may not disturb someone else.
    b. we all exhibit symptoms of discomfort when we are unhappy, so we might all be considered mentally ill.
    c. the criterion is concerned only with the person performing the behavior, not the person experiencing the discomfort.
    d. some people are not aware of the severe problems their behaviors create and, thus, do not experience any discomfort.
    Answer: d   LO: 2; conceptual   page: 9

15. The criterion of abnormality that views the behaviors as diseases is referred to as the ____ criterion:
    a. mental health
    b. mental illness
    c. psychophysiological
    d. psychosomatic
    Answer: b   LO: 2; factual, conceptual   page: 9

Chapter 1

16. The mental health criterion for sees abnormality as:
    a. an extension of the classic mind-body question.
    b. a disease that can be diagnosed through medical tests.
    c. a disease process that can be cured biologically.
    d. a physical problem that can be diagnosed and cured medically.
    Answer: c   LO: 2; factual, conceptual   page: 9

17. One reason the American Psychiatric Association removed homosexuality from its list of psychological disorders in 1973 is because:
    a. it was more important for gays and lesbians to focus on other psychological problems they may have than on their sexual orientation.
    b. gays and lesbians argued that their sexual orientation does not cause them discomfort and they have no wish to change it.
    c. research over the past 25 years has indicated that the range of "normal" sexual orientations is so broad that homosexuality is no more deviant than heterosexuality.
    d. a person's homosexual orientation may cause discomfort for that person, but most mental health professionals currently view it within a healthy range of sexual practices.
    Answer: b   LO: 2; factual, conceptual   page: 9

18. A problem with the mental illness criterion of abnormality is that the term:
    a. implies a clear, identifiable physical process of deviance from "health" that leads to specific behaviors or symptoms, when in fact this clarity does not exist.
    b. is a legal one, and cannot be used appropriately when trying to diagnose or treat a person with a mental disorder.
    c. does not refer to some identifiable physical entity.
    d. provides no hope that persons with psychological disorders can ever be cured.
    Answer: a   LO: 2; conceptual   page: 9

19. Which of the following criterion *best* helps a mental health professional determine whether a behavior is abnormal?
    a. subjective discomfort
    b. statistical deviance
    c. cultural norms
    d. maladaptiveness
    Answer: d   LO: 2; factual   page: 9

Looking at Abnormality

20. John has been sent by his wife for therapy. Following the death of his father last year, John has begun to sleep all day, he barely eats, he tells his wife about the voices he hears that order him to burn his arms and feet with cigarettes, and he has been unable to work for the past six months. Most likely a therapist today would describe John's behavior as:
    a. statistically deviant.
    b. subjectively uncomfortable.
    c. mentally ill.
    d. maladaptive.
    Answer: d   LO: 2; applied   pages: 9-10

21. Theories that view mental disorders as similar to physical diseases caused by the breakdown of a bodily system are:
    a. natural theories.
    b. supernatural theories.
    c. psychological theories.
    d. stress-related theories.
    Answer: a   LO: 2; factual   page: 10

22. Andromeda has been sad and unable to eat lately. She has sleep disturbances, and her friends are concerned for her welfare. Dr. Galen decides to treat her with hot mineral baths, infusions of medicinal concoctions, use of magnets to return her internal organs to their proper location, and blood letting. We could assume that Dr. Galen accepts which type of theory of mental disorders?
    a. natural
    b. supernatural
    c. psychological
    d. stress-related
    Answer: a   LO: 4; applied   page: 10

23. Which theories discussed in the text would view mental disorders as the result of divine intervention, demonic possession, or personal sin?
    a. religious theories
    b. cultural theories
    c. supernatural theories
    d. cosmic theories
    Answer: c   LO: 4; conceptual   page: 10

Chapter 1

24. Recently, Greta has been expressing bizarre ideas in an odd voice contorting her face, and moving her arms about as she speaks. Her family has become frightened of her strange behavior and called Dr. Schneider for advice. He has said Greta needs to undergo exorcism to rid her of her disorder and suggested the family call in the parish priest. We might logically assume that Dr. Schneider accepts which type of theories of mental disorders?
    a. natural theories
    b. supernatural theories
    c. psychological/Stress-related theories
    d. theocratic theories
    Answer: b   LO: 4; applied   page: 10

25. Thelma's extraordinary sadness, unceasing crying, and loss of interest in eating and grooming has greatly worried her family and friends. They have insisted that she get professional help, so she finally agrees. After talking with Thelma for a while, Dr. Fromm advises Thelma to take a cruise around the Greek Isles, try to relax and play while on the cruise, and to learn better ways to deal with her problems. This remedy would suggest that Dr. Fromm accepts which type of theories of mental disorders?
    a. natural theories
    b. supernatural theories
    c. psychological/Stress-related theories
    d. psychodynamic theories
    Answer: c   LO: 4; applied   page: 10

26. Because of his bizarre behavior, Gideon was ostracized from his town and told never to return unless he could return his behavior to normal. This type of treatment would reflect _____ _____ of mental disorders.
    a. natural
    b. supernatural
    c. psychological/Stress
    d. political
    Answer: b   LO: 4; applied   page: 11

27. The notion that the human body contains a positive force and a negative force that must be balanced in order for the individual to be healthy best represents which ancient theory of mental health?
    a. Chinese
    b. Egyptian
    c. Hebrew
    d. Greek
    Answer: a   LO: 5; factual   page: 11

Looking at Abnormality

28. The early belief that a woman's mental disorders is often caused by a wandering uterus was held by the:
    a. Greeks and the Chinese.
    b. Egyptians and Chinese.
    c. Egyptians and the Greeks.
    d. Egyptians and the Hebrews.
    Answer: c LO: 5; factual pages: 11-12

29. From the Old Testament, it seems likely that the ancient Hebrews believed that madness:
    a. was a punishment from God.
    b. was punishable by stoning.
    c. could not be cured.
    d. required compassion and forgiveness.
    Answer: d LO: 5; factual page: 12

30. The Greek physician Hippocrates attributed mental illness to:
    a. an affliction from the gods.
    b. punishment for sins.
    c. an imbalance in the body's humors (fluids).
    d. severe emotional shock.
    Answer: c LO: 5; factual page: 12

31. The Greek physician Hippocrates believed that mental illness should be treated by requiring:
    a. the afflicted person to retreat to a temple for healing ceremonies.
    b. atonement, fasting, and possibly ostracism or death.
    c. bleeding, rest, change of diet, or removal from the family.
    d. the afflicted person to talk about the traumatic event in order to reduce its effects.
    Answer: c LO: 5; factual page: 12

32. During the period of the Inquisition, persons accused of witchcraft often confessed to various supernatural acts. While these confessions were likely coerced through torture, it is also possible that they resulted from:
    a. mental illness expressed through delusions and/or hallucinations.
    b. malnutrition, leading to poor health and a desire to gain acceptance (and thus be fed) by the Church.
    c. a desire by the people to remove all forms of evil from society.
    d. a total sense of helplessness that led people to want to die rather than continue living in poverty and oppression.
    Answer: a LO: 6; factual pages: 13-14

Chapter 1

33. During the period of the Inquisition, many people accused of witchcraft often confessed to holding conversations with the devil and flying with witches. Based on the symptoms described, it is possible that these unfortunates may have suffered from:
    a. hysteria.
    b. obsessive-compulsive disorder.
    c. schizophrenia.
    d. a personality disorder.
    Answer: c   LO: 6; factual   pages: 13-14

34. The group of persons most likely to be accused of being witches in sixteenth to seventeenth century England were:
    a. male bankers and merchants because others were envious and wanted their fortune.
    b. older, unmarried, poor women who begged and were often considered disgusting by their neighbors.
    c. older, rich widows whose children wished to inherit their wealth.
    d. pious married women who instilled jealousy in their neighbors for their virtuousness.
    Answer: b   LO: 6; factual   page: 14

35. It is clear from the writings of various authors during the Inquisition, as well as from the witch hunts in our own history and in modern cultures that accept a belief in witchcraft that:
    a. madness invariably leads to witchcraft.
    b. witchcraft invariably leads to madness.
    c. madness and witchcraft are two distinct entities.
    d. madness and witchcraft are one and the same.
    Answer: c   LO: 6; factual   page: 14

36. Our modern word *bedlam* derives from:
    a. beds in hospitals set aside for mad persons.
    b. the practicing of beating violent mentally ill persons until they became subdued.
    c. lamps that burned 24 hours a day by the straw beds of the mentally ill.
    d. the Hospital of St. Mary of Bethlehem in London where mentally ill were housed.
    Answer: d   LO: 7; factual   page: 15

37. As noted in the text, Shakespeare wrote in King Lear (Act II, Scene iii), "Bedlam beggars, who, with roaring voices. . . . Sometimes with lunatic bans, sometimes with prayers enforce their charity." In this declaration, he was referring to:
    a. the ostracism of the mentally ill.
    b. the practice of forcing the mentally ill to beg in the streets.
    c. the practice of forcing the mentally ill to atone for their sins.
    d. the deranged behavior of the mentally ill as expressed by their shouting.
    Answer: b   LO: 7; conceptual   page: 15

Looking at Abnormality

38. Up until the late eighteenth century, typical treatment of the mentally ill in Europe included:
    a. chaining and beating them.
    b. use of medicinal herbs to cure them.
    c. providing rest and relaxation to ease their distress.
    d. considering their ramblings as valid prophecies.
    Answer: a   LO: 7; factual   page: 15

39. A common practice at mental hospitals throughout Europe in the sixteenth to eighteenth centuries was to:
    a. keep patients isolated, with no visits from family or friends.
    b. encourage family and friends to visit the mentally ill.
    c. exhibit the patients to the public for a fee.
    d. unchain them periodically so they could get exercise.
    Answer: c   LO: 7; factual   page: 15

40. The first *Act for Regulating Madhouses*, which was aimed at improving conditions of private madhouses, was passed in:
    a. Hamburg in 1375.
    b. England in 1547
    c. England in 1774.
    d. the United States in 1775.
    Answer: c   LO: 7; factual   pages: 15-16

41. Compared with asylums in Europe during the eighteenth century, conditions in American asylums were:
    a. much worse.
    b. somewhat worse.
    c. about the same.
    d. much better.
    Answer: c   LO: 7; factual   pages: 15-16

42. The asylum that Benjamin Franklin helped to establish in 1756, with wards for the mentally ill, was:
    a. the Pennsylvania Hospital in Philadelphia.
    b. the Public Hospital in Williamsburg.
    c. St. Mary's of Bethlehem.
    d. the Franklin Institute in Boston.
    Answer: a   LO: 7; factual   page: 16

Chapter 1

43. The first hospital in America exclusively for the mentally ill was:
    a. the Pennsylvania Hospital in Philadelphia, Pennsylvania.
    b. the Public Hospital in Williamsburg, Virginia.
    c. Reikers Hospital in New York.
    d. Bellevue Hospital in New York.
    Answer: b   LO: 7; factual   page: 16

44. Treatment of patients in early mental hospitals in America, consisting of electrical shocks, bleeding, plunging them into ice water or hot water, starvation, and use of restraints was designed to:
    a. drive out the evil spirits.
    b. frighten patients into a cure.
    c. restore health.
    d. punish their inappropriate behaviors.
    Answer: c   LO: 7; factual   page: 16

45. The term *moral management* refers to:
    a. providing patients with a pleasant setting, good food, social activities, and therapy.
    b. ensuring that the patients pray, atone for their sins, and learn proper ways to behave.
    c. keeping patients confined so they cannot cause harm to society.
    d. beating patients whenever their behavior harms another but rewarding them for acceptable behaviors.
    Answer: a   LO: 7; factual   page: 16

46. The moral management of mental hospitals was:
    a. widespread in the United States, but not in Europe.
    b. widespread in Europe, but not in the United States.
    c. widespread in Europe and the United States.
    d. only accepted on a limited basis in both Europe and the United States.
    Answer: c   LO: 7; factual   page: 16

47. Among the things for which Dorothea Dix crusaded was:
    a. ensuring that the mentally ill be treated humanely.
    b. keeping the mentally ill isolated.
    c. establishing treatment residences for the mentally ill poor.
    d. ensuring effective in-home care for the mentally ill.
    Answer: a   LO: 7; factual   page: 16

Looking at Abnormality

48. The approach to psychological disorders that supplanted the moral management movement in the late nineteenth century was the:
    a. behavioral movement.
    b. mental hygiene movement.
    c. stress reduction movement.
    d. mental illness approach.
    Answer: b   LO: 7; factual   page: 16

49. The major difference between the moral management and mental hygiene movements is that:
    a. moral management stresses religion and believes that prayer and atonement are important for treating mental illness.
    b. mental hygiene states that mental disorders are medical diseases and should be treated biologically.
    c. mental hygiene believes that the mentally ill need a clean, comfortable environment in order to improve.
    d. There is no difference--they are basically synonymous.
    Answer: b   LO: 7; conceptual   page: 16

50. One of the reasons the mental hygiene movement gained support in the late nineteenth century is because:
    a. other treatments were not working.
    b. there were more psychologists to practice these methods.
    c. there had been major advances in preventing major medical diseases.
    d. it was endorsed by the American Psychological Association.
    Answer: c   LO: 7; factual   pages: 16-17

51. A founder of the mental hygiene movement, Clifford Beers, was particularly interested in the medical basis of mental illness after he had:
    a. been institutionalized and saw that it worked for him.
    b. been institutionalized and found that the moral management approach did not work for him.
    c. been institutionalized, beaten, placed in strait jackets, and locked in a padded cell.
    d. seen how effective some forerunners to this treatment had been for his brother.
    Answer: c   LO: 7; factual   page: 17

Chapter 1

52. In his 1908 book, *A Mind That Found Itself*, Clifford Beers:
    a. outlined his plan for preventing mental illness and reforming the treatment of the mentally ill.
    b. wrote a satire about the mental health movement as it existed at that time.
    c. explained his own bout with mental illness and stated that it takes hard work and determination by the afflicted person to overcome the disorder.
    d. talked about the power of prayer and devotion for learning what it is that causes mental discomfort and how to overcome it.
    Answer: a   LO: 7; factual   page: 17

53. As a champion of the mental hygiene movement, Clifford Beers advocated:
    a. public education about mental illness.
    b. keeping the mentally ill isolated from the rest of society.
    c. "re-educating" the mentally ill to rid them of their unclean thoughts.
    d. treating the mentally ill with rest and relaxation to effect a cure.
    Answer: a   LO: 7; factual   page: 17

54. With the advent of the mental hygiene movement:
    a. there was rapid improvement in many forms of treatment for the mentally ill.
    b. the poor often remained warehoused in overcrowded, isolated institutions.
    c. medical advances for treatment of mental disorders became increasingly rapid.
    d. rich and poor patients were now able to receive effective treatment.
    Answer: b   LO: 7; factual   page: 17

55. The term *psychic epidemic* is the same as:
    a. insanity.
    b. witchcraft.
    c. mental illness.
    d. mass madness.
    Answer: d   LO: 7; factual   page: 17

56. Psychic epidemics:
    a. are a relatively recent phenomenon in abnormality.
    b. have been found across the recorded history of abnormality.
    c. are generally restricted to particular demographic groups.
    d. were much more common in early history than in later times.
    Answer: b   LO: 7; factual   page: 17

Looking at Abnormality

57. The term used when large numbers of people appear to be afflicted with the same set of bizarre behavioral symptoms and may seem to lose touch with reality is:
    a. mass hypnosis.
    b. psychic epidemics.
    c. a psychotic breakdown.
    d. multiple mania.
    Answer: b   LO: 7; factual   page: 17

58. The earliest recorded information of dance frenzies were noted in:
    a. 365 B.C. in Greece.
    b. 1374 in Germany.
    c. 1428 in Russia.
    d. 1518 in Spain.
    Answer: b   LO: 6; factual   page: 17

59. Persons described as "abused by the devil" to such an extent that they dance themselves to death have been noted to suffer from:
    a. dance frenzy.
    b. mass mania.
    c. dance fever.
    d. demonic dancing.
    Answer: a   LO: 6; factual   pages: 17-18

60. A form of dance frenzy that occurred in 1518 at a chapel in Hohlenstein, where over 400 people were alleged to have danced during a 4-week period, was called:
    a. Hohlenstein fever.
    b. chapel frenzy.
    c. St. Vitus' dance.
    d. psychic fever.
    Answer: c   LO: 6; factual   page: 18

61. Tarantism is a form of psychic epidemic in which people:
    a. dance until they drop in order to rid the farms of tarantulas.
    b. develop mass hysteria about tarantulas and spend days tracking them down and beating them out of their hiding places.
    c. develop acute pain that they attribute to tarantula bites, jump around and dance wildly, and beat each other with whips.
    d. fear their towns are being overrun by giant spiders, so they burn down their own houses to rout them out.
    Answer: c   LO: 6; factual   page: 18

Chapter 1

62. Teresa develops acute pain, which she attributes to being bitten by a tarantula. She then begins to jump about wildly, dance feverishly, tear at her clothes, dig a hole in the ground and roll in it. She is not alone in these activities since there are many other people engaging in similar behaviors. It is likely that they are suffering from:
    a. paranoia.
    b. St. Vitus' dance.
    c. tarantella.
    d. tarantism.
    Answer: d   LO: 6; applied   page: 18

63. Many religious sects over the ages have practiced behaviors similar to dance frenzies in performing their religious services. Often participants are so emotionally charged that they jerk violently, run, sing, scream, and dance. These activities are most likely to be seen in groups that are:
    a. affluent and feel compelled to express their devotion and appreciation.
    b. in the middle income groups, feeling strongly connected to their roots.
    c. suffering from economic and social deprivation and alienation.
    d. economically mixed, since there is no particular correlation between these activities and economic status.
    Answer: c   LO: 6; factual, conceptual   page: 18

64. A likely adaptive purpose of performing the extreme dancing, jumping, jerking, screaming, and other behaviors exhibited in expressions of psychic epidemics is:
    a. reduction of stress and tension.
    b. crying out for help.
    c. wanting to be accepted.
    d. There appears to be no adaptive purpose--these are maladaptive behaviors.
    Answer: a   LO: 6; factual   page: 18

65. In today's world, mass hysteria tends to focus on:
    a. modern concerns.
    b. fear of specific wildlife.
    c. war.
    d. financial concerns.
    Answer: a   LO: factual   page: 18

Looking at Abnormality

66. Based on information in the text, which common fear would be *least likely* in modern times to arouse mass hysteria concerns?
    a. war
    b. environmental toxins
    c. terrorist plots
    d. serial murders
    Answer: c LO: factual page: 18

67. A common underlying cause of psychic epidemics across the ages and cultures appears to be:
    a. the vulnerability of youth.
    b. religious beliefs.
    c. chronic stress.
    d. excessive affluence.
    Answer: c LO: factual page: 18

68. Which of the following statements *best* reflects current thinking about supernatural theories of abnormality?
    a. These theories are now rejected by most societies around the world.
    b. These theories are currently rejected by most industrial societies but are accepted by many developing nations.
    c. These theories are currently accepted by many industrial societies but are rejected by most developing nations.
    d. These theories continue to be accepted by many societies around the world, both industrial and developing.
    Answer: b LO: 4; factual page: 19

69. Psychological theories of abnormality view the mentally ill as:
    a. social and emotional creatures who have been affected by events and people around them.
    b. having a major defect in their minds that makes it difficult for them to interact appropriately with their environment.
    c. possessing certain gifts from their environments that others are incapable of understanding, which causes them great stress.
    d. needing to find the right balance between their religious views and their society in order to reduce their symptoms.
    Answer: a LO: 4; factual page: 19

Chapter 1

70. Which of the following is the most realistic potential threat of the biological theories of mental illness at the present time?
    a. An inability to help the mentally ill
    b. Using an argument that a group of persons is biologically inferior as a justification to harm them
    c. Warehousing the mentally ill in institutions while attempting different methods of treatment on them
    d. There are no realistic potential threats to this theory; it offers excellent promise for eventual (or current) cure
    Answer: b   LO: 4; factual   page: 19

71. In the mainstream of current research and practice, the dominant theories are:
    a. natural and psychological.
    b. psychological and supernatural.
    c. biological and natural.
    d. biological and psychological.
    Answer: d   LO: 4; factual   page: 19

72. The current thinking among many mental health workers today is to take an integrated approach toward abnormality. This is called:
    a. the integrative approach.
    b. biopsychosocial integration.
    c. biogenetic integration.
    d. the eclectic approach.
    Answer: b   LO: 4; factual, conceptual   page: 19

73. Currently, _____ cultures have some type of spiritual healers.
    a. many
    b. few
    c. no
    d. restricted
    Answer: a   LO: 4; factual   page: 19

74. In cultures where healers do not subscribe to supernatural theories of abnormality:
    a. these theories find no place in treating people with psychological problems.
    b. these theories may influence treatment because of a client's beliefs.
    c. serious therapists discourage clients from allowing such theories to influence treatment.
    d. these theories rarely surface, but if they do they have no serious effect on treatment.
    Answer: b   LO: 4; factual   page: 19

Looking at Abnormality

75. One major difference between psychiatrists and psychologists is:
    a. psychologists focus more on psychological disorders than psychiatrists do.
    b. psychiatrists have an M.D. degree, psychologists do not.
    c. psychologists are more likely than psychiatrists to prescribe medications.
    d. psychiatrists are less likely than psychologists to use a medical approach.
    Answer: b   LO: 8; factual   page: 20

76. Dr. Malorie has been treating patients for the emotional problems for 15 years. She specializes in difficult psychological disorders, such as schizophrenia, bipolar disorder, and major depression. Due to the severity of these illnesses, many of her patients are taking medications; thus, she works closely with other mental health professionals who prescribe and monitor the patients' medications. Based on these facts, we would expect Dr. Malorie to be a:
    a. psychiatrist.
    b. psychologist.
    c. psychiatric nurse.
    d. psychiatric social worker.
    Answer: b   LO: 8; applied   page: 20

77. Clinical psychologists typically:
    a. have a Psy.D. in psychology and often prescribe medications.
    b. have a Ph.D. in psychology but do not prescribe medications.
    c. prescribe medications but refer clients to psychiatrists for further therapy.
    d. have the same type of training that psychiatrists have.
    Answer: b   LO: 8; factual   page: 20

78. The text states that clinical social workers:
    a. have a Bachelors degree in social work and a Masters degree in psychology.
    b. have a Bachelors degree in social work and provide clients with psychotherapy.
    c. have a Masters degree in social work and help clients overcome social conditions that contribute to psychological problems.
    d. have a Masters degree in social work, provide psychotherapy, and can prescribe medications for certain clients.
    Answer: c   LO: 8; factual   page: 20

79. John works at an inpatient psychiatric facility where he delivers medical care to patients, as well as certain forms of psychotherapy such as group therapy. It is likely that he is a:
    a. psychologist.
    b. psychological assistant.
    c. clinical social worker.
    d. psychiatric nurse.
    Answer: d   LO: 8; applied   page: 20

Chapter 1

80. As discussed in the text, students who begin to study and read about abnormal psychology:
    a. become extremely good at analyzing themselves, their friends, and their family.
    b. often see many signs of abnormality in themselves, their friends, and their family.
    c. become less anxious about their own issues of being "normal."
    d. are less likely to label themselves and others with some type of psychological disorder than those who don't study the subject.
    Answer: b LO: factual page: 21

81. "Medical student's disease" is the tendency:
    a. to see signs of abnormality in oneself and others.
    b. of students of abnormal psychology to develop certain disorders.
    c. to begin solving the problems of people around you.
    d. to become ill because you are subjected to so many disorders.
    Answer: a LO: conceptual page: 21

82. Feeling that one's life is "out of control" is:
    a. common for those between 18 and 25, but a sign of abnormality for older people.
    b. common for most people of all ages from time to time.
    c. a sign that a person should tune into because it indicates a need for therapy.
    d. extremely rare for most people who have a solid support system.
    Answer: b LO: factual page: 21

83. Sally is a sophomore at a prestigious eastern college. Although she has always done well in school, runs around the track every morning, and maintains a healthy diet, mid-way through her abnormal psychology class, she began to realize that she has many of the symptoms that are characteristic of major depression. As she looks around at the people in her life, she notices that they, too, can be easily labeled with certain psychological disorders. Sally likely has:
    a. medical student's disease.
    b. major depression.
    c. misinterpreted the symptoms of depression.
    d. delusions of grandeur.
    Answer: a LO: applied page: 21

Looking at Abnormality

84. Randy has just begun the second semester of his freshman year. His grades for the first semester were much lower than he had expected, and the work was much harder. His parents are unhappy with his performance and are pressuring him to improve his grades so he can become a lawyer and join father's legal practice. Randy believes he is a failure and has had recent thoughts of "not living anymore" so that he won't embarrass himself or his family any further. He has problems sleeping and is losing weight because his appetite is depressed. He also finds it difficult to get out of bed to go to his morning classes. If you were Randy's roommate, you might:
    a. suggest he drop out of school and go home.
    b. go to the student counseling center with him so he can talk to a therapist.
    c. tell him to cheer up because things are bound to get better.
    d. call his parents and tell them what's going on.
    Answer: b   LO: applied   page: 21

Essay Questions

85. You have been hired by the American Psychiatric Association and the American Psychological Association to find a term to apply to abnormal behavior that avoids stigmatizing persons with these behaviors. First, describe all of the factors involved in determining whether a behavior is considered to be abnormal. Second, state what term you believe would satisfy these two organizations, and explain how your term would avoid the stigma of current labels.

    First, the answer must include a discussion of the role that context, gender, and culture play in determining whether a behavior is considered abnormal. Second, the student should attempt to find a term that avoids the stigma of any of the current labels, and explain how this term avoids that stigma.

86. Imagine that you are the director of a mental health facility and you are trying to educate your personnel with respect to issues of sensitivity. You understand that there are different ways to define abnormality and want to find the one that is least offensive. Discuss with your staff the evidence supporting and disputing the five proposed ways of defining abnormality presented in the text.

    Cultural relativism: judgment on societal norms; but some behaviors are universally abnormal, and concern for labeling any unpopular views as abnormal as a form of control.
    Statistical deviance: rare/unusual behaviors are abnormal; problems with clarity of definition, and not all rare behaviors--such as creativity--are abnormal.
    Subjective discomfort: cause the person to be in distress; but a person is not always

Chapter 1

aware of the problems with his or her behavior, or the behaviors may cause others distress but not the person with the disorder.
Mental illness: hypothetically provides a way to deal with the disorders, but too much ambiguity in definition.
Maladaptive: Cause distress and prevent a person from functioning appropriately, but manifestation and designation of abnormality as a label are influenced by gender and culture.

87. Discuss how the supernatural, natural, and psychological theories of abnormality have influenced our attitudes toward and treatment of psychological disorders over the years. Include both the humane and inhumane treatment of the mentally ill over the ages in terms of all three perspectives.

Natural: mental illness results from breakdown in physical processes; Supernatural: mental illness results from divine intervention; Psychological: mental illness results from negative life events/chronic stress. Based on the source of the problem, each theory suggests different causes of abnormality and what it considers to be appropriate remedies. All of the theories have been applied both humanely and inhumanely throughout history. While natural and psychological theories predominate in the more developed societies today, supernatural theories still have influence, even in the technologically developed societies.

88. You have been invited to speak for 20 minutes at the local Lions Club about ancient beliefs about abnormality and its treatment. Provide an overview of your presentation. How would you introduce the topic? What would you cover? How would you conclude?

Chinese: *Yin/yang* balance of positive and negative forces, what causes them to be out of balance, and the results of imbalance; vital air flow on various body organs affects specific emotions.
Egyptians: Mental functioning in brain; hysteria due to wandering uterus that interferes with body's functioning.
Greeks: Also believed hysteria is due to wandering uterus that interrupts proper functioning of the body; lay people believed the gods were involved in mental illness, but the physicians, who developed a system for classifying mental disorders, believed they were due to an imbalance of the four basic body humors (fluids).
The Hebrews: Although mental illness is God's punishment for sinning and breaking the commandments, physicians could at least comfort, if not cure the disorders.

Looking at Abnormality

89. Your friend is unclear about the similarities and differences in terms of training and responsibilities for psychologists, psychiatrists, social workers, and psychiatric nurses. Give your friend an understandable explanation of each based on what you learned from the text.

    Psychiatrists: M.D. with specialty in treating physical and psychological problems; prescribe medication
    Clinical Psychologists: Ph.D. in psychology specializing in dealing with psychological problems; often do research on causes/treatment of psychological problems; do not currently prescribe medication
    Clinical social workers: LCSW, focus on helping clients overcome social conditions that contribute to psychological problems
    Psychiatric Nurses: Nursing degree, often work on inpatient psychiatric wards, deliver medications, perform certain types of therapy, such as group therapy.

90. Discuss the various difficulties in coming up with a completely satisfactory definition of abnormality. What term would you use? Explain how this term would be appropriate for describing all aspects of abnormal behavior.

    Incorporate all five ways of describing abnormal behavior, plus effects of gender and culture; then incorporate a thoughtful discussion of the student's own perspectives and rationale.

Chapter 2   Assessing and Diagnosing Abnormality

1. The process of gathering information about what is wrong with a person and the possible causes of his or her symptoms is called:
    a. diagnosis.
    b. syndrome.
    c. assessment.
    d. prognosis.
    Answer: c   LO: 1; factual   page: 24

2. An assessment:
    a. pinpoints the specific nature and cause(s) of a person's psychological problems.
    b. gathers information about what is wrong with a person and the possible causes of the symptoms.
    c. tells the therapist the most appropriate treatment for a person's psychological problems.
    d. is an educated guess about what is causing a person to have psychological problems.
    Answer: b   LO: 1; factual, conceptual   page: 24

3. A diagnosis is:
    a. a prediction of how well an individual is expected to progress during the course of treatment.
    b. information about what is wrong with a person and possible causes of the symptoms.
    c. a set of procedures to follow for treating a person with physical or psychological problems.
    d. a label attached to a set of symptoms that tend to occur with one another.
    Answer: d   LO: 1; factual, conceptual   page: 24

4. Which of the following is a ***danger*** inherent in diagnosing a person with a psychological disorder?
    a. Labeling someone with a psychiatric diagnosis can have stigmatizing effects for the person.
    b. A diagnosis allows mental health professionals to communicate with each other about a person's problem.
    c. A diagnosis assists mental health professional to do research on psychological problems.
    d. The psychiatric diagnosis guides a therapist in treating an individual for the diagnosed problem.
    Answer: a   LO: 1; factual, conceptual   page: 24

Assessing and Diagnosing Abnormality

5. In learning about a person's current symptoms, a therapist will initially want to gather information about their:
   a. ambiguity or clarity.
   b. severity and chronicity.
   c. usefulness and value.
   d. severity and usefulness.
   Answer: b   LO: 1; conceptual   page: 25

6. The most often used criteria for diagnosing most of the major psychological disorders:
   a. require that the symptoms be so severe and pervasive that they interfere with a person's ability to function in daily life.
   b. suggest that symptoms that are sufficiently pervasive to cause the patient discomfort will justify such a diagnosis.
   c. vary from each other, so there is no set pattern for determining individual diagnoses and it must be done on an individual basis.
   d. require that symptoms be so severe as to cause discomfort for the patient in order to justify such a diagnosis.
   Answer: a   LO: 1; conceptual   page: 25

7. When gathering information about recent events in a person's life, the therapist:
   a. will focus more on the negative events (such as death of a loved one) than on the positive events (such as promotion at work).
   b. will focus more on the positive events (such as promotion at work) than on the negative events (such as death of a loved one).
   c. is concerned with both positive and negative events that result in change in the person's life.
   d. is not actually concerned about whether the symptoms have a specific triggering event or come "out of the blue" for purposes of diagnosis.
   Answer: c   LO: 1; factual   pages: 25-26

8. During Mr. Brown's initial interview with Dr. Rose, the therapist asked the client to see his physician for a complete physical examination. Most likely Dr. Rose did this because:
   a. she did not want to be held responsible if Mr. Brown had a heart attack or stroke while under her care.
   b. she thought he looked ill and was concerned for his well being.
   c. she needed to determine if he had a medical condition that might cause psychological symptoms.
   d. it is required to be included on the diagnostic information by insurance companies.
   Answer: c   LO: 1; applied   page: 26

Chapter 2

9. A physical examination in conjunction with the initial psychological assessment process can provide the therapist with information concerning:
   a. whether a medical disease is causing psychological symptoms.
   b. a person's ability to work well in a therapeutic setting.
   c. whether a person is in sufficiently good health to endure psychotherapy.
   d. whether the person is "faking" his or her symptoms.
   Answer: a   LO: 1; factual   page: 26

10. With respect to a client's use of drugs:
    a. in order to respect the client's issues of confidentiality, the psychologist should not probe until the client has opened up the topic.
    b. a psychologist needs to know both legal and illegal use since many drugs can cause psychological symptoms.
    c. the psychologist's main concern is whether the client is taking illegal drugs, since this would affect the diagnosis.
    d. the psychologist needs to know about prescription drugs, since there may be a drug interaction with medications she prescribes.
    Answer: b   LO: 1; factual   page: 26

11. With regard to a client's past history of psychological problems, it is:
    a. irrelevant to current treatment since the past cannot be changed.
    b. irrelevant to current treatment since the focus is now on "where do we go from here?"
    c. relevant to current treatment since knowing the history can help the therapist change how the client views the world.
    d. relevant to current treatment since knowing the history can help the therapist form a diagnosis.
    Answer: d   LO: 1; factual   page: 26

12. Jackson Andrews presents himself in Dr. Candy's office, complaining that space aliens are sharing with him their plan to attack San Francisco. During the initial interview, Dr. Candy asks Mr. Andrews about any past history of psychological problems he might have had. Her major reason for asking this is to help her:
    a. make a differential diagnosis.
    b. decide if she should take the case.
    c. decide if he should be hospitalized.
    d. determine if he will cooperate in therapy.
    Answer: a   LO: 1; applied   page: 26

Assessing and Diagnosing Abnormality

13. When making a differential diagnosis, a therapist is determining:
    a. whether a client actually needs therapy.
    b. how consistent a client's symptoms are.
    c. which of two or more disorders a client has.
    d. how extreme the client's symptoms are.
    Answer: c   LO: 1; conceptual   page: 26

14. One important reason for asking a client about his or her family history of psychological disorders is to:
    a. assist the therapist in making a differential diagnosis.
    b. assist the therapist in assessing the client's support system.
    c. help the client feel more comfortable, knowing the problem is not unique.
    d. assist the client in understanding the origins of his or her problem.
    Answer: a   LO: 1; factual, conceptual   page: 26

15. Concerning assessment of a client's family history of psychological disorders:
    a. many therapists have objected to this since there is little consistency in these disorders from one family member to another.
    b. therapists find this information useful because it helps them determine whether they can count on the client's family as a resource for his or her social support.
    c. therapists find this information useful because it helps them work with the client's family, which is the likely source of the client's problem.
    d. therapists find this information useful in forming a differential diagnosis since some disorders seem to run in certain families.
    Answer: d   LO: 1; factual, conceptual   page: 26

16. Which of the following *best* helps a therapist determine if a client is experiencing neurological disorders?
    a. family history of psychological disorders
    b. recent events in client's life
    c. intellectual and cognitive functioning
    d. current symptoms
    Answer: c   LO: 1; factual, conceptual   page: 27

17. Which of the following *best* help the therapist form a differential diagnosis?
    a. current symptoms and family history of psychological disorders
    b. current symptoms and prior diagnoses
    c. recent events and drug use
    d. current symptoms and physical condition
    Answer: a   LO: 1; factual   pages: 25-27

Chapter 2

18. Which of the following ***best*** assesses a client's coping style?
    a. "Are you close with any members of your family?"
    b. "What do you believe is your most pressing problem?"
    c. "How do you generally handle problems in your life?"
    d. "What do you think would be the best treatment for your symptoms?"
    Answer: c   LO: 1; applied   page: 27

19. It is important for the therapist to assess a client's social resources because:
    a. being close with family and friends is important for effective therapeutic results.
    b. living alone causes a client to feel isolated and impairs therapeutic effectiveness.
    c. even when family members cause conflict, they are important to therapy.
    d. the quality of a client's relationships with family and friends can affect therapeutic results.
    Answer: d   LO: 1; conceptual   page: 27

20. A person's belief about his or her ability to overcome the presenting symptoms:
    a. is a measure of the client's concept of symptoms.
    b. reflects the client's sense of self-efficacy.
    c. demonstrates the client's self-concept.
    d. is a measure of the client's self-esteem.
    Answer: b   LO: 1; conceptual   page: 27

21. A client's sociocultural background:
    a. helps streamline therapy because it provides the therapist with important ideas of what to expect from a client.
    b. assists the therapist in providing information concerning particular risk factors the client may be facing.
    c. is not particularly helpful because it is inappropriate for a therapist to stereotype or generalize on the basis of sociocultural background.
    d. adds some information that can be useful but is not of major importance since each client has a different level of acculturation.
    Answer: b   LO: 1; conceptual   page: 28

22. Acculturation reflects the:
    a. number of generations a family has been in the country to which their ancestors immigrated.
    b. level of education that an immigrant has achieved in his or her adopted country.
    c. extent to which a person feels alienated from his or her culture of origin or from the mainstream culture.
    d. extent to which a person identifies with his or her culture of origin or with the mainstream culture.
    Answer: d   LO: 1; conceptual   page: 28

Assessing and Diagnosing Abnormality

23. Knowledge of a client's level of acculturation:
    a. assists the therapist in understanding how clients experience psychological distress and how they will respond to therapeutic interventions.
    b. assists the therapist in deciding which medications should be prescribed, since acculturation will affect how clients react to drugs.
    c. is a deterrent to effective therapy because therapists are not sufficiently trained in cultural diversity.
    d. is a deterrent to effective therapy because it is difficult for therapists to overcome the tendency to stereotype.
    Answer: a   LO: 1; conceptual   page: 28

24. Wanda was extremely nervous when she came to Dr. Rose's office for her first therapy session, but she soon feels very much at ease and almost felt like she was having a "normal" conversation because Dr. Rose asked her questions like, "Tell me about yourself," and Wanda was able to say everything that was on her mind. This initial session is an example of:
    a. a formal interview.
    b. an open-ended interview.
    c. an unstructured interview.
    d. a comfortable interview.
    Answer: c   LO: 2; applied   pages: 28-29

25. Whether a test actually measures what it says it measures is an issue of the test's:
    a. reliability.
    b. generalizability.
    c. construction.
    d. validity.
    Answer: d   LO: 5; conceptual   page: 29

26. If a test appears to measure what it is supposed to measure, we can say it has _____ validity.
    a. face
    b. content
    c. concurrent
    d. construct
    Answer: a   LO: 5; factual, conceptual   page: 29

27. If a test assesses all important aspects of a phenomenon, we can say it has _____ validity.
    a. face
    b. content
    c. concurrent
    d. construct
    Answer: b   LO: 5; factual, conceptual   page: 29

Chapter 2

28. _____ is an indicator of the test's consistency.
    a. Validity
    b. Reliability
    c. Generalizability
    d. Concurrence
    Answer: b   LO: 5; factual, conceptual   page: 29

29. Construct validity is concerned with whether a test:
    a. assesses all important aspects of a phenomenon.
    b. yields the same results as other measures of the same behavior, thoughts, feelings.
    c. predicts the behavior it is supposed to measure.
    d. measures what it is supposed to measure and not something else.
    Answer: d   LO: 5; factual, conceptual   page: 30

30. _____ reliability is an indicator of how consistent the results of a test are over time.
    a. Test-retest
    b. Alternate form
    c. Internal
    d. Interrater
    Answer: a   LO: 5; factual, conceptual   page: 30

31. Which biological test consists of narrow X-ray beams that are passed through a person's head from a variety of angles?
    a. Computerized tomography (CT)
    b. Magnetic resonance imaging (MRI)
    c. Positron emission tomography (PET)
    d. Electroencephalogram (EEG)
    Answer: a   LO: 2; factual   page: 31

32. A major limitation of using a single CT scan is:
    a. that it cannot use sufficient amounts of X ray to get a clear picture.
    b. it can reveal brain injury, but not tumors or structural abnormalities.
    c. it cannot provide an image of activity in the brain.
    d. it can only provide a two-dimensional image of the brain.
    Answer: c   LO: 3; factual   page: 31

Assessing and Diagnosing Abnormality

33. Which test involves injecting a patient with radioactive isotopes to show differences in activity levels of specific areas of the brain?
    a. Computerized tomography (CT)
    b. Magnetic resonance imaging (MRI)
    c. Positron emission tomography (PET)
    d. Electroencephalogram (EEG)
    Answer: c   LO: 2; factual   page: 31

34. Researchers use magnetic resonance imaging (MRI) to study:
    a. magnetic fields in the brain.
    b. functional and structural brain abnormalities.
    c. thought processes in the brain.
    d. intellectual differences among patients.
    Answer: b   LO: 2; factual   pages: 31-33

35. The biological testing tool that is safe to use and provides detailed pictures of brain anatomy, activity, and functioning is:
    a. computerized tomography (CT)
    b. magnetic resonance imaging (MRI)
    c. positron emission tomography (PET)
    d. electroencephalogram (EEG)
    Answer: b   LO: 2; factual   pages: 31-33

36. As demonstrated by a recording from an Electroencephalogram (EEG), during a normal waking state, EEG activity:
    a. typically exhibits theta waves.
    b. predominately exhibits the large delta waves.
    c. predominately exhibits beta waves.
    d. alternates between alpha and beta waves.
    Answer: d   LO: 2; factual   pages: 33-34

37. Event-related potentials (ERPs) allow researchers to examine the extent and nature of electrical activity associated with a stimulus. They are currently particularly helpful in identifying:
    a. schizophrenia.
    b. depression.
    c. attentional problems.
    d. serotonin levels.
    Answer: c   LO: 2, 3; factual   page: 34

Chapter 2

38. A current limitation on the use of biological assessment devices is that, for the most part, they:
    a. can only identify gross structural or functional abnormalities.
    b. cannot differentiate between the brains of people with psychological disorders and those without such disorders.
    c. can only identify major brain disturbances, such as tumors.
    d. cannot diagnose specific psychological disorders of individual patients.
    Answer: d   LO: 3; factual   page: 34

39. In addition to biological tests, which of the following tests is used to assess possible brain damage?
    a. neuropsychological
    b. projective
    c. intelligence
    d. personality
    Answer: a   LO: 2; factual   page: 35

40. The Bender-Gestalt Test assesses a client's:
    a. sensorimotor skills.
    b. personality development.
    c. intelligence.
    d. personality disorders.
    Answer: a   LO: 2; factual   page: 35

41. When reproducing a drawing from the Bender-Gestalt:
    a. it is common even for normal clients to omit parts of the drawing.
    b. a client with brain damage may rotate or change parts of the drawing.
    c. a normal client will find all of the drawings equally as easy or difficult.
    d. a person's specific type of brain damage will be detected.
    Answer: b   LO: 2; factual   page: 35

42. Typically, a therapist will rely on _____ to make a determination that a client has some type of brain damage.
    a. biological tests
    b. neuropsychological tests
    c. biological and neuropsychological tests
    d. cognitively based intelligence tests
    Answer: c   LO: 2; factual, conceptual   page: 35

Assessing and Diagnosing Abnormality

43. The Halstead-Reitan and the Luria-Nebraska Test are batteries of test that:
    a. assess a client's intelligence.
    b. pinpoint the type of brain damage a client has.
    c. pinpoint the type of psychological disorder a client has.
    d. assess a client's ability to function socially.
    Answer: b   LO: 2; factual   pages: 35-36

44. An IQ score of 100 on the WAIS-R indicates that:
    a. the person performed much higher than other people of similar age.
    b. the person performed similarly to the average performance of people of similar age.
    c. the person performed much lower than other people of similar age.
    d. there may have been something wrong with administering the test, since this is an atypical score on an IQ test.
    Answer: b   LO: 2; factual, conceptual   page: 36

45. Intelligence tests are designed to measure:
    a. how smart someone is.
    b. basic intellectual abilities.
    c. a person's motivation.
    d. how much a person knows.
    Answer: b   LO: 2; conceptual   page: 36

46. One criticism of intelligence tests is they are biased in favor of:
    a. middle- and upper-class Anglo-Americans.
    b. persons who are highly creative.
    c. persons with exceptional musical ability.
    d. lower socioeconomic status minorities.
    Answer: a   LO: 3; factual   page: 36

47. A major limitation of most intelligence tests is that they fail to address:
    a. individual differences.
    b. cultural differences.
    c. intellectual potential.
    d. social awareness.
    Answer: b   LO: 3; factual   pages: 36-37

Chapter 2

48. Which of the following statements *best* addresses universal concepts of intelligence?
    a. It would only be possible to make meaningful cross-cultural comparisons if a culture-fair test were created.
    b. On the basis of the culture-fair tests that we now have, psychologists have begun to understand how the concept of intelligence is viewed around the world.
    c. Even if a universal test were created, general statements about intelligence would be difficult to make because notions of intelligence vary around the world.
    d. There is a generally accepted, universal understanding of what constitutes intelligence and it is often being tested and compared cross-culturally.
    Answer: c   LO: 4; conceptual   page: 37

49. When Jill first saw Dr. Kennedy, she was asked to tell him about the symptoms she was currently experiencing, as well as any symptoms she had experienced in the past. She noticed that Dr. Kennedy asked her very specific questions and seemed to be checking things off on a checklist. Most likely Dr. Kennedy was conducting a(n) _____ with Jill.
    a. unstructured clinical interview
    b. structured clinical interview
    c. informal interview
    d. preliminary assessment
    Answer: b   LO: 2; applied   pages: 38-39

50. The therapist asks the client a series of specific, standardized questions about the client's symptoms, both past and present, and the responses are scored according to concrete criteria in:
    a. an unstructured clinical interview.
    b. a structured clinical interview.
    c. a symptom questionnaire.
    d. a battery of tests.
    Answer: b   LO: 2, 6; factual, conceptual   pages: 38-39

51. Which of the following is a structured clinical interview?
    a. The Bender-Gestalt
    b. The MMPI-2
    c. The Behavior Checklist
    d. The Diagnostic Interview Schedule
    Answer: d   LO: 2; factual   page: 38

Assessing and Diagnosing Abnormality

52. One benefit of a standard set of questions and scoring system for structured clinical interviews is that it:
    a. increases the reliability of information gathered.
    b. allows the client to express himself or herself freely.
    c. allows the client to get used to the therapist before opening up.
    d. increases validity in terms of future clinical research.
    Answer: a   LO: 3, 6; factual   page: 39

53. A common symptom questionnaire that asks the client to indicate which of four levels of a given symptom best describe the client's feelings in the last two weeks is the:
    a. Anti-Depressant Scale (ADS)
    b. Beck Depression Inventory (BDI)
    c. Breckenridge Inventory of Depression Scale (BIDS)
    d. Sadness and Depression Scale (SADS)
    Answer: b   LO: 2; factual   page: 39

54. One way that the Child Behavior Checklist (CBCL) differs from other symptom questionnaires is that:
    a. parents are asked to fill it out.
    b. the language is much simpler.
    c. it is not as apparent from the questions what is being assessed.
    d. it is considerably shorter than other symptom questionnaires.
    Answer: a   LO: 2; factual   page: 40

55. A questionnaire used to assess people's typical ways of thinking, feeling, and behaving is called:
    a. a symptom questionnaire.
    b. an intelligence test.
    c. a personality inventory.
    d. a neurological test.
    Answer: c   LO: 2; factual   page: 40

56. The personality inventory that is most widely used around the world is the:
    a. Beck Depression Inventory (BDI).
    b. Minnesota Multiphasic Personality Inventory (MMPI).
    c. California Personality Inventory (CPI).
    d. Rorschach test.
    Answer: b   LO: 2; factual   page: 40

Chapter 2

57. Milton's psychologist has asked him to undergo a battery of psychological tests. One of the tests contains 566 true/false questions such as, "I would rather win than lose in a game," and "I am afraid of losing my mind." We might expect that Milton is taking the:
    a. Beck Depression Inventory (BDI)
    b. Minnesota Multiphasic Personality Inventory (MMPI)
    c. California Personality Inventory (CPI)
    d. Thematic Apperception Test (TAT)
    Answer: b   LO: 2; applied   page: 40

58. Which of the following scales was added to the MMPI-2?
    a. vulnerability to eating disorders
    b. vulnerability to homosexuality
    c. social introversion
    d. the lie scale
    Answer: a   LO: 2; factual   page: 40

59. Items on the MMPI were selected in terms of their ability to differentiate people with specific psychological disorders from those without psychological disorders. As a result, it has a high level of:
    a. test-retest reliability.
    b. predictive validity.
    c. construct validity.
    d. concurrent validity.
    Answer: d   LO: 5; conceptual   pages: 40-41

60. The major criticisms of the MMPI seem to center around its use with people who are:
    a. extremely psychopathic.
    b. mildly depressed.
    c. culturally diverse.
    d. socially withdrawn.
    Answer: c   LO: 3; conceptual   page: 41

61. One advantage of direct behavioral observations over self-report data is that:
    a. high interrater reliability is achieved.
    b. the observer's subjective analysis is obtained.
    c. the client's subjective interpretation is avoided.
    d. more time can be spent gathering data.
    Answer: c   LO: 3, 6; factual   page: 42

Assessing and Diagnosing Abnormality

62. _____ tests are used to uncover a person's unconscious issues or motives.
    a. Objective
    b. Subjective
    c. Neurological
    d. Projective
    Answer: d   LO: 2; factual, conceptual   page: 43

63. _____ tests are based on the assumption that a person will interpret ambiguous stimuli in a way that reflects their current concerns, feelings, relationships with others, and conflicts or desires.
    a. Objective
    b. Subjective
    c. Projective
    d. Intelligence
    Answer: c   LO: 2; conceptual   page: 43

64. Jason was shown a series of cards that looked like blots of ink. His psychologist asked him to look at the cards and tell her what it looks like and what it could be. Jason was taking a _____ Test.
    a. Thematic Apperception
    b. Rorschach
    c. Bender Gestalt
    d. California Personality Inventory
    Answer: b   LO: 2; applied   page: 43

65. The psychologist might be particularly interested in a client's Rorschach response if the client:
    a. responds to the inkblot as a whole.
    b. looks at each card for a long time before responding.
    c. responds very quickly to each card.
    d. considers color as well as shape in responding.
    Answer: b   LO 2; conceptual   page: 43

66. The client is asked to make up a story about what is happening in a series of pictures in the:
    a. Rorschach Test.
    b. Bender-Gestalt.
    c. MMPI.
    d. Thematic Apperception Test.
    Answer: d   LO: 2; factual   page: 43

Chapter 2

67. The Thematic Apperception Test is given in an attempt to have the client:
    a. become more relaxed in the therapeutic setting.
    b. demonstrate his or her ability for creativity.
    c. express his or her concerns, wishes, and motives.
    d. demonstrate aspects of verbal intelligence.
    Answer: c   LO: 2; factual   page: 43

68. Compared to the Rorschach and Thematic Apperception Test, the Sentence Completion Test is:
    a. interpreted more subjectively.
    b. interpreted less subjectively.
    c. less structured.
    d. more structured.
    Answer: d   LO: 2; factual   pages: 43-44

69. When working with children, therapists often have the children play with toys or make drawings and then talk about them. What specifically would a therapist be looking for in observing the child?
    a. the child's intelligence level
    b. specific styles of play
    c. specific themes that emerge
    d. the child's level of creativity
    Answer: c   LO: 2; factual, conceptual   page: 44

70. From the psychoanalytic perspective, which of the following is an advantage of using projective tests?
    a. They help assess conflicts and concerns about which the client may be unaware.
    b. They have been found to be highly reliable assessment tools.
    c. They have been found to show fairly high content validity.
    d. They help assess a client's ability to work well in a therapeutic setting.
    Answer: a   LO: 3, 6; conceptual   pages: 43-45

71. Which of the following is a major criticism of projective tests?
    a. There is not enough research to determine their usefulness.
    b. They are not helpful in uncovering an individual's unconscious conflicts.
    c. They are extremely difficult to administer.
    d. Their interpretation is highly subjective and open to interpretive bias.
    Answer: d   LO: 3; factual, conceptual   page: 44

Assessing and Diagnosing Abnormality

72. Gregory was brought to therapy by his parents who are concerned about his lack of cooperation in school and at home. Gregory does not want to be in therapy and sits through his entire 50-minute sessions every week saying nothing. In therapeutic terms, this is an example of:
    a. transference.
    b. counter-transference.
    c. rebellion.
    d. resistance.
    Answer: d   LO: 2; applied   page: 45

73. Robert had been seeing a Dr. Melody for two months about the break-up of his marriage. They had been working on ways that Robert could get on with his life but continue to play a major parenting role with his two teenage sons with whom he was extremely close. Suddenly, Dr. Melody's husband left her, and now she is trying to convince Robert that he should return to his wife for the sake of keeping his family together. This is an example of:
    a. transference.
    b. counter-transference.
    c. ethical misconduct.
    d. resistance.
    Answer: b   LO: 3; applied   pages: 45-46

74. When a therapist's feelings about a significant person affect interaction with a client, it is called:
    a. resistance.
    b. transference.
    c. counter-transference.
    d. bias.
    Answer: c   LO: 3; factual, conceptual   pages: 45-46

75. A problem therapists can encounter when working with children is that children often:
    a. lie to protect themselves.
    b. lie to protect someone else.
    c. have difficulty articulating feelings.
    d. overuse their imaginations.
    Answer: c   LO: 3, 6; factual   page: 46

Chapter 2

76. According to the text, which of the following is the *most* correct statement?
    a. Parents are the most accurate source of information about their children.
    b. Parents may bring children to therapy as a way of seeking treatment for themselves.
    c. Parents have a relatively accurate perception of their children, even if they do not always provide accurate information to the therapist.
    d. Despite their own personal issues, parents tend to have and relate a relatively accurate perception of their children to the therapist.
    Answer: b   LO: 2; factual   pages: 46-47

77. In terms of comparing parents' and teachers' assessments of children, they are:
    a. usually highly consistent with each other.
    b. often discrepant with each other.
    c. rarely, if ever, consistent with each other.
    d. teachers usually have a clearer picture than parents of the child's problems.
    Answer: b   LO: 2; factual   page: 47

78. Vera was taken to the Student Health Services on her campus because in class she talked about her experiences, some very recently, of communicating with spirits. Professor Camptom became concerned, especially because Vera is a good student who has been under a great deal of pressure lately. Vera had told Professor Camptom that her mother in Brazil was very ill and the spirits had spoken of the older woman's impending death. When she spoke with the college therapist about her concerns and experiences, the therapist determined that Vera was experiencing a psychotic break due to excessive stress in her life. Something that undoubtedly influenced the therapist's diagnosis is:
    a. counter-transference.
    b. resistance.
    c. cultural bias.
    d. stereotyping.
    Answer: c   LO: 4; applied   pages: 47-48

79. Which of the following is not a problem of cultural bias in terms of diagnosing clients' psychological disorders?
    a. The therapist may overdiagnose disorders based on cultural differences.
    b. The therapist may underdiagnose disorders due to clients' culture.
    c. The therapist may misdiagnose disorders due to a client's cultural background.
    d. The therapist may diagnose different disorders depending on a client's culture.
    Answer: d   LO: 4; factual, conceptual   pages: 47-49

Assessing and Diagnosing Abnormality

80. European Americans tend to express more _____ symptoms compared to other cultural groups.
    a. somatic
    b. emotional
    c. behavioral
    d. neurological
    Answer: a   LO: 4; factual   page: 49

81. Despite training about cultural differences, therapists may still experience difficulties when dealing with clients from diverse cultures because of:
    a. individual differences.
    b. cultural norms.
    c. subtle stereotypes.
    d. ineffective techniques.
    Answer: a   LO: 4; factual   page: 49

82. A set of symptoms that occur together is referred to as a:
    a. diagnosis.
    b. syndrome.
    c. model.
    d. symptomatology.
    Answer: b   LO: 7; factual   page: 49

83. A classification system is:
    a. a group of symptoms that occur together.
    b. a technique for placing similar symptoms together.
    c. a set of rules to explain how particular symptoms fit a given classification.
    d. a set of syndromes and rules to determine if a person's symptoms fit that set.
    Answer: d   LO: 7; factual   page: 50

84. One of the first persons to devise a classification system for psychological symptoms was:
    a. Galen.
    b. Freud.
    c. Hippocrates.
    d. Socrates.
    Answer: c   LO: 7; factual   page: 50

Chapter 2

85. The official manual that has been used for over 40 years in the United States for diagnosing psychological disorders is the:
    a. Diagnostic and Statistical Manual of Mental Disorders of the American Psychiatric Association (DSM).
    b. Psychological Assessment Scales of the American Psychological Association (PAS).
    c. Current Procedural Terminology Codes of the American Psychiatric Association (CPTC).
    d. International Classification of Diseases, 9th Revision, Clinical Modification (ICD-9-CM).
    Answer: a	LO: 7; factual	page: 50

86. A problem with early versions of the DSM was:
    a. it was so large that it was difficult for clinicians to use effectively.
    b. descriptions of disorders were so abstract that reliability of diagnoses was low.
    c. it was not used by all clinicians, and thus reliability of diagnoses was low.
    d. there was not sufficient theory to allow clinicians to make appropriate diagnoses.
    Answer: b	LO: 8; factual	page: 50

87. In the later revisions of the DSM:
    a. there is more theory than in early editions.
    b. diagnostic criteria require interference with ability to function.
    c. more credence is given to Freudian theory than before.
    d. diagnostic criteria are less stringent than in early editions.
    Answer: b	LO: 8; factual	page: 51

88. The length of time a disorder typically lasts and the likelihood of future relapse is the _____ _____ of a disorder.
    a. prediction
    b. prognosis
    c. diagnosis
    d. course
    Answer: d	LO: 7; factual	page: 51

89. The term *prevalence* refers to the number of people who:
    a. ever had a specific psychological disorder.
    b. had a specific psychological disorder during a specified period of time.
    c. might be expected to develop a specific psychological disorder.
    d. might be expected to develop any psychological disorder.
    Answer: b	LO: 7; factual, conceptual	page: 52

Assessing and Diagnosing Abnormality

90. _____ refers to the number of new cases of a disorder that develop during a specific period of time.
    a. Prevalence
    b. Occurrence
    c. Incidence
    d. Expectancy
    Answer: c   LO: 7; factual   page: 52

91. A problem with DSM-III and DSM-IIIR that was expected to be overcome in DSM-IV was:
    a. low reliability of diagnoses.
    b. low validity of diagnoses.
    c. high dependence on theory.
    d. difficult criteria to understand.
    Answer: a   LO: 8; factual   page: 52

92. In an effort to increase reliability of diagnoses in the DSM-IV, researchers:
    a. redefined each of the characteristics used as criteria for a disorder.
    b. conducted numerous field trials in clinical and research settings.
    c. increased reliance on specific clinical theories of psychopathology.
    d. reevaluated research over the past 100 years to refine criteria for each disorder.
    Answer: b   LO: 8; factual   page: 52

93. With respect to the five axes used in the DSM to evaluate a client's behavior:
    a. only the first axis lists actual disorders and criteria needed for a diagnosis.
    b. only the first two list actual disorders and criteria needed for a diagnosis.
    c. the first two provide information about what may affect a person's mental health.
    d. each axis lists the disorders and criteria needed for a diagnosis, as well as other information about what may affect a person's mental health.
    Answer: b   LO: 7; factual   pages: 52-53

94. Soon after Sam retired, his wife died. After 55 years of marriage, they anticipated his retirement as time to "get to know each other" again. Sam's children are worried he may be suicidal. They found a gun on his dresser, although as they were growing up, he consistently preached to them about the dangers of weapons. Over the past six months, he has lost 20 lbs, and he no longer enjoys playing with his grandchildren. His daughter took him to his doctor, who said there is nothing physically wrong with Sam but suggested he be evaluated by a psychologist. Which DSM Axis would be used to determine his *psychological diagnosis*?
    a. Axis I
    b. Axis III
    c. Axis IV
    d. Axis V
    Answer: a   LO: 7; applied   pages: 52-53

Chapter 2

95. Soon after Sam retired, his wife died. After 55 years of marriage, they anticipated his retirement as time to "get to know each other" again. Sam's children are worried he may be suicidal. They found a gun on his dresser, although as they were growing up, he consistently preached to them about the dangers of weapons. Over the past six months, he has lost 20 lbs, and he no longer enjoys playing with his grandchildren. His daughter took him to his doctor, who said there is nothing physically wrong with Sam but suggested he be evaluated by a psychologist. Which DSM Axis would be used to assess the *types of stressors* Sam is facing in order to develop a useful treatment plan?
   a. Axis I
   b. Axis III
   c. Axis IV
   d. Axis V
   Answer: c   LO: 7; applied   page: 54

96. A person diagnosed with Borderline Personality Disorder would receive that diagnosis on
   a. Axis I
   b. Axis II
   c. Axis III
   d. Axis IV
   Answer: b   LO: 7; factual   pages: 53-54

97. A person's problem with diabetes would be indicated on which Axis of the DSM?
   a. Axis I
   b. Axis II
   c. Axis III
   d. Axis V
   Answer: c   LO: 7; factual   pages: 53-54

98. One of the concerns about using DSM-IV relates to its:
   a. difficulty of use.
   b. continuing ambiguity.
   c. low interrater reliability.
   d. potential cultural bias.
   Answer: d   LO: 4, 7; factual   pages: 57-58

99. The debate over whether a diagnosis of Masochistic Personality Disorder should be included in DSM-IIIR is an example of _____ influences.
   a. political
   b. cultural
   c. legal
   d. individual
   Answer: a   LO: 8; factual   page: 57

Assessing and Diagnosing Abnormality

100. A criticism of the DSM-IV is that it:
    a. presents the Western male as a standard of mental health.
    b. presents Western females as a standard of mental health.
    c. does not address cultural diversity in mental health.
    d. presents so many cultural variations that it is confusing.
    Answer: a   LO: 7; factual, conceptual   pages: 57-58

101. A major critic of psychiatry, who is particularly concerned that labeling persons as "mentally ill" is a social judgment, is:
    a. Susan Nolen-Hoeksema.
    b. David Wechsler.
    c. Thomas Szasz.
    d. David Rosenhan.
    Answer: c   LO: 9; factual   page: 58

102. The psychologist who created a huge shake-up in the mental health field by having participants admitted to mental hospitals after falsely stating they heard voices saying the words "empty," "hollow," and "thud," and denying any other symptoms, is:
    a. David Wechsler.
    b. David Rosenhan.
    c. Martin Seligman.
    d. Thomas Szasz.
    Answer: b   LO: 9; factual   pages: 58-60

103. In his research on "sane" people being admitted to mental hospitals, David Rosenhan noted that:
    a. the hospital personnel quickly determined that the pseudopatients were "faking it."
    b. the behavior of the pseudopatients was interpreted in terms of their diagnosis.
    c. the pseudopatients were able to fool even the real patients on the wards.
    d. after being discharged, records of the pseudopatients indicated they were "normal."
    Answer: b   LO: 9; factual   pages: 58-60

104. A potential danger of labeling someone as having a psychological problem is:
    a. it may jeopardize the person's ability to receive appropriate medical care.
    b. the person may be unable to receive helpful therapy to overcome the problem.
    c. it causes others to ignore the person's behavior entirely.
    d. it affects how other people behave toward that person.
    Answer: d   LO: 9; conceptual   page: 58

Chapter 2

105. When evaluating self-assessment questionnaires on the market today, the consumer should remember that the information:
    a. provides an excellent profile if the person filling out the form is honest.
    b. is suggestive of possible problems, but is not conclusive.
    c. is pretty much like astrology and should be used only for amusement.
    d. must be interpreted by a professional in order to be reliable.
    Answer: b   LO: 3, 6; conceptual   page: 62

Essay Questions

106. Ann comes to see Dr. Maas because she states that she has had no energy for several months, and the problem has become increasingly worse over the past three weeks. She can think of no particular trigger either for the original onset or for the worsening of her symptoms. She indicates on her intake form that her father died many years ago, when Ann was a teenager, and that she and her mother have had problems since that time, particularly with respect to "setting boundaries." What steps would you take to assess Ann's problem(s), and what diagnosis would you give her?

The student should discuss the various assessment tools to be used to diagnose Ann's problem, *including* a referral for a physical examination by her treating physician to rule out any biological causes of her decline in energy levels. Once any physical basis for her problems is eliminated, a battery of tests could include the Bender-Gestalt, to assess any neurological problems; the WAIS-R to assess intellectual functioning; and the TAT, Draw-a-Person, and MMPI to look at various underlying personality traits and attitudes that may relate to her presenting problems.

The student then needs indicate the type of interview the student feels would be effective for gathering information on Axes III-V of DSM-IV in order to assess other factors relevant to Ann's current problem; then, depending on what the student indicates with respect to the foregoing, a diagnosis can be made on Axis I, and if applicable, Axis II.

Assessing and Diagnosing Abnormality

197. As stated in the acknowledgments section of DSM-IV, over 1,000 people were involved in preparing the manual. This included the DSM-IV Task Force members and many mental health professionals who participated in work groups. Their intent was to come up with a manual that would make diagnosing mental disorders a relatively consistent and effective process for providing help. Discuss how they have achieved those goals, and discuss what problems continue to exist in terms of diagnosing people with psychological disorders.

    The student will need to discuss issues of improved interrater reliability and how that affects diagnosis and communication among mental health professionals; how reducing ambiguity improves in diagnoses and thus treatment; and how attention to issues of cultural and gender diversity reduces bias in those areas. However, cultural and gender bias remain, interrater reliability still remains to be seen; and the issues of labeling and stigmatizing individuals must be addressed.

108. Thomas Szasz has criticized the mental health profession for labeling persons as "mentally ill," which he states is a "myth" and a social judgment. Discuss both sides of this argument in terms of the appropriateness and dangers of diagnosing a person with a mental disorder.

    The student may note that there are some universally accepted behaviors (as pointed out in Chapter 1) that are agreed upon as being abnormal. Further, behaviors that are dangerous to oneself or to others need to be dealt with in order to maximize the individual's own life and to protect society. The dangers of labeling are most apparent in terms of others' perceptions and behaviors toward a person who has been labeled, and Rosenhan's (1973) research on "Being Sane in Insane Places" would be appropriate in this discussion, as would Harris et al.'s (1992) research on labeling a child as having a behavior problem. Another danger lies in the politicization of labeling someone who has unpopular beliefs (a major concern of Szasz).

Chapter 2

109. Vera was taken to the Student Health Services on her campus because in class she talked about her experiences, some very recently, of communicating with spirits. Professor Camptom became concerned, especially because Vera is a good student who has been under a great deal of pressure lately. Vera had told Professor Camptom that her mother in Brazil was very ill and the spirits had spoken of the older woman's impending death. When she spoke with the college therapist about her concerns and experiences, the therapist determined that Vera was experiencing a psychotic break due to excessive stress in her life, and she was diagnosed with Schizophrenia, Paranoid Type. Discuss the factors that you believe influenced the therapist's diagnosis. How would you go about assessing Vera's current emotional situation, and how would you apply the five axes of DSM-IV?

    First the student must discuss cultural issues and the fact that it is not uncommon in Brazil for people to see and communicate with spirits; thus, the therapist's diagnosis is premature. Discuss the assessment tools the student believes, from reading the text, would be appropriate for gathering information about Vera's state and the type of information necessary for making a complete diagnosis on the five axes of DSM-IV.

110. Discuss the purpose of the *Diagnostic and Statistic Manual of Mental Disorders of the American Psychiatric Association* and its evolution over the past 45 years, including its present format.

    The student should discuss the importance of having an unambiguous classification system that aids in communication among mental health professionals, ease of diagnosis, and relationship between a consistent diagnosis and effective treatment modalities. The evolution from the first and second editions that relied heavily on psychoanalytic theory to more specific diagnostic criteria based on observations in DSM-III and DSM-IIIR, and on extensive field studies in DSM-IV should then follow. Also, the student should discuss the use of the five axes, beginning with DSM-III. The issues of cultural and gender bias and the political influences in its development should be addressed.

Chapter 3   Approaching and Treating Abnormality

1. A theoretical approach is defined in the text as a:
   a. set of assumptions about the likely causes and appropriate treatments of abnormality.
   b. set of criteria used to determine the appropriate diagnostic assessment tools.
   c. way of determining which is the correct way to analyze a potential client's problems.
   d. mutually exclusive set of criteria used for diagnosis, assessment, and treatment.
   Answer: a   LO: 1; factual, conceptual   page: 66

2. A clinician who looks for structural or functional deficits in the brain would be taking which approach to abnormality?
   a. biological
   b. psychosocial
   c. behavioral
   d. sociocultural
   Answer: a   LO: 1; conceptual   page: 66

3. A psychologist who takes a biological approach to abnormality would most likely look at:
   a. structural or functional deficits in the brain, biochemical imbalances, or genetics.
   b. early childhood experiences, recent traumas, thinking styles, or personality traits.
   c. the client's typical ways of behaving in or reacting to specific situations.
   d. the impact of societal factors on the client's psychological well being.
   Answer: a   LO: 1; conceptual   page: 66

4. The psychosocial approach to abnormality focuses on:
   a. structural or functional deficits in the brain, biochemical imbalances, or genetics.
   b. early childhood experiences, recent traumas, thinking styles, or personality traits.
   c. the client's typical ways of behaving in or reacting to specific situations.
   d. the interaction between biological and psychological factors.
   Answer: b   LO: 2; conceptual   page: 66

5. When Cynthia first came to see Dr. Fields, Dr. Fields primarily asked about her early childhood experiences and recent events that have occurred in her life. We might expect that Dr. Fields takes a _____ approach to abnormality.
   a. biological
   b. sociocultural
   c. psychosocial
   d. behavioral
   Answer: c   LO: 1; applied   page: 66

Chapter 3

6. The construction foreman who, in 1848, had a tamping iron thrust through his brain, causing a drastic change in personality, although no other apparent changes, was:
   a. Phineas Fogg
   b. Lord Rutland
   c. Phineas P. Gage
   d. Galen P. Green
   Answer: c   LO: 2; factual   page: 67

7. Studies indicate that damage to the area of the frontal lobe as experienced by Phineas Gage in the mid-nineteenth century, typically experience changes in their:
   a. ability to learn new information, but they retain old memories unhampered.
   b. ability to make rational decisions in personal and social matters.
   c. ability to reason abstractly and perform complex calculations.
   d. long-term memory, although their short-term memory remains intact.
   Answer: b   LO: 2; factual   page: 67

8. The cerebrum:
   a. regulates many complex human activities.
   b. is divided into three sections.
   c. is the primary visual area of the brain.
   d. is located within the deep structure of the brain.
   Answer: a   LO: 2; factual   page: 68

9. The left hemisphere of the brain is involved in:
   a. spatial perception.
   b. pattern recognition.
   c. processing of emotion.
   d. language.
   Answer: d   LO: 2; factual   page: 68

10. The right hemisphere of the brain is involved in:
    a. spatial perception.
    b. language.
    c. logic.
    d. mathematical computations.
    Answer: a   LO: 2; factual   page: 68

Diagnosing and Treating Abnormality

11. Stimulation of certain areas of the _____ produces sensations of pleasure, while stimulation of others areas produces sensations of pain.
    a. thalamus
    b. pituitary
    c. hypothalamus
    d. reticular articulating device
    Answer: c   LO: 2; factual   page: 69

12. Damage to the limbic system has been seen to:
    a. result in chronically aggressive behavior.
    b. cause excessively compulsive behavior.
    c. have little effect on expressive behavior.
    d. cause tinnitus.
    Answer: a   LO: 2; factual   page: 69

13. Jesse is a highly emotional man, prone to gorging himself, with an apparent inability to control his aggressive and sexual urges. From a biological perspective, a psychologist might consider that Jesse has damage to his:
    a. limbic system.
    b. ventricles.
    c. thalamus.
    d. parietal lobe.
    Answer: a   LO: 2; factual   page: 69

14. Chemical compounds that facilitate sending signals from one neuron to another are called:
    a. axons.
    b. dendrites.
    c. neurotransmitters.
    d. synapses.
    Answer: c   LO: 2; factual   page: 70

15. The *best* definition of a neurotransmitter is a:
    a. compound that facilitates sending signals from one neuron to another.
    b. brain wave that transmits ideas from the brain to other parts of the body.
    c. mechanical device that researchers use to stimulate brain activity.
    d. type of sound equipment used by neurosurgeons to locate damaged sections of the brain.
    Answer: a   LO: 2; factual   page: 70

Chapter 3

16. The _____ sends messages and the _____ receives messages.
    a. synapse; axon
    b. dendrite; axon
    c. axon; synapse
    d. axon; dendrite
    Answer: d   LO: 2; factual   page: 70

17. The amount of a given neurotransmitter released from the terminal button is affected by the processes of:
    a. axons and dendrites.
    b. reuptake and degradation.
    c. sending and blocking.
    d. sending and receiving.
    Answer: b   LO: 2; factual   page: 70

18. _____ is the process in which the initial neuron that releases a neurotransmitter into the synapse reabsorbs the neurotransmitter, decreasing the amount of neurotransmitter left in the synapse.
    a. Degradation
    b. Bondage
    c. Absorption
    d. Reuptake
    Answer: d   LO: 2; factual   page: 70

19. _____ is the process in which the receiving neuron releases an enzyme into the synapse that breaks down the neurotransmitter into other biochemicals.
    a. Degradation
    b. Bondage
    c. Absorption
    d. Reuptake
    Answer: a   LO: 2; factual   page: 70

20. Having less than the normal amount of reuptake or degradation results in _____ levels of neurotransmitters in the synapse.
    a. abnormally high
    b. slightly higher
    c. slightly lower
    d. abnormally low
    Answer: a   LO: 2; factual   page: 70

Diagnosing and Treating Abnormality

21. Reuptake and degradation are _____ processes of the brain.
    a. abnormal
    b. abnormal, but not harmful
    c. atypical, but not harmful
    d. normal
    Answer: d   LO: 2; factual   page: 70

22. Hormones are chemicals that:
    a. travel from neuron to neuron.
    b. are released directly into the blood.
    c. are extremely rare in very young and very old individuals.
    d. have relatively little influence on mood.
    Answer: b   LO: 2; factual   page: 70

23. Chemicals that may affect a person's mood, energy levels, and stress reactions are:
    a. neurons.
    b. DNA.
    c. hormones.
    d. hemotomes.
    Answer: c   LO: 2; factual   page: 70

24. Which of the following is *most likely* to cause biochemical systems to work improperly and can also cause major structural anomalies in the brain?
    a. the parasympathetic system
    b. the sympathetic system
    c. genetic abnormalities
    d. reuptake and degradation
    Answer: c   LO: 2; factual, conceptual   page: 71

25. The area of research that concerns genetic studies of personality and abnormality is called:
    a. molecular genetics.
    b. DNA research.
    c. abnormal genetics.
    d. behavior genetics.
    Answer: d   LO: 2; factual   page: 71

Chapter 3

26. Psychologists who take a biological approach believe that abnormal brain structure, biochemical imbalances, and _____ cause psychopathology.
    a. genetic anomalies
    b. genetic transmission
    c. neurotransmission
    d. neuronal reuptake
    Answer: a   LO: 2; factual   page: 71

27. The area of study that is interested in knowing the extent to which behaviors are inherited is:
    a. behavior therapy.
    b. behavior genetics.
    c. behavior research.
    d. behavioral medicine.
    Answer: b   LO: 2; factual   page: 71

28. At conception, the normal fertilized embryo has:
    a. 23 chromosomes
    b. 21 pairs of chromosomes
    c. 46 chromosomes
    d. 46 pairs of chromosomes
    Answer: c   LO: 2; factual   page: 71

29. If a child receives an X chromosome from the mother and an X chromosome from the father, that child will:
    a. probably be a girl.
    b. definitely be a girl.
    c. probably be a boy.
    d. definitely be a boy.
    Answer: b   LO: 2; factual   page: 71

30. William is the captain of his high school football team. He has always been very athletic and very comfortable with being the only boy in a family that has six daughters. We can safely assume that William received _____ from his mother and _____ from his father.
    a. an X; an X
    b. a Y; a Y
    c. a Y; an X
    d. an X; a Y
    Answer: d   LO: 2; conceptual; applied   page: 71

Diagnosing and Treating Abnormality

31. When chromosome 21 is present in triplicate (there are three chromosomes) instead of the usual pair, we would expect the child:
    a. to be a boy.
    b. to be a girl.
    c. to have Down syndrome.
    d. to have exceptional intelligence.
    Answer: c   LO: 2; factual   page: 72

32. A child receives _____ of a parent's total genes.
    a. all
    b. one-half
    c. one-quarter
    d. one-eighth
    Answer: b   LO: 2; factual   page: 72

33. Typically, physical disorders (such as diabetes or epilepsy) and psychological disorders result from:
    a. monogenic processes.
    b. homogenic processes.
    c. heterogenic processes.
    d. polygenic processes.
    Answer: d   LO: 2; factual   page: 72

34. According to behavior geneticists, most disorders result from:
    a. a single faulty gene.
    b. a specific faulty gene.
    c. a combination of altered genes.
    d. a single faulty chromosome.
    Answer: c   LO: 2; factual   page: 72

35. Family history studies, twin studies, and adoption studies are often used to learn about:
    a. various forms of biological therapies.
    b. ways to mediate the effect families have on their offspring.
    c. the family systems approach to therapy.
    d. heritability of psychological disorders.
    Answer: d   LO: 2; factual, conceptual   pages: 73-75

Chapter 3

36. When scientists conduct family history studies, the persons known to have the particular disorder are called:
   a. controls.
   b. sources.
   c. probands.
   d. targets.
   Answer: c   LO: 2; factual   page: 73

37. A major problem with family history studies is that several family members could have a particular disorder because:
   a. they are related and are thus more likely to be exposed to the faulty gene.
   b. they share the same environmental stresses.
   c. each might "cover" for the others in denying that they have the disorder.
   d. researchers have difficulty separating boundaries among family members.
   Answer: b   LO: 2; conceptual   page: 73

38. Identical twins are called _____ twins.
   a. dizygotic
   b. monozygotic
   c. fraternal
   d. concordance
   Answer: b   LO: 2; factual   page: 73

39. Georgine and Geraldine are sisters who share the same birthdate. They look, act, and sound so much alike that they are able to fool their friends by switching places with each other at different social events, and no one can tell the difference. It's safe to assume that they are _____ twins.
   a. monozygotic
   b. dizygotic
   c. fraternal
   d. concordance
   Answer: a   LO: 2; conceptual, applied   page: 73

40. _____ twins are likely to share, on average, 50% of their genes.
   a. Monozygotic
   b. Dizygotic
   c. Identical
   d. All
   Answer: b   LO: 2; factual, conceptual   page: 73

Diagnosing and Treating Abnormality

41. The probability that both twins of a monozygotic pair will have a disorder if one of those twins has the disorder is called the:
    a. genetic risk.
    b. known risk factor.
    c. dominance rate.
    d. concordance rate.
    Answer: d   LO: 2; factual   page: 73

42. A major stumbling block in family history studies and twin studies is:
    a. the heritability of genetic disorders.
    b. teasing out environmental factors.
    c. dealing with enmeshed families.
    d. differentiating between MZ and DZ siblings.
    Answer: b   LO: 2; conceptual   page: 73

43. The studies that offer the best means for separating genetic from environmental influences are:
    a. family history studies.
    b. twin studies.
    c. adoption studies.
    d. individual studies.
    Answer: c   LO: 2; factual, conceptual   pages: 74-75

44. The twin studies conducted at the University of Minnesota have provided evidence that:
    a. some personality traits are substantially influenced by genetics.
    b. personality is determined almost exclusively by environment.
    c. personality is determined almost exclusively by genetics.
    d. there is no conclusive way of determining how much is genetics and how much environment.
    Answer: a   LO: 2; factual   page: 74

45. The term Freud used to describe psychical energy that derives from physiological drives and processes is the:
    a. limbic system.
    b. libido.
    c. id.
    d. unconscious.
    Answer: b   LO: 3; factual   page: 76

Chapter 3

46. According to Freud, all behaviors and thoughts, whether normal or abnormal, result from:
    a. our interactions with our environment.
    b. biological processes.
    c. physiological drives.
    d. our early socialization.
    Answer: c   LO: 3; factual, conceptual   page: 76

47. The three systems of the human psyche that regulate the libido are the:
    a. id, ego, and superego.
    b. conscious, preconscious, and unconscious.
    c. oral, anal, and phallic.
    d. internal, external, and lateral.
    Answer: a   LO: 3; factual   page: 76

48. The system from which the libido emanates is the:
    a. id.
    b. ego.
    c. superego.
    d. limbic.
    Answer: a   LO: 3; factual   page: 76

49. The storehouse of rules and regulations that we learn from our parents and society is the:
    a. id.
    b. ego.
    c. superego.
    d. libido.
    Answer: c   LO: 3; factual   page: 76

50. The part of the psyche that attempts to release libidinal energy, satisfy impulses and drives, stick within the constraints of reality, and maintain norms of acceptable behavior is the:
    a. id.
    b. ego.
    c. superego.
    d. libido.
    Answer: b   LO: 3; factual   page: 76

51. The three levels of awareness described by Freud are the:
    a. sensory register, short term, and long term.
    b. conscious, preconscious, and unconscious.
    c. conscious, preconscious, and subconscious.
    d. id, ego, and superego.
    Answer: b   LO: 3; factual   page: 76

Diagnosing and Treating Abnormality

52. According to Freud, most of what drives human thought and behavior occurs in the:
    a. conscious.
    b. preconscious.
    c. unconscious.
    d. subconscious.
    Answer: c   LO: 3; factual   page: 76

53. The conflict among the id, ego, and superego usually take place in the:
    a. conscious.
    b. preconscious.
    c. unconscious.
    d. subconscious.
    Answer: c   LO: 3; factual   page: 76

54. When unconscious wishes, needs, and memories are unacceptable to a person or to society, the _____ pushes them back into the unconscious in a process called _____.
    a. conscious; anxiety
    b. conscious; repression
    c. superego; suppression
    d. ego; repression
    Answer: d   LO: 3; factual   page: 76

55. When unacceptable thoughts, ideas, or memories attempt to surface from the unconscious, this produces:
    a. anxiety.
    b. id arousal.
    c. preconscious arousal.
    d. a therapeutic response.
    Answer: a   LO: 3; factual   pages: 76-77

56. Amy was five years old when her brother Billy was born. Although she had been completely toilet trained for three years, soon after Billy arrived Amy was having "accidents" and her parents threatened to put her back in diapers. Besides this, Amy also insisted that she wanted to suck on a bottle again, just like Billy. This would demonstrate the defense mechanism of:
    a. repression.
    b. regression.
    c. displacement.
    d. denial.
    Answer: b   LO: 3; applied   page: 77

Chapter 3

57. Henry goes out on a binge every month when he gets his paycheck, and he doesn't come back home until his money is gone. When he does come home, he smells from liquor. Maggie, his wife, finally got him to go to AA, which he did just to get her off his back. After everyone else at the meeting got up and introduced themselves, saying something to the effect of, "Hi. I'm Bill, and I'm an alcoholic," it was finally Henry's turn. He got up and said, "Hi. I'm Henry, and I'm a normal drinker." Henry is exhibiting which defense mechanism?
    a. suppression
    b. regression
    c. displacement
    d. denial
    Answer: d   LO: 3; applied   page: 77

58. This morning when Rose came to work, she discovered that her boss, Linda, had gotten into her computer and had put her own name on all of the tables and charts that Rose had created over the past two years that they worked together. Although many people in the office don't like Linda, it appears that the director of the office does, so Rose is afraid to confront Linda with what she did. Instead, when Rose goes home that night she yells at her daughter when the daughter asked if she could go to her best friends house for dinner. This is an example of which defense mechanism?
    a. intellectualization
    b. rationalization
    c. displacement
    d. reaction formation
    Answer: c   LO: 3; applied   page: 77

59. Gail's doctor tells her she has a lump in her breast and will need a biopsy to determine if the lump is malignant. After discussing the matter with her doctor, Gail immediately goes to Barnes & Noble bookstore and purchases every recent book on breast cancer. She reads through the night and is still reading the next morning when it's time for her to go to work. At work, she discusses with her co-workers the meeting she had with her doctor, and then shares with them all she has learned about breast cancer, its causes, its treatments, as well as diet, wellness groups, and everything else she read. Surprisingly, however, she does not seem terribly upset that she may have breast cancer. The defense mechanism she is exhibiting is:
    a. reaction formation.
    b. rationalization.
    c. intellectualization.
    d. denial.
    Answer: c   LO: 3; applied   page: 77

Diagnosing and Treating Abnormality

60. When Sam comes home "late from work," he snoops around the house as if he's trying to find something. His wife asks what he's looking for, and he responds, "I know you had a man here. I can smell his cologne." Sally says Sam must have had a drink too many in the office, because after she came home from work she cleaned the house, paid the bills, then made dinner, which he missed because he said he had a business meeting. Sam insists that Sally is hiding someone and begins looking in closets and under the bed. After checking every possible hiding place in the house and yard, he relents, but says, "Don't you ever let me find you with him." The defense mechanism Sam is most likely using is:
    a. reaction formation.
    b. projection.
    c. denial.
    d. rationalization.
    Answer: b   LO: 3; applied   page: 77

61. Shortly after Sarah was born, Cynthia began to resent her baby. She hated all the time and attention Sarah demanded, and most of all she hated the crying and fussing. Sarah is now 35 years old and Cynthia calls her four times a day to check on her. She is so solicitous and protective of her daughter that Sarah feels totally controlled and has described it to her therapist as feeling "strangled." Sarah's therapist suggests that this may be a demonstration of _____ on Cynthia's part.
    a. reaction formation
    b. sublimation
    c. denial
    d. rationalization
    Answer: a   LO: 3; applied   page: 77

62. Patty Randolph was kidnapped when she was a freshman in college. Her captors locked her in a dark closet, starved her for days on end, made her publicly state that her parents were murderers of young children, and forced her to commit felonious crimes. After six months of this treatment, she came to believe that the people who had kidnapped her had opened up new and wonderful worlds for her, that they were kind people who intended to make the world a better place if only they could get rid of the capitalist oppressors. This is an example of:
    a. reaction formation.
    b. identification.
    c. projection.
    d. sublimation.
    Answer: b   LO: 3; applied   page: 77

Chapter 3

63. Pablo had a violent temper as a child, for which he was often punished. He also had wild sexual fantasies, but when he described them to his mother, she turned purple with rage and told him these thoughts were evil and she should beat them out of his head. As a teenager, Pablo began to paint using vivid colors to display intense feelings and riotous themes. By the time he was an adult, he was world famous and internationally acclaimed as one of the world's foremost artists. Critics and the public alike appreciated his extraordinary talent. Pablo's painting is the defense mechanism called:
   a. reaction formation.
   b. intellectualization.
   c. projection.
   d. sublimation.
   Answer: d   LO: 3; applied   page: 77

64. Freud believed that personality development:
   a. stopped at the end of childhood.
   b. stopped at the beginning of young adulthood.
   c. continued throughout a person's life.
   d. was irrelevant to lifetime experiences.
   Answer: a   LO: 3; factual, conceptual   page: 78

65. According to Erik Erikson, personality development:
   a. ends at the completion of childhood.
   b. ends after an adolescent achieves a sense of identity.
   c. continues into early adulthood.
   d. continues throughout the lifespan.
   Answer: d   LO: 3; conceptual   page: 78

66. According to Erik Erikson, as personality develops, we:
   a. are faced with a series of conflicts that must be resolved.
   b. continue to resolve the same set of conflicts over and over.
   c. become more fixated on previous stages of development.
   d. become increasingly better at resolving crises.
   Answer: a   LO: 3; conceptual   page: 78

67. The theory that focuses on the role of early interpersonal relationships in the development of self-concept is:
   a. psychosexual.
   b. psychosocial.
   c. object relations.
   d. self-actualization.
   Answer: c   LO: 3; factual   pages: 78-79

Diagnosing and Treating Abnormality

68. One of the proponents of the object relations school was:
    a. Sigmund Freud.
    b. Melanie Klein.
    c. Erik Erikson.
    d. Alfred Adler.
    Answer: b   LO: 3; factual   page: 78

69. Which psychoanalytic school of thought is concerned with the concept of developing a sense of self in relation to other?
    a. psychosexual
    b. psychosocial
    c. object relations
    d. Adlerian
    Answer: c   LO: 3; factual   page: 78

70. In object relations theory, when a person fails to resolve the second and third stages of development and thus comes to see himself or herself AND others as either all good or all bad, it is referred to as:
    a. paradox.
    b. vacillation.
    c. splitting.
    d. dichotomous.
    Answer: c   LO: 3; conceptual   page: 79

71. According to object relations theory, two common symptoms of the borderline personality are:
    a. splitting and lack of boundaries.
    b. vacillation and demanding boundaries.
    c. dichotomous thinking and vacillation.
    d. ambiguity and ambivalence.
    Answer: a   LO: 3; factual   page: 79

72. Which approach to personality developed as an attempt to provide explanations for human behavior that could be tested scientifically?
    a. cognitive
    b. behavioral
    c. classical
    d. humanistic
    Answer: b   LO: 4; factual   page: 79

Chapter 3

73. Behaviorists focus on:
    a. unconscious conflicts that drive human behavior.
    b. observable, replicable relationships between events and behavior.
    c. maladaptive behaviors that stem from dysfunctional assumptions.
    d. the individual's capacity for self-definition and self-direction.
    Answer: b   LO: 4; conceptual   page: 79

74. Learning that is acquired through association of a neutral stimulus with a stimulus that naturally produces a response (an unconditioned stimulus) is:
    a. operant conditioning.
    b. Skinnerian conditioning.
    c. instrumental conditioning.
    d. classical conditioning.
    Answer: d   LO: 4; factual   page: 80

75. When a heroin addict merely sees a syringe, he or she may experience physiological responses similar to those experienced when the addict actually uses heroin. This is explained in terms of:
    a. classical conditioning.
    b. operant conditioning.
    c. instrumental conditioning.
    d. observational learning.
    Answer: a   LO: 4; applied   page: 80

76. E. L. Thorndike noted in _____ that behaviors that are followed by a reward are strengthened.
    a. classical conditioning
    b. the law of effect
    c. reinforcement theory
    d. reward theory
    Answer: b   LO: 4; factual   page: 81

77. Behaviors that are paired with reward every time they occur are on:
    a. a continuous reinforcement schedule.
    b. a partial reinforcement schedule.
    c. an extinction schedule.
    d. a paired punishment/reward schedule.
    Answer: a   LO: 4; factual   page: 81

Diagnosing and Treating Abnormality

78. Extinguishing a behavior is more difficult when it was learned using a:
    a. continuous reinforcement schedule.
    b. a fixed ratio schedule.
    c. a fixed interval schedule.
    d. a partial reinforcement schedule.
    Answer: d   LO: 4; conceptual   page: 81

79. The process of getting rid of a behavior is called:
    a. acquisition.
    b. spontaneous recovery.
    c. extinction.
    d. association.
    Answer: c   LO: 4; factual   page: 81

80. Anita occasionally gives her cocker spaniels, Baby and Destiny, a treat when she is preparing her own meals at the kitchen counter. They have learned to stand next to her when she prepares her meals. She always gives them treats if they come running to greet her when she comes home at night, and so they come running to greet her every night when she comes home. Which behavior will be more resistant to extinction?
    a. Both would be equally as difficult to extinguish.
    b. Begging in the kitchen would be harder to extinguish.
    c. Greeting her at the door would be harder to extinguish.
    d. Neither would be difficult to extinguish.
    Answer: b   LO: 4; applied   page: 81

81. The person most logically connected with Social Learning Theory is:
    a. Ivan Pavlov.
    b. E. L. Thorndike.
    c. B. F. Skinner.
    d. Albert Bandura.
    Answer: d   LO: 5; factual   page: 82

82. A major difference between observational learning and classical or operant conditioning is:
    a. observational learning acknowledges the importance of cognitive events.
    b. classical and operant conditioning acknowledge the importance of cognitive events.
    c. observational learning is acquired through association of stimuli.
    d. inconsequential--there are no major differences, only different explanations of how behavior occurs.
    Answer: a   LO: 5; conceptual   page: 82

Chapter 3

83. Jenny is thinking about throwing a rock at her younger sister, Sally, but as she picks up the rock, she thinks about what she saw yesterday--when her brother, Billy, threw a doll at Sally, their mother said he could not play with his Nintendo game for the next week, and Billy got sent to his room. Slowly, Jenny puts the rock down and walks away from the little girl. We might assume that Jenny is demonstrating:
   a. classical conditioning.
   b. operant conditioning.
   c. observational learning.
   d. consequential learning.
   Answer: c   LO: 5; applied   page: 82

84. Cognitive theories address the importance of:
   a. thoughts and beliefs.
   b. observable behaviors.
   c. testable behaviors.
   d. stimuli and responses.
   Answer: a   LO: 6; conceptual   page: 82

85. The explanations we offer for why an event took place are:
   a. control beliefs.
   b. causal attributions.
   c. faulty assumptions.
   d. automatic thoughts.
   Answer: b   LO: 6; conceptual   page: 82

86. The belief a person has about his or her ability successfully to execute the behaviors required to accomplish a goal is:
   a. self-concept.
   b. self-esteem.
   c. self-efficacy.
   d. self-image.
   Answer: c   LO: 6; factual   page: 83

87. As stated in the text, the belief that "I should be loved by everyone for everything I do" is a(n):
   a. dysfunctional assumption.
   b. automatic thought.
   c. reasonable assumption.
   d. reasonable expectation.
   Answer: a   LO: 6; factual   pages: 83-84

Diagnosing and Treating Abnormality

88. The difference between dysfunctional beliefs and automatic thoughts is that automatic thoughts are:
    a. about a specific situation we are facing.
    b. global evaluations of all situations.
    c. healthier than dysfunctional beliefs.
    d. less intrusive than dysfunctional beliefs.
    Answer: a   LO: 6; factual, conceptual   page: 84

89. Which approach to personality developed, in large part, as a reaction to the pessimistic and deterministic psychodynamic theories?
    a. cognitive
    b. behavioral
    c. classical
    d. humanistic
    Answer: d   LO: 7; factual   page: 84

90. The _____ perspective focuses on the capacity that humans have for self-definition and self-direction.
    a. behavioristic
    b. psychodynamic
    c. humanistic
    d. cognitive
    Answer: c   LO: 7; factual, conceptual   page: 84

91. Who would be most likely to believe that, without undue pressure from others, a person would naturally move toward personal growth, self-acceptance, and self-actualization?
    a. Erik Erikson
    b. B. F. Skinner
    c. Melanie Klein
    d. Carl Rogers
    Answer: d   LO: 7; factual, conceptual   page: 84

92. According to Maslow's theory, with respect to an individual's hierarchy of needs,
    a. physiological needs must be met before self-actualization can occur.
    b. esteem needs must be met before physiological needs can be met.
    c. aesthetic needs must be met before esteem needs can be met.
    d. there is no exact order, since we attempt to meet all of our needs as we can.
    Answer: a   LO: 7; factual, conceptual   page: 85

Chapter 3

93. When comparing humanistic and existential theories:
    a. humanistic theories take a more positive view of human abilities than existential theories.
    b. existential theories take a more positive view of human abilities than humanistic theories.
    c. both theories hold positive views of human abilities.
    d. both theories hold negative views of human abilities.
    Answer: a   LO: 7; conceptual   pages: 84-85

94. Chlorpromazine has been used most successfully for:
    a. reducing delusions, hallucinations, and severe disorganization of thoughts.
    b. reducing anxiety brought about by social interactions.
    c. elevating mood for persons suffering from depression.
    d. curing the most significant symptoms of schizophrenia.
    Answer: a   LO: 8; factual   page: 86

95. Antidepressant drugs, such as MAO inhibitors, tricyclic antidepressants, and SSRIs have been used successfully for treatment of:
    a. depression only.
    b. schizophrenia only.
    c. depression, anxiety, and eating disorders.
    d. depression and personality disorders.
    Answer: c   LO: 8; factual   page: 86

96. When Ginny arrived (early) for her appointment with her psychoanalyst, Dr. Rose, the receptionist said that the doctor was running a few minutes late and would be with her shortly. As Dr. Rose opened her office door at five minutes after the hour to ask Ginny to come in, the client began to rant and rave about how rude and unprofessional it was for a therapist to keep a client waiting. Dr. Rose might consider this an example of:
    a. Ginny's irrational behavior.
    b. transference.
    c. counter-transference.
    d. resistance.
    Answer: b   LO: 9; applied   page: 88

97. When comparing Interpersonal Therapy (IPT) with traditional psychodynamic therapy,
    a. they are actually synonymous.
    b. traditional psychodynamic therapy is more structured and directive.
    c. IPT is more structured and directive.
    d. IPT is more structured, by traditional psychodynamic therapy is more directive.
    Answer: c   LO: 9; conceptual   page: 88

Diagnosing and Treating Abnormality

98. The psychotherapy that is most likely to focus on the individual discovering his or her potentialities and place in the world is:
    a. psychodynamic.
    b. humanistic-existential.
    c. behavioral.
    d. cognitive.
    Answer: b   LO: 9; factual, conceptual   pages: 88-89

99. Which of the following techniques is *least* likely to be used by a client-centered therapist?
    a. unconditional positive regard
    b. confrontation
    c. genuineness
    d. empathic understanding
    Answer: b   LO: 9; conceptual   pages: 86-92

100. The method used to gradually extinguish anxiety responses and their accompanying maladaptive behaviors is:
    a. systematic desensitization.
    b. aversion therapy.
    c. flooding.
    d. response shaping.
    Answer: a   LO: 9; factual   pages: 89-90

101. Sam suddenly was having a problem with his job responsibilities. As a repair person for the phone company, he must climb telephone poles. He now has developed an extreme fear of heights. Because Sam needs to overcome the problem quickly, a behavior therapist might use:
    a. a technique to uncover unconscious conflicts.
    b. reinforcement therapy.
    c. flooding.
    d. client-centered therapy.
    Answer: c   LO: 9; application   page: 89

102. Anita asked her brother, Larry, to loan her money for a program to help her quit smoking by using techniques like shock, pictures of black lungs from people who died from smoking-related illnesses, and having smokers chain smoke for hours on end. This program uses:
    a. distraction techniques.
    b. flooding.
    c. aversion therapy.
    d. systematic desensitization.
    Answer: c   LO: 9; application   pages: 89-90

Chapter 3

103. A therapy that has been used in mental hospitals that is credited, together with drug therapy and deinstitutionalization, for greatly reducing the inpatient populations is:
    a. psychodynamic therapy.
    b. client-centered therapy.
    c. token economies.
    d. systematic desensitization.
    Answer: c LO: 9; factual pages: 90-91

104. The three steps that a client may expect to cycle through with a cognitive therapist are:
    a. identify maladaptive behaviors, understand the causes of the behaviors, develop ways to change the behaviors.
    b. identify irrational thoughts, challenge irrational thoughts, face the client's worst fears about these thoughts.
    c. identify the client's most pressing problems, understand what causes the problems, work on ways to eliminate the problems.
    d. complete a questionnaire to assess typical ways of responding, go through the results with the therapist, decide which behaviors need to change.
    Answer: b LO: 9; factual, conceptual pages: 91-92

105. The therapist most likely to attempt to "join" the family in order to exert influence over the processes each family member uses to interact with the others would subscribe to which type of family therapy?
    a. Carl Rogers
    b. Fritz Perls
    c. Virginia Satir
    d. Salvador Minuchin
    Answer: d LO: 10; factual, conceptual page: 92

106. Among the strategies of family therapists is to challenge:
    a. the family's belief that "the problem" is an individual family member.
    b. the family's importance as a unit.
    c. the notion that family members interact in important ways.
    d. all the ways that family members have of interacting with each other.
    Answer: a LO: 10; conceptual pages: 92-93

107. When comparing treatment effectiveness for children, what outcome is most commonly supported?
    a. Behavioral therapies produce a larger and more reliable effect than talking therapies.
    b. Talking therapies produce a larger and more reliable effect than behavioral therapies.
    c. Behavioral therapies and talking therapies both have similar positive effects.
    d. Behavioral therapies and talking therapies both seem to have slightly negative effects.
    Answer: a LO: 11; factual page: 95

Diagnosing and Treating Abnormality

108. Among the best predictors of successful therapy are:
    a. the type of therapy that is used and length of time in therapy.
    b. positive relationship between client and therapist and a belief that it will work.
    c. the type of drugs used combined with the type of therapy used.
    d. the client's gender and the therapist's training.
    Answer: b   LO: 12; factual   pages: 97-98

109. In terms of the cultural and gender issues in therapy:
    a. there has been a great deal of support for the notion that women prefer therapies that focus on interpersonal relationships and expression of emotion.
    b. there has been a great deal of support for the notion that women prefer therapies that focus on challenging their beliefs and teaching new ways to behave.
    c. there has been a great deal of rigorous research conducted on the variable of gender in therapy, but not a large number of studies with respect to cultural influences.
    d. there has not been enough rigorous research conducted on gender or culture to support specific preferences on the basis of those variables
    Answer: d   LO: 12; factual   pages: 98-100

110. George is being treated for depression. Part of his treatment involves prayers, songs, dances, emphasis on cultural heritage, and some herbal medicines. The focus of the treatment is on reintegrating George into his community. Based on this type of treatment, we might expect that George is:
    a. Native American.
    b. Asian American.
    c. African American.
    d. Mexican American.
    Answer: a   LO: 12; applied   page: 101

111. Rita has consulted a folk healer for her feelings of anxiety. She believes that perhaps a jealous neighbor has put a curse on her. The healer uses prayers, holy palm, and incantations, and applies healing ointments and oils, as she has Rita drink special herbal medicines. It is likely that Rita is from a _____ culture.
    a. Asian
    b. Hispanic
    c. Jamaican
    d. Native American
    Answer: b   LO: 12; applied   page: 101

Chapter 3

112. When making a decision about choosing a therapist for one's own personal problems,
    a. it is inappropriate to "shop" for a therapist.
    b. it is helpful to ask about the therapist's religious beliefs.
    c. it is helpful to learn about the therapist's specialty areas.
    d. it is best to work with a therapist who already knows your family.
    Answer: c   LO: 12; factual   page: 103

Essay Questions

113. Imagine that you are a world-renown psychologist, well known for your research, writing, and clinical experience working with persons suffering from the entire range of abnormal behaviors. You have been asked to talk to a group of undergraduates who are now studying abnormal psychology. In order to help them understand the different theories of abnormality, consider how you will compare and contrast the similarities and differences among the fundamental assumptions about the causes of and appropriate treatments for abnormality.

    Address (a) biological approach in terms of structural deformities of the brain, biochemical imbalances, and genetic factors; and the use of drug therapies as the most effective treatments; and (b) psychosocial approach covering psychological and social factors, including maladaptive thoughts, unconscious conflicts, dysfunctional family systems, and negative interpersonal relationships as causes; and various forms of psychotherapy (psychodynamic, behavioral, cognitive, humanistic, family systems) for treating the problems, considering what each says in terms of the causes of abnormality and the specific techniques used for treating it.

114. As an upper division student, you have been asked to simplify the behavioristic theories for students in an Introductory Psychology class. Describe how you will explain the major differences among classical conditioning, operant conditioning, and observational learning, being sure to describe the specific elements involved in each. Give appropriate examples of each, then consider and discuss the amount of overlap among the three theories and give an example of this overlap.

    Discuss the pairing of the neutral stimulus with the UCS and the UCS/UCR/CS/CR paradigm; the roles that reinforcement and punishment, as well as different schedules of reinforcement play in repetition and extinction of behavior; and learning through observing the behavior and consequences of those behaviors performed by others, as well as the impact of the observed person's status. Explore how these differences are not always clear-cut--an example may be in the development and maintenance of phobias that are classically conditioned by maintained by avoidance that reduces anxiety, while therapy may include watching someone else interact with the phobic object.

Diagnosing and Treating Abnormality

115. You have recently become fascinated with Albert Bandura's Social Learning Theory because you have begun watching how young children learn. You have noticed that they learn a variety of behaviors (good and bad) from seeing them on television. To help the children's parents effectively guide their children, describe how you would explain to the parents how Social Learning Theory applies to both behavioral and cognitive theories.

    Include issues of reinforcement and punishment, but the cognitive processes of observing, perceiving, and making a determination about the behavior of another and the consequences of the behavior.

116. After taking courses in abnormal psychology, child development, and family systems, Jenny has decided she wants to become a psychotherapist. However, she has become overwhelmed with all the different theories to explain what causes psychological disorders and all the different types of therapy that are used to treat these disorders. She has asked you to help her sort these issues out. Explain how you would explain this information by comparing and contrasting the various forms of psychotherapy, looking not only at how they differ from each other in terms of causative factors and treatment, but also addressing how they overlap.

    In terms of how they overlap, the most apparent issue is that each attempts to help the individual (or family) live a happier and healthier life. Also, many therapists use a combination of approaches, depending on the client and the particular issue(s) involved. Differences that need to be discussed include what each approach considers to be the cause of the problem(s) and the methods and techniques used for treating the problem(s), as well as the role of the client and the therapist.

117. You are a therapist who has just received a phone call from a distraught father saying that he can't take his son's outrageous behavior any longer. For the past month the child has been urinating behind the television set in the living room. How would you, as therapist, approach the problem?

    This would entail having the whole family involved in therapy as a unit, since the son appears to be the "identified patient" or the family "symptom bearer" or "scapegoat." Discuss both conjoint and structural family therapy techniques for dealing with the family in order to eliminate the symptoms of the child, enhance communication in the family, and realign family structure and dynamics. Give examples of what the student (as therapist) would do.

Chapter 3

118. Discuss the issues of culture and gender that are important for effective therapy outcomes.

The major issue here is sensitivity to differences while maintaining an awareness of individual differences--not overgeneralizing or stereotyping while not imposing the therapist's own values. The student should discuss how individuals from different cultures may exhibit different symptoms for the various disorders, talk about some of the disorders that may be unique to a particular culture, address different beliefs about the causes of abnormality and how to treat it, including rituals, herbal remedies, and healers. Also, the student should discuss issues of matching in terms of gender and culture, and why/when it may or may not be desirable.

Chapter 4   Anxiety Disorders

1. The fears of a person with an anxiety disorder are:
   a. similar in degree to those of persons without the disorder.
   b. similar in duration to those of persons without the disorder.
   c. greater in both degree and duration to those of persons without the disorder.
   d. similar in degree, but greater in duration to those of persons without the disorder.
   Answer: c   LO: 1; factual   page: 108

2. When William goes to his doctor complaining of dizziness, shaking, and ringing in his ears, the doctor determines that these are _____ symptoms of anxiety.
   a. somatic
   b. emotional
   c. cognitive
   d. behavioral
   Answer: a   LO: 1; applied   pages: 108-109

3. Andrew is constantly worrying that something bad will happen to him, such as getting fired, his girlfriend leaving him, or a piano dropping on his head. He constantly fears he is losing control of his life. This is likely a _____ symptom of anxiety.
   a. somatic
   b. emotional
   c. cognitive
   d. behavioral
   Answer: c   LO: 1; applied   pages: 108-109

4. The evolutionary response that our bodies have developed to deal with threats to our safety is called the _____ response.
   a. anxiety
   b. fight or flight
   c. fear
   d. stand or run
   Answer: b   LO: 2; factual   pages: 108-109

5. As stated in the text, an important difference between a person's adaptive fear response and anxiety is that in adaptive fear:
   a. the response subsides when the threat ends.
   b. the individual worries about the present, but not the future.
   c. there is no concern about future events.
   d. the fear may exceed the threat, but ends when the threat is over.
   Answer: a   LO: 2; factual   page: 109

Chapter 4

6. Chronic anxiety:
   a. interferes with daily living.
   b. increases medical illness.
   c. increases appetitive responding.
   d. leads to other psychological disorders.
   Answer: a   LO: 2; factual   page: 109

7. A person who suffers from chronic anxiety:
   a. probably will not suffer from other mental disorders.
   b. may also suffer from other mental disorders.
   c. probably had a serious mental disorder in the past.
   d. is equally as likely as anyone else to suffer from other mental disorders.
   Answer: b   LO: 2; factual   pages: 109-110

8. Short, intense periods of anxiety involving heart palpitations, trembling, feeling of choking, fear of having a heart attack, and fear that you are going crazy are symptoms of:
   a. phobias.
   b. agoraphobia.
   c. panic attack.
   d. post-traumatic stress disorder.
   Answer: c   LO: 3; conceptual   page: 110

9. Panic attacks are most likely to occur:
   a. specifically and consistently in certain situations.
   b. "out of the blue," without a specific trigger.
   c. in certain situations, although they don't always occur in those situations.
   d. in any situation, but with predictable triggers.
   Answer: c   LO: 3; factual   page: 110

10. According to the text, _____ % of the U. S. population suffers from occasional panic attacks:
    a. 1 to 2
    b. 2 to 6
    c. 8 to 12
    d. 9 to 15
    Answer: c   LO: 3; factual   page: 110

11. A person who has recurrent, unexpected panic attacks is suffering from:
    a. overanxiety.
    b. generalized anxiety.
    c. agoraphobia.
    d. panic disorder.
    Answer: d   LO: 3; factual   page: 111

Anxiety Disorders

12. Most panic disorders develop during:
    a. early adolescence.
    b. the adolescent period.
    c. late adolescence to mid-30s.
    d. early adulthood to mid-40s.
    Answer: c   LO: 3; factual   page: 111

13. A person who fears places where she or he might be unable to escape during a panic attack suffers from:
    a. claustrophobia.
    b. agoraphobia.
    c. acrophobia.
    d. generalized anxiety.
    Answer: b   LO: 4; factual   page: 111

14. Which of the following *is false* about agoraphobia?
    a. Anywhere from one-third to one-half of people diagnosed with panic disorder develop agoraphobia.
    b. The majority of people who suffer from agoraphobia experience either full-blown or moderate panic attacks.
    c. Agoraphobia occurs in people who do not have panic attacks.
    d. Agoraphobia usually occurs within three months of the onset of recurrent panic attacks.
    Answer: d   LO: 4; factual   page: 111

15. Which of the following *are not* stimuli that agoraphobics fear?
    a. busy, crowded places
    b. enclosed spaces
    c. wide open spaces
    d. people
    Answer: d   LO: 4; factual   page: 112

Chapter 4

16. When she was 23 years old, "Aunt Sally" was "stood up at the altar." Her fiancé didn't show up at the wedding, although Sally and 200 guests did. This was so devastating for her that she began to choke, sob, and shake, and thought she was having a heart attack on the spot. She was so embarrassed by the experience that she refused to see anyone but close family members for months. Then, from that day until the day she died, Aunt Sally would not go beyond sight of her house. The mere suggestion she do so caused such extreme agitation that her doctor would have to give her medication to calm her down. Her refusal to go out of sight of her home indicates that Aunt Sally has:
    a. social phobia.
    b. agoraphobia.
    c. panic attacks.
    d. high anxiety.
    Answer: b LO: 4; applied page: 112

17. According to biological theories, people who are prone to panic attacks have:
    a. a hypersensitivity to carbon monoxide.
    b. a poor balance between the autonomic nervous system and sympathetic nervous system.
    c. more serotonin, GABA, and norepinephrine in the brain.
    d. lower levels of activity in the limbic areas of their brains.
    Answer: a LO: 5; factual page: 113

18. Which of the following statements is *true* about biological treatments for panic and agoraphobia?
    a. Tricyclic antidepressants, such as imipramine, can reduce panic attacks in 60 to 90% of patients.
    b. Benzodiazepines, such as alprazolam, work by suppressing the central nervous system.
    c. Selective serotonin reuptake inhibitors (SSRIs) can reduce panic attacks and general symptoms of anxiety in 60 to 80% of patients.
    d. Both benzodiazepines and tricyclic antidepressants can be physically addictive.
    Answer: b LO: 5; factual page: 114

19. Which of the following *is false* concerning findings from the family studies on panic disorder?
    a. There appears to be a biological vulnerability to panic disorder.
    b. Vulnerability to panic disorder may be transmitted through disordered genes.
    c. The concordance rate of dizygotic twins for panic disorder is almost as high as that of monozygotic twins.
    d. Approximately 25% of first-degree relatives of persons with panic disorder have a history of that disorder.
    Answer: c LO: 6; factual page: 114

Anxiety Disorders

20. Which of the following is *false* about cognitive-behavioral treatments for panic and agoraphobia?
    a. They can greatly reduce the risk of relapse among patients undergoing benzodiazepine treatment.
    b. They have been found to bring about complete relief from panic and agoraphobia in 85 to 90% of patients within 12 weeks.
    c. They often involve inducing the symptoms of a panic attack deliberately.
    d. They have been found to require long-term therapy of at least 6 months in order to be effective.
    Answer: d   LO: 6; factual   page: 114-119

21. Which model of panic disorder states that people prone to panic attacks pay close attention to bodily sensations and misinterpret those sensations in a negative way?
    a. biological
    b. cognitive
    c. behavioral
    d. psychodynamic
    Answer: b   LO: 6; factual   page: 114

22. According to Seligman and Binick's (1977) research on the *safety signal hypothesis*, persons with panic disorder reduce the frequency of their attacks by:
    a. seeking out people and places that are associated with a low risk of panic attacks.
    b. becoming aware of what it is that triggers their attacks and being prepared with calming thoughts.
    c. having a person they feel comfortable with go with them to the places they believe cause their panic attacks.
    d. preparing cards with "safe thoughts" on them to read whenever they are feeling a panic attack is about to happen.
    Answer: a   LO: 7; conceptual   page: 115

23. Of the biological treatments used for panic disorder and agoraphobia:
    a. tricyclic antidepressants are preferred because they have the longest lasting results with the fewest side effects.
    b. benzodiazepines are preferred because it works quickly to reduce symptoms and is nonaddictive.
    c. the selective serotonin reuptake inhibitors (SSRIs) are preferred because they are both strong and have few known side effects.
    d. the selective serotonin reuptake inhibitors (SSRIs) are being tried for panic disorder because they have been effective in treating anxiety.
    Answer: d   LO: 7; factual   page: 116-117

Chapter 4

24. Which of the following psychological treatments has been the most effective in eliminating panic and agoraphobia?
   a. biological
   b. cognitive
   c. behavioral
   d. cognitive-behavioral
   Answer: d   LO: 7, 8; factual   page: 117

25. Sandra complained of dizziness, heart palpitations, chills and sweats, and a sense that she was losing control and going crazy whenever she went to the mall. Dr. Harris has been teaching Sandra a series of relaxation and breathing exercises, which Sandra says have given her a new sense of control in her life. Dr. Harris now has Sandra keeping a journal in which she writes down her thoughts about her bodily sensations, their intensity, and when these sensations occur. Dr. Harris is using which therapeutic approach?
   a. psychological
   b. biological
   c. cognitive-behavioral
   d. psychodynamic
   Answer: c   LO: 8; applied   page: 117

26. When Sam told Dr. Field that he was so overwhelmed by his panic symptoms that he could not think about anything else, Dr. Field had Sam spin around and around until he became so dizzy he almost collapsed. Dr. Field was probably:
   a. doing something potentially harmful to her client.
   b. inducing panic so she can help him look at his thoughts.
   c. getting him so tired he becomes exhausted and stops thinking about his panic.
   d. helping him to relax so his panic state will be reduced.
   Answer: b   LO: 8; applied   page: 117

27. Which of the following *is not* a technique used in cognitive-behavioral therapy for treatment of panic disorder?
   a. relaxation training
   b. systematic desensitization
   c. challenging catastrophic thoughts
   d. triggering safety signals
   Answer: d   LO: 8; factual   pages: 118-119

Anxiety Disorders

28. A strong, persistent fear of a specific object or situation, beyond the actual threat it presents, is:
    a. a panic attack.
    b. a phobia.
    c. an obsession.
    d. a compulsive object.
    Answer: b   LO: 9; factual   page: 119

29. Specific phobia and social phobia are similar in that they both involve:
    a. changing one's life to avoid the feared object or situation.
    b. not thinking about the feared object or situation.
    c. fear of inanimate objects or situations.
    d. fear of objects or situations that concern people or other living creatures.
    Answer: a   LO: 9; factual   page: 119

30. Which of the following *is not* one of the most common types of specific phobia?
    a. animal
    b. situational
    c. blood-injection-injury
    d. water
    Answer: d   LO: 9; factual   page: 120

31. Which is the most common of the animal type phobias in the United States?
    a. spiders
    b. cockroaches
    c. dogs
    d. snakes
    Answer: d   LO: 9; factual   page: 120

32. Which type of phobia decreases, rather than increases, heart rate and blood pressure, and is more likely to run in families?
    a. animal
    b. natural environment
    c. situational
    d. blood-injection-injury
    Answer: d   LO: 9; factual   page: 121

Chapter 4

33. When Howard went to visit friends in Japan, they took him out to dinner at one of the finest restaurants in Tokyo. After a few glasses of sake he began to feel quite warm. When he began eating his sushi, Howard found himself unable to control his fingers and proceeded to drop his food in his lap. The young ladies who were with Howard began to giggle, and he became so embarrassed that he will no longer eat in public. In fact, after he returned to the United States he quit his job because he was no longer able to attend business lunches. It is likely that Ken has:
   a. agoraphobia.
   b. simple phobia.
   c. social phobia.
   d. xenophobia.
   Answer: c   LO: 10; applied   pages: 121-122

34. Social phobia most likely to occur during:
   a. early childhood
   b. middle childhood
   c. adolescence
   d. early adulthood
   Answer: c   LO: 10; factual   page: 122

35. According to Freud, phobias develop as a result of:
   a. fear of the opposite sex parent, who is seen as a rival.
   b. displacement of unconscious anxiety onto the phobic object.
   c. fear of the opposite sex parent, who is seen as a love object.
   d. identification with the same sex parent, who shares the same fear.
   Answer: b   LO: 11; conceptual   page: 122

36. The case of "Little Hans" is used by psychoanalytic theory to explain:
   a. simple phobias.
   b. social phobias.
   c. agoraphobia.
   d. generalized anxiety.
   Answer: a   LO: 11; factual   page: 123

37. Behavioral theories of phobias explain their development as a result of:
   a. classical conditioning.
   b. operant conditioning.
   c. classical conditioning.
   d. instrumental conditioning.
   Answer: a   LO: 11; factual   page: 123

Anxiety Disorders

38. Behavioral theories of phobias explain their maintenance as a result of:
    a. classical conditioning.
    b. operant conditioning.
    c. observational learning.
    d. social learning.
    Answer: b   LO: 11; factual   page: 123

39. The case of "Little Albert" is used to demonstrate:
    a. the acquisition of a simple phobia.
    b. the acquisition of social phobia.
    c. the extinction of a simple phobia.
    d. counter-conditioning.
    Answer: a   LO: 11; factual   page: 123

40. One semester Jessica enrolled in a class in the Social Science building, which is located at the top of her campus. As it happens, there are rattlesnakes that sometimes come down from the hills above campus, and thus signs are posted alerting students to "Beware of Rattlesnakes." Although Jessica never saw a snake, seeing the sign was enough to have her drop the class and never take another in that building. What could be say about Jessica's behavior and its relation to her ophidiophobia?
    a. By associating the thought of the sign with her phobia, she gets positive reinforcement and maintains the phobia.
    b. By avoiding the feared object, she gets reinforcement and maintains the phobia.
    c. By avoiding the feared object, she gets positive reinforcement and maintains the phobia.
    d. By avoiding the feared object, she is reducing her anxiety and thus working toward extinguishing her phobia.
    Answer: b   LO: 11; applied   page: 123

41. "Prepared classical conditioning" would make which item most likely to be feared?
    a. a gun
    b. a knife
    c. heights
    d. a one-eyed man
    Answer: c   LO: 11; factual   page: 124

Chapter 4

42. Research on "training" persons to become phobic by shocking them as they viewed particular pictures:
    a. supported the theory of prepared classical conditioning because participants came to fear snakes faster than flowers, and their fears to flowers were extinguished more easily than to snakes.
    b. supported the theory of prepared classical conditioning because participants came to fear snakes faster than flowers, although it was equally as difficult to extinguish both phobias.
    c. did not support the theory of prepared classical conditioning, because participants came to fear snakes faster than flowers, and their fears to flowers were extinguished more easily than to snakes.
    d. did not support the theory of prepared classical conditioning, because participants came to fear guns and knives faster than snakes, and all phobias were resistant to extinction.
    Answer: a   LO: 11; factual   page: 124

43. When James was a little boy he was playing on the kitchen floor with a little mouse. His mother came into the kitchen, screamed, grabbed a broom, killed the mouse, and began to shake and cry. Ever since, James has been phobic of mice. His phobia could be best explained by:
    a. operant conditioning.
    b. observational learning.
    c. biological theories.
    d. psychoanalytic theory.
    Answer: b   LO: 11; applied   page: 125

44. On the basis of the evidence in the text, the development of phobias is best explained by:
    a. biological theory.
    b. behavioral theory.
    c. psychodynamic theory.
    d. cognitive theory.
    Answer: b   LO: 11; factual   page: 125

Anxiety Disorders

45. Which of the following case examples from the text provides support for the behavioral theories of phobias?
    a. Little Hans, who developed a fear of horses after his anxiety was displaced onto a neutral object (a horse, in this case).
    b. Little Albert, who developed a fear of snakes after observing his mother reacting with extreme fright to the sight of a snake.
    c. Little Albert, who developed a fear of white rats and other white objects after having these objects become conditioned stimuli when paired with a loud noise.
    d. Little Hans, whose mother comforted him every time he expressed anxiety and punished him when he failed to show fears of objects that she feared.
    Answer: c   LO: 11; factual   page: 126

47. After attending a few sessions with his therapist, Andrew was asked to determine what he feared most, and then to think about what he feared almost that much, and then to think of something else that would be third in his ranking of fears, and to continue in this way until he had a list of about six items, going from his most feared to something that caused no fear at all. His therapist then taught him relaxation techniques, and then began to have Andrew relax as the items on his list were brought to mind, beginning with the least feared object. This type of therapy is referred to as:
    a. relaxation therapy.
    b. a hierarchy of fears.
    c. systematic desensitization.
    d. in vivo sensitization.
    Answer: c   LO: 12; applied   page: 126

48. When John, a telephone line man, came to Dr. Henderson for therapy, John said he needed to be "cured quickly" because he was on the verge of losing his job. John had quite suddenly developed acrophobia and was thus unable to climb telephone poles without developing vertigo and obvious concerns for falling and injuring himself. Although it is a frightening technique, Dr. Henderson decided that the best one to use would be
    a. systematic desensitization.
    b. relaxation therapy.
    c. modeling.
    d. flooding.
    Answer: d   LO: 12; applied   page: 126

49. As noted in the text, a useful approach for treating social phobia is:
    a. applied tension technique in one-on-one sessions.
    b. applied tension and systematic desensitization in a group setting.
    c. systematic desensitization, modeling, and flooding in a group setting.
    d. systematic desensitization, modeling, and flooding in one-on-one sessions.
    Answer: c   LO: 12; factual   page: 126

Chapter 4

50. Which of the following has been the *least* effective for treatment of specific phobias and social phobia?
    a. behavioral therapy
    b. cognitive therapy
    c. cognitive-behavioral therapy
    d. drug therapy
    Answer: d   LO: 12; factual   page: 127

51. A person who repeatedly reexperiences an agonizing event, whether by intrusive images, nightmares, or flashbacks; who feels numb and detached from others; and who always feels on guard against the event recurring is suffering from:
    a. panic attack.
    b. agoraphobia.
    c. post-traumatic stress disorder (PTSD).
    d. obsessive-compulsive disorder (OCD).
    Answer: c   LO: 13; factual   page: 128

52. Which of the following *is not* a symptom of post-traumatic stress disorder (PTSD) described in the text?
    a. reexperiencing the traumatic event
    b. emotional numbing
    c. hypervigilance
    d. excessive attachment
    Answer: d   LO: 13; factual   pages: 128-129

53. Which of the following *is not* a way in which children tend to manifest symptoms of post-traumatic stress disorder (PTSD) differently than adults?
    a. Children express their distress through aches, pains, and other somatic symptoms.
    b. Children try to act more like adults or their older siblings in order to deal with the trauma.
    c. Children's anxiety tends to generalize to more situations.
    d. Children tend to play out the trauma repetitively with dolls or other toys.
    Answer: b   LO: 13; factual   page: 129

Anxiety Disorders

54. When William was in Vietnam, his outfit fell under enemy fire. Only he and three other men survived, and he watched and could do nothing as his best friend was blown up. After returning home, he hid his medals away and refused to talk about them or the war. For years, now, he has been having nightmares in which he sees himself and his friends being blown apart; the dreams cause him to wake up screaming and in a cold sweat. Before going to Vietnam he seldom drank alcohol, but now he is either drunk or high on marijuana most of the day, which he says is the only way he can make it through without exploding. He is constantly on the look out for enemies, who now include not only the Viet Cong, but the U.S. government as well. William is suffering from:
    a. panic disorder.
    b. post-traumatic stress disorder (PTSD).
    c. obsessive compulsive disorder (OCD).
    d. social phobia.
    Answer: b   LO: 13; applied   page: 129

55. According to the text, which of the following is *most correct* with respect to post-traumatic stress disorder (PTSD)?
    a. A child is more likely than an adult to develop PTSD as the result of a natural disaster.
    b. Suffering as a community makes the survivors more likely to develop PTSD because the trauma seems more dramatic.
    c. Human made traumas are more likely to cause PTSD than natural disasters.
    d. Children are more vulnerable than adults to developing PTSD.
    Answer: c   LO: 13; factual   pages: 129-130

56. Mary is a survivor of date rape that took place last week. She reported the rape to the police, who have arrested the perpetrator. She has also been through a rape examination and has been tested for sexually transmitted diseases and HIV. Based on the statistics presented in the text, we might expect that Mary will experience post-traumatic stress symptoms severe enough to qualify for a diagnosis of PTSD for at least another week. If she is like 50% of other rape survivors, she may continue to experience such severe symptoms for:
    a. three more months.
    b. one more year.
    c. three more years.
    d. five more years.
    Answer: a   LO: 13; applied   page: 130

Chapter 4

57. In terms of recovery from PTSD:
    a. most people suffering from PTSD recover within 3 months of the trauma.
    b. about one-quarter of those suffering from PTSD recover within 3 months of the trauma; another quarter within 12 months; but some never recover.
    c. about one-half of those suffering from PTSD recover within 3 months; others continue for at least a year or longer.
    d. recovery rate from PTSD is very poor, with most people never completely recovering.
    Answer: c   LO: 13; factual   page: 130

58. Research by Schlenger, Kulka, Fairbank, and Hough (1992) found that _____ veterans suffered the highest rates of PTSD and _____ veterans suffered the lowest rates as a result of the Vietnam War.
    a. Hispanic; white
    b. Hispanic; African-American
    c. white; Hispanic
    d. African-American; Hispanic
    Answer: a   LO: 13; factual   page: 131

59. Which of the following individuals would be *most* likely to develop PTSD?
    a. A woman who witnessed her best friend's murder (due to gunshot), who lives with her husband and two children, and who has a ruminative coping style.
    b. A man who was tortured while a prisoner-of-war (POW) in Vietnam, who lost several friends during the war, who is married and has an active coping style.
    c. A woman whose child was severely injured during a class field trip, who has few friends, and who has an active coping style.
    d. A man who left his family behind in his native country to try to find work in the United States, who has been mugged and discriminated against since his arrival, and who lives alone and has a ruminative coping style.
    Answer: d   LO: 13; applied   page: 132

60. The most powerful predictors of a person's reaction to trauma are:
    a. personality factors and severity of the trauma.
    b. severity and duration of the trauma, and proximity of the person to the trauma.
    c. the number of other people involved in the trauma.
    d. whether it was a "natural" or "human" made trauma.
    Answer: b   LO: 14; factual   page: 132

Anxiety Disorders

61. Which of the following are important factors in determining a person's ability to handle trauma?
    a. social support and coping style
    b. physical health and financial resources
    c. social support and financial resources
    d. government intervention and social support
    Answer: a   LO: 14; factual   pages: 132-133

62. Psychodynamic and existential therapists suggest that people who _____ their trauma may be less likely to develop PTSD.
    a. are in denial about
    b. minimize
    c. can make sense of
    d. keep talking about
    Answer: c   LO: 14; factual   page: 134

63. Which of the following *is not* a treatment goal for PTSD?
    a. exposing clients to what they fear in order to extinguish that fear
    b. challenging distorted cognitions that contribute to the symptoms
    c. helping clients manage their daily life problems to reduce stress in their life
    d. helping clients learn how not to think about the trauma to reduce the stress
    Answer: d   LO: 15; factual   page: 134

64. Emelda was violently raped one evening by a man she knew and believed she could trust. The rape took place over a period of several hours, during which time he held a knife to her throat and kept threatening to kill her if she didn't do all that he told her to do. Her therapist is now having her identify the thoughts and events that now cause her anxiety and ranking them from most anxiety-provoking to least. Using relaxation techniques, Emelda's therapist is taking her through this hierarchy to imagine the event to its smallest detail in order to help Emelda challenge her distorted thoughts, such as guilt, and to reduce the anxiety produced by the traumatic rape. This form of working through the event is:
    a. systematic desensitization.
    b. flooding.
    c. confrontation.
    d. aversion therapy.
    Answer: a   LO: 15; applied   page: 135

Chapter 4

65. If a PTSD survivor cannot find meaning in the triggering traumatic event, one way to deal with the intrusive thoughts is to:
   a. try to find meaning in the event.
   b. yell "no!" loudly when the thoughts intrude.
   c. try to relax whenever the thoughts intrude.
   d. focus on the thoughts and think about why they are there.
   Answer: b   LO: 15; factual   page: 135

66. One of the most effective treatments found so far for PTSD is:
   a. use of benzodiazepines.
   b. use of antidepressants.
   c. systematic desensitization.
   d. problem solving.
   Answer: c   LO: 15; factual   page: 135

67. The best use of drugs for treating PTSD appears to be to:
   a. calm the survivor down so the symptoms can subside.
   b. quell the symptoms so the survivor can more easily face his or her memories.
   c. help the survivor stop thinking about the traumatic events.
   d. eliminate the memories by working on specific areas of the brain where they are stored.
   Answer: b   LO: 15; factual   page: 136

68. The Navajo treatment for combat veterans suffering from PTSD that involves the veteran, his family, community members, and a tribal healer participating in ritual songs for 7 days and 7 nights to return balance and harmony to the veteran and the community is called the:
   a. Warrior's Absolution.
   b. Tribal Healing Ceremony.
   c. Sun Dance.
   d. Enemy Way.
   Answer: d   LO: 15; factual   page: 136

69. The major difference between generalized anxiety disorder (GAD) and the other anxiety disorders is that:
   a. in GAD there is a specific situation that causes anxiety to occur all the time.
   b. the other anxiety disorders are triggered by a specific object or event.
   c. people with GAD have a few specific fears, such as job performance or their health.
   d. the other anxiety disorders are much more diffuse in terms of what triggers them.
   Answer: b   LO: 16; factual   page: 137

Anxiety Disorders

70. Generalized anxiety disorder (GAD):
    a. is a relatively rare disorder.
    b. is so common it is called the "common cold of psychological disorders."
    c. is a relatively common disorder.
    d. has such vague symptoms that it's difficult to determine how many people have it.
    Answer: c   LO: 16; factual   page: 137

71. In terms of understanding GAD:
    a. more is known about its causes and appropriate treatments than the other anxiety disorders.
    b. less is known about its causes and appropriate treatments than the other anxiety disorders.
    c. as much is known about its causes and appropriate treatments as the other anxiety disorders.
    d. it has not been sufficiently differentiated from the other anxiety disorders to determine whether its causes and treatments are similar or dissimilar.
    Answer: b   LO: 16; factual   page: 137

72. What evidence says that people with GAD focus on detecting possible threats in the environment at even an unconscious level?
    a. Teaching people with GAD relaxation exercises lowers their anxiety by quelling their unconscious fears of losing control.
    b. People with GAD unconsciously avoid processing threatening information and thus do not think through events they fear long enough to consider how they might cope if these events actually happened.
    c. When asked to recite a list of words, people with GAD recite words that contain threatening content slower than a matched group without GAD, even when these words are presented at a speed too quickly to be consciously processed.
    d. When asked to recite a list of words that are a certain color, people with GAD name the color of words that are threatening more slowly than people without GAD, even when these words are presented at a speed too quickly to be consciously processed.
    Answer: d   LO: 17; factual   page: 138

73. One way that people with GAD are self-defeating is that:
    a. they worry so much about what might happen that they overprepare for emergencies.
    b. by avoiding fully processing images of what they worry about, they do not consider ways to cope if the event does happen.
    c. they are so vigilant that they are on constant guard to keep all negative thoughts out of their heads, so they keep positive thoughts out as well.
    d. they are so tense so much of the time that the only way they can cope is to relax, which they tend to overdo.
    Answer: b   LO: 17; factual   page: 138

Chapter 4

74. Use of benzodiazepines for treating GAD has been found to:
    a. produce no relief.
    b. produce short-term relief.
    c. produce long-term relief.
    d. be the most effective therapy.
    Answer: b   LO: 17; factual   page: 138

75. With respect to the anxiety disorders:
    a. there appear to be few, if any, gender differences.
    b. men are more likely to be diagnosed with these disorders than women are.
    c. women are more likely to be diagnosed with these disorders than men are.
    d. men are more likely to be diagnosed with PTSD, but women are more likely to be diagnosed with the other anxiety disorders.
    Answer: c   LO: 18; factual   page: 138

76. In terms of anxiety disorders, which of the following is *most* accurate?
    a. Female relatives of people with panic disorder are more likely than male relatives to have the disorder also.
    b. Female relatives of people with panic disorder are more likely than male relatives to suffer from alcohol abuse and dependence disorders.
    c. Male relatives of people with panic disorder are more likely than female relatives to have the disorder also.
    d. The male and female relatives of a person with panic disorder are equally likely to have the disorder also.
    Answer: a   LO: 18; factual   page: 138

77. A syndrome similar to the anxiety disorders that is reported in Hispanic cultures is described by Guarnaccia et al. (1996) as including "trembling, heart palpitations, a sense of heat in the chest rising into the head... loss of consciousness... dizziness, faintness, and spells." The person may also swear, shout, or hit people, and then fall to the ground in convulsions. This syndrome is called:
    a. *la belle indifference.*
    b. *ataque de nervios.*
    c. running amok.
    d. *loco-loca.*
    Answer: b   LO: 19; factual   page: 140

Anxiety Disorders

78. When comparing PTSD in other cultures with those in the United States:
    a. PTSD is more common in the United States than elsewhere.
    b. Puerto Ricans involved in the 1985 floods actually suffered from depression, not PTSD.
    c. Southeast Asians may be especially vulnerable to PTSD due to the chronic and severe nature of the traumas they experience.
    d. in the United States, PTSD is more common among upper-middle-class whites than among members of disadvantaged minorities.
    Answer: c LO: 19; factual pages: 140-141

79. In terms of diagnosing PTSD:
    a. the symptoms are extremely similar from one culture to another.
    b. survivors in the United States are more likely to report somatic symptoms than survivors in some other cultures.
    c. Asian survivors are more likely than those in the United States to report psychological symptoms.
    d. Asian survivors are more likely than those in the United States to report somatic symptoms.
    Answer: d LO: 19; factual page: 140

80. When seeking treatment for PTSD, a person from southeast Asia is:
    a. more likely than someone from the United States to discuss the primary symptoms of startle reactions, nightmares, reexperiencing the trauma, and irritability.
    b. much less likely than someone from the United States to discuss dissociative experiences, such as hallucinations or loss of physical functioning.
    c. less likely than someone from the United States to discuss the primary symptoms of startle reactions, nightmares, reexperiencing the trauma, and irritability.
    d. equally as likely as someone from the United States to talk about the traumas he or she experienced.
    Answer: c LO: 19; conceptual page: 141

81. When working with a trauma survivor from southeast Asia who suffers from PTSD, the therapist:
    a. must avoid talking about the trauma for several sessions because of cultural taboos.
    b. will need to interrogate the survivor in-depth, since that is the only way to get the entire story and begin the healing process.
    c. must challenge the survivor's distorted beliefs about the traumatic event and the survivor's part in it.
    d. needs to be highly sensitive and supportive in getting the survivor's story to avoid further traumatizing the survivor.
    Answer: d LO: 19; conceptual page: 141

Chapter 4

82. Which of the following *is not likely* to be a reason for minority status war veterans to be more vulnerable to PTSD than white veterans?
    a. genetic weaknesses
    b. sociocultural conditions
    c. preexisting chronic stress
    d. social support networks
    Answer: a   LO: 20; conceptual   pages: 141-142

83. Obsessive-compulsive disorder (OCD) is a disorder in which anxiety results from:
    a. obsessional thoughts that cannot be relieved by carrying out a compulsive behavior.
    b. compulsive thoughts that cannot be relieved by carrying out an obsessive behavior.
    c. obsessional thoughts, even if the compulsive behavior is carried out.
    d. compulsive thoughts, even if the obsessive behavior is carried out.
    Answer: a   LO: 21; conceptual   page: 142

84. Thoughts, images, or impulses that are persistent, that intrude on a person's consciousness without control, and that cause significant anxiety or distress are called:
    a. compulsions.
    b. fixations.
    c. phobias.
    d. obsessions.
    Answer: d   LO: 21; conceptual   page: 144

85. The most common obsession across cultures appears to be:
    a. death.
    b. contamination.
    c. sexual thoughts.
    d. immoral impulses.
    Answer: b   LO: 21; factual   page: 144

86. How does obsessive-compulsive disorder (OCD) differ across cultures and gender?
    a. People in developing countries are more likely to experience obsessions that focus on repeated bouts; men are more likely to experience OCD compared to women.
    b. People in industrialized countries are more likely to develop OCD; women are more likely than men to experience OCD, as they are more likely to experience all of the anxiety disorders.
    c. OCD is manifested so differently across cultures and gender that it may be soon declassified as an anxiety disorder due to its low diagnostic reliability.
    d. OCD is similar across cultures and gender, except in its peak age of onset, which is at a younger age for men compared to women.
    Answer: d   LO: 21; factual   pages: 144-145

87. Howard is so fanatic about germs that he has his room sterilized twice a day, and anyone entering his room must wear surgical rubber gloves. He will not take a bath but showers five hours a day, scrubbing to the point that he has rubbed off his skin and is covered with sores. Howard appears to be suffering from:
   a. post-traumatic stress disorder (PTSD).
   b. panic disorder.
   c. obsessive-compulsive disorder (OCD).
   d. xenophobia.
   Answer: c   LO: 21; applied   pages: 142-145

88. Repetitive behaviors or mental acts an individual feels he or she must perform are called:
   a. phobias.
   b. obsessions.
   c. compulsions.
   d. stereotypic acts.
   Answer: c   LO: 21; conceptual   page: 144

89. Which of the following is *most* accurate?
   a. There is no way to reduce the anxiety brought about by obsessional thoughts.
   b. Compulsive behaviors serve their purpose of reducing anxiety from obsessional thoughts.
   c. Compulsive behaviors never serve their purpose of reducing anxiety from obsessional thoughts.
   d. Compulsive behaviors temporarily serve their purpose of reducing anxiety from obsessional thoughts.
   Answer: d   LO: 21; conceptual   page: 145

90. With respect to the link between the specific obsession the person has and the specific compulsion that helps dispel the obsession, that link:
   a. is clearly discernible.
   b. is easily "uncoded."
   c. is often not discernible.
   d. does not exist.
   Answer: c   LO: 21; factual   page: 145

91. The apparent purpose of the compulsive behavior is to:
   a. reduce the anxiety of the obsessive thoughts.
   b. directly play out the obsessive thoughts in actions.
   c. gain attention and thereby find support in reducing the obsessive thoughts.
   d. engage in them for their own sake, without concern for the obsessive thoughts.
   Answer: a   LO: 21; conceptual   page: 145

Chapter 4

92. Persons afflicted with OCD:
   a. generally have no other psychological disorders--this one's enough!
   b. often suffer from depression as well, but typically not from other anxiety disorders.
   c. often suffer from other anxiety disorders, but not from other psychological disorders.
   d. often suffer from depression as well as other anxiety disorders.
   Answer: d   LO: 21; factual   page: 145

93. With respect to gender differences for OCD:
   a. females are much more likely than males to be diagnosed with OCD.
   b. males are much more likely than females to be diagnosed with OCD.
   c. onset appears to be much earlier for males than for females.
   d. onset appears to be much earlier for females than for males.
   Answer: c   LO: 21; factual   page: 145

94. Some of the most promising recent research on OCD views it as:
   a. neurologically based.
   b. unconsciously based.
   c. based on faulty beliefs.
   d. developed through operant conditioning.
   Answer: a   LO: 22; factual   page: 146

95. Biological theories of OCD suggest that it is:
   a. a neurological disorder caused by hyperactivation of a brain circuit.
   b. excessive amounts of serotonin that hyperactivate the brain circuitry.
   c. a neurological disorder caused by previously undetected lesions on the frontal cortex.
   d. a neurological disorder caused by underactivation of a brain circuit.
   Answer: a   LO: 22; factual   page: 146

96. Edress was 21 years old when her son was born. At first she was excited, but after a few days of changing diapers, running whenever he cried, and no longer being able to go out with her friends, she began to resent him. She had frequent thoughts of killing him, but everyone who saw him said, "What a beautiful baby--how happy you must be. You're going to be a wonderful mother with such a darling baby!" So she came to believe he really was a blessing. Soon after his first birthday, Edress began to see dead fetuses lying in the street whenever she took her son for a walk. She had to cross the street 13 times in order to reduce the anxiety she felt when she saw these horrible objects. This connection between her OCD and its origins would most likely come from the _____ perspective.
   a. biological
   b. behavioral
   c. cognitive
   d. psychodynamic
   Answer: d   LO: 22; applied   pages: 146-147

Anxiety Disorders

97. In terms of treating OCD:
    a. antidepressant drugs have been extraordinarily successful.
    b. cognitive-behavioral therapy has been seen to have long-term results in reducing symptoms.
    c. psychodynamic therapy is most effective because it gets at the root of the problem.
    d. there is no universally effective therapy.

    Answer: d   LO: 22; factual   page: 149

Essay Questions

98. After studying the chapter on anxiety disorders, you have suddenly noticed that many of the people you know are exhibiting a number of symptoms that you think may fit within the diagnostic criteria for these disorders. To determine exactly which disorder these people may have, you will need to name and describe the various anxiety disorders described in the text, being specific in terms of symptoms of each, theories of how each disorder may develop, and how they are similar to and different from each other. Remembering that these people are near and dear to you, you want to find the best treatment for them, so for each disorder, which type of therapy will result in the optimal outcome?

    Students should include the following disorders: panic attacks, panic disorder, agoraphobia, simple phobias, social phobia, post-traumatic stress disorder, generalized anxiety disorder, and obsessive-compulsive disorder, presenting the somatic, behavioral, and cognitive aspects of each. Appropriate theories--classical conditioning, operant conditioning, biological, cognitive (and psychodynamic would also be nice)--should be discussed as most appropriate for each specific disorder. Blood-injection-injury phobia should be distinguished from the other phobias in terms of physiological responses and treatment; generalized anxiety disorder should be distinguished in terms of its pervasive anxiety rather than specific situations or objects; and obsessive-compulsive disorder should be specifically differentiated from the other anxiety disorders in terms of the need to perform the compulsive behaviors to reduce the anxiety and the vagueness of its origins as compared with the other anxiety disorders. While cognitive-behavioral therapy works effectively for most of these disorders by challenging distorted beliefs; behavior therapy has been effective particularly with respect to systematic desensitization, modeling, and when indicated, flooding; drug therapy is also indicated in many cases; and psychodynamic therapy has been helpful in some instances. The harmful side effects of medications needs to be addressed as well.

Chapter 4

99. Imagine that you have been asked to give two different presentations to two different business organizations to help their members understand and avoid developing anxiety disorders. One presentation will be to a men's group, the other to a women's group. Discuss the difference in prevalence and symptomatology between men and women with respect to the anxiety disorders. What explanation can you give for these differences? What would you suggest to each of these groups to help them deal with their anxiety and to reduce their chances of developing an anxiety disorder?

    Address the fact that women are more often diagnosed with these disorders than men, however, men are more likely to succumb to alcohol and drug addiction. Explanations should include discussions of the argument that women may have greater genetic vulnerability to panic with agoraphobia and the criticisms of that argument; the role that progesterone may (or may not) play in increasing women's vulnerability; the psychodynamic beliefs that women's self-concepts and resulting behaviors can increase their risk for these disorders. Explanations should include the evidence that exists, criticisms of the evidence, and what still needs to be tested. Also discuss the effects of different coping styles in developing, maintaining, and overcoming these disorders. Appropriate therapies for each should address biological therapies for short-term help and cognitive-behavioral therapies for long-term reduction of symptoms.

100. You are training a group of students who will work as peer counselors on a campus with a diverse student population. Explain to them the cross-cultural experiences of the anxiety disorders; discuss the general similarities and the specific differences in symptoms and treatment. Include a discussion of how *ataque de nervios* is similar and different, how it might be diagnosed differently according to DSM-IV, and why it is not. Also address the special issues noted in the text for southeast Asian refugees.

    In addition to the basic psychological symptoms, the student should include the description of "trembling, heart palpitations, a sense of heat in the chest rising into the head. . . loss of consciousness...dizziness, faintness, and spells" and that the person may also swear, shout, or hit people, and then fall to the ground in convulsions. The student should discuss why it would be inappropriate to give the diagnosis of depression rather than panic attack. Cultural differences that include family taboos about talking about psychological problems should be included in the description of southeast Asian refugees, as well as the severity of the trauma and the somatic symptoms. In terms of treatment, discuss the ritualistic approach of the Puerto Ricans, with the herbal remedies, dancing, and healer; note the need for sensitivity in terms of family taboos and concern about becoming too intrusive (frightening) in learning about the refugee's background and problems.

Anxiety Disorders

101. Janice has called your office to discuss with you her problem of agoraphobia. After several incidents of panic attack while driving on the freeway or shopping at the mall, she is now totally unable to leave her house. It is becoming increasingly problematic for her because members of her family are constantly insisting that she "get out of the house," and they become angry with her for not coming to family get-togethers. Also, she had to take a loss in income because she could not keep her job as a receptionist. How would you treat Janice to get her back into a normal lifestyle?

    If the student suggests use of drugs (tricyclic antidepressants, benzodiazepines, and SSRIs), these should be used as an adjunct only to cognitive-behavioral therapy because they do not have long-lasting effects, and they do have serious side effects. The student should discuss the five components of cognitive-behavioral therapy: relaxation and breathing exercises, identifying catastrophizing cognitions, combine relaxation and breathing exercises while experiencing panic symptoms, challenging catastrophizing thoughts, and use of systematic desensitization (which should be explained in detail, with examples).

102. After reading the chapter on anxiety disorders and listening to class lectures, you have come to realize that it's not all a matter of *"nature OR nurture,"* but a combination of both. You have started to realize that it's time to look at what's going on in your own life. From that perspective, consider the vulnerability-stress models of anxiety, then discuss what creates the vulnerability in the first place, and what is necessary to produce a full-blown disorder?

    Discuss the biological preparedness of fight-or-flight syndrome for responding to threatening situations and the types of impairment that can lead to oversensitivity and overresponding. Then, discuss differences in what is perceived as threatening and how that can lead to arousal. Poorly regulated autonomic nervous system, chronic, mild anxiety or depression, or a genetic predisposition may be innate but will not create a problem unless the person tends to catastrophize, think in perfectionist ways, and be hypervigilant for signs of threat. With respect to certain disorders, such as PTSD, a triggering traumatic event must also occur.

Chapter 5   Mood Disorders

1. The most common emotion in depression is:
   a. grief.
   b. sadness.
   c. anhedonia.
   d. loss of energy.
   Answer: b   LO: 1; factual   page: 157

2. The term *anhedonia* is used to describe some symptoms of depression. With respect to depression, this term refers to losing:
   a. interest in everything in life.
   b. interest in pleasure.
   c. the ability to eat.
   d. the desire to have sex.
   Answer: a   LO: 1; factual   page: 159

3. Which of the following is not a typical symptom of depression?
   a. change in appetite
   b. change in sleep patterns
   c. change in self-concept
   d. change in activity levels
   Answer: c   LO: 1; conceptual   page: 159

4. With respect to the depressed person's activity levels, which is the **most accurate** statement?
   a. A typical symptom of depression is lack of energy and chronic fatigue, but some depressed people become physically agitated.
   b. The most significant symptom of depression is intense lack of energy and chronic fatigue.
   c. While many depressed individuals state they can barely move their bodies out of bed, it is more common that they become physically agitated.
   d. Slightly more than half of all individuals suffering from depression experience extreme lack of energy and chronic fatigue, the other half become physically agitated.
   Answer: a   LO: 2; factual   page: 159

5. A person who experiences depressed mood, plus two other symptoms of depression for at least a 2-year period during which the depressive symptoms do not remit for more than 2 months, would be diagnosed as having:
   a. double depression.
   b. cyclothymic disorder.
   c. major depression.
   d. dysthymic disorder.
   Answer: d   LO: 1; factual   page: 160

Mood Disorders

6. A person who experiences depressed mood, plus four other symptoms of depression chronically for at least 2 weeks, and the symptoms interfere with the person's ability to function in everyday life would be diagnosed as having:
   a. double depression.
   b. cyclothymic disorder.
   c. major depression.
   d. dysthymic disorder.
   Answer: c   LO: 1; factual   page: 160

7. Compared to major depression, dysthymic disorder is _____ severe and is _____ chronic.
   a. less; more
   b. less; less
   c. more; less
   d. more; more
   Answer: a   LO: 1 factual   page: 160

8. Since the birth of her last child, Sumi has been haunted by evil spirits who threaten to take over her body and kill her. She sees hearses following her whenever she has the energy to walk to the park with her children. She tires easily, so doesn't stay in the park for long. After a suicide attempt, her husband brought her to see Dr. Vahdi, who has diagnosed her with:
   a. depression with catatonic features.
   b. depression with psychotic features.
   c. depression with melancholic features.
   d. depression with atypical features.
   Answer: b   LO: 1; applied   page: 161

9. Richard is described by his friends as one of the "walking wounded." Although he reacts positively to positive events, he has gained 30 lbs in the last year, sleeps most of the day, and is hypersensitive to any type of perceived rejection--whether by a woman he's interested in or by some act of a friend. At times he seems suicidal. It is likely that Richard has:
   a. depression with catatonic features.
   b. depression with psychotic features.
   c. depression with melancholic features.
   d. depression with atypical features.
   Answer: d   LO: 1; applied   pages: 161-162

Chapter 5

10. A common occurrence that passes within 2 weeks of a child's birth and may be due to hormonal changes and/or sleep deprivation and the stress of a new baby is:
    a. postpartum depression.
    b. postpartum blues.
    c. baby blues.
    d. major depression with melancholia.
    Answer: b   LO: 1; conceptual   page: 162

11. Three weeks ago, Cynthia gave birth to a beautiful, healthy baby boy. She "knows" she should feel happy and excited but instead is extremely depressed, crying for hours every day, and she can barely motivate herself to care for her son or herself. She feels guilty about being depressed and about resenting her son. It is likely that Cynthia is experiencing:
    a. postpartum depression.
    b. postpartum blues.
    c. baby blues.
    d. dysthymia.
    Answer: a   LO: 1; applied   page: 162

12. Which of the following is *most correct* about seasonal affective disorder (SAD)?
    a. In the United States, SAD is more likely to occur during summer than during winter.
    b. The mood changes accompanying SAD are related not only to the weather, but also to other environmental events.
    c. A person who lives in Minnesota is more likely to get SAD than someone living in Louisiana.
    d. Although they exhibit many fewer symptoms, persons afflicted with SAD, nonetheless, show residual effects of the disorder during the summer.
    Answer: c   LO: 1; factual, conceptual   pages: 162-163

13. Harold, a 30-year-old businessman, has experienced anhedonia for about the past month. He frequently wakes up very early in the morning, during which time his symptoms are especially debilitating. He feels extremely guilty about many things and has lost a significant amount of weight since the onset of his symptoms. With which subtype of depression would Harold be diagnosed?
    a. depression with catatonic features
    b. depression with melancholic features
    c. depression with seasonal pattern
    d. depression with atypical features
    Answer: b   LO: 2; applied   page: 162

Mood Disorders

14. Which of the following statements is *false* about gender and age differences in depression?
    a. Women are twice as likely as men to be diagnosed with depression, but rates among children do not show this gender difference.
    b. Rates of depression are highest among those between the ages of 15 and 24.
    c. Due possibly to cohort effects or an increase in their coping skills with age, people who are age 85 or older show lower rates of depression than those aged 55-70.
    d. An increasing number of children are developing depression by the time they reach mid-adolescence.
    Answer: c   LO: 3; factual   pages: 163-164

15. Which of the following *is not* associated with a tendency to have more frequent and persistent depressive episodes?
    a. having less than a high school education level
    b. being African American
    c. having an unstable marital history
    d. being female
    Answer: b   LO: 3; factual   pages: 163-166

16. Which of the following is an accepted explanation of the lower rates of depression among the elderly?
    a. Due to cohort effects, the elderly are better able to hide their signs of depression.
    b. Depressed people tend to be more realistic about their self-perceptions, so others do not interpret their behaviors as signs of depression.
    c. Depression appears to interfere with physical health; consequently, depressed people are more likely to die before they get old.
    d. Having gone through the Great Depression and four wars, the elderly have gotten used to "living without," so other things don't bother them as much.
    Answer: c   LO: 3; conceptual   page: 164

17. With respect to age of onset of depression, which of the following is correct?
    a. The earlier the onset, the better the lifetime prognosis.
    b. The earlier the onset, the worse the lifetime prognosis.
    c. Lifetime prognosis for chronic depression is not related to age of onset.
    d. We have insufficient data to predict differences in prognosis.
    Answer: b   LO: 3; factual   page: 166

18. According to Blazer et al. (1994), which group had the highest rates of depression?
    a. African-Americans
    b. Asians
    c. Hispanics
    d. whites
    Answer: c   LO: 3; factual   page: 166

Chapter 5

19. Cross-cultural studies of depression have found:
    a. industrialized nations have lower rates of depression than nonindustrialized countries.
    b. industrialized nations have higher rates of depression than nonindustrialized countries.
    c. rates of depression are about the same in both industrialized and nonindustrialized countries, but for different reasons.
    d. researchers are not able to determine differences because people around the world exhibit different symptoms of depression.
    Answer: b   LO: 3; factual   page: 167

20. Which of the following is *false* about the course of depression?
    a. Approximately half of the people who have an episode of depression will relapse.
    b. If a person does relapse into a further episode of depression, it will most likely be within a year of recovering from the previous episode.
    c. The more previous episodes of depression people have had, the more likely they are to relapse into further episodes of depression.
    d. People who have inadequate social support from friends and family are more likely to relapse into new episodes of depression.
    Answer: b   LO: 3; factual   page: 168

21. Richard was buzzing with ideas. Every possible problem that humanity has ever faced came racing through his head, and he frantically solved each of them, writing down his solutions on whatever slip of paper was handy. He was so deeply involved in the importance of his work and its value to the world that he charged thousands of dollars worth of travel on his charge cards, traveling to see the leaders of the major nations, although he could not get an audience with any of them. He finally returned home from his travels, shredded and burned his notes, refused to speak to his friends or family members, and was barely able to move himself out of bed for days on end. Richard is suffering from:
    a. Bipolar I Disorder.
    b. Bipolar II Disorder.
    c. cyclothymic disorder.
    d. major depression.
    Answer: a   LO: 4; applied   page: 169-170

22. In _____ disorder, people experience more severe depression and only milder periods of mania; in _____ disorder, people experience more severe manic episodes and only milder periods of depression.
    a. Bipolar II Disorder; cyclothymic disorder
    b. Bipolar I Disorder; cyclothymic disorder
    c. Bipolar I Disorder; Bipolar II Disorder
    d. cyclothymic disorder; Bipolar II Disorder
    Answer: b   LO: 4; factual   page: 170

Mood Disorders

23. Bipolar disorder is:
    a. more common than unipolar depression.
    b. equally as common as unipolar depression.
    c. less common than unipolar depression.
    d. more often seen in men than in women.
    Answer: c   LO: 4; factual   page: 170

24. A diagnosis of rapid cycling bipolar disorder requires that a person experience:
    a. at least four manic-depressive cycles a day.
    b. at least one manic-depressive cycle a day.
    c. at least four manic-depressive cycles a month.
    d. at least four manic-depressive cycles a year.
    Answer: d   LO: 4; factual   page: 170

25. The example given in the text about how a person from the Amish community would manifest manic symptoms indicates that:
    a. the behaviors exhibited would be very similar to the DSM diagnostic criteria for the disorder as applied to other persons.
    b. the behaviors exhibited would likely be considered "normal" if performed by someone not from the Amish community.
    c. the behaviors exhibited would be more extreme and pronounced than manic behaviors performed by someone not from the Amish community.
    d. there are no recorded cases of a member of the Amish community being diagnosed with bipolar disorder.
    Answer: b   LO: 5; conceptual   page: 171

26. Which of the following is a true statement concerning bipolar disorder?
    a. Bipolar I disorder occurs only in highly industrialized nations, but Bipolar II Disorder has been found cross-culturally.
    b. Because of the extra energy that people experience during their manic episodes, most people with the disorder appreciate it.
    c. Some of the most influential people in history have both suffered and benefitted from bipolar disorder.
    d. Although persons going through a manic state believe their ideas are magnificently brilliant, the reality is that these ideas make no sense at all.
    Answer: c   LO: 6; factual   page: 171

Chapter 5

27. Storr (1988), in his biography of Sir Winston Churchill, determined that:
    a. Churchill's depression was a greater asset to him than his mania.
    b. Churchill's cyclothymic disorder played no part in his greatness.
    c. Churchill's manic behaviors earned him respect and support for his brilliant ideas.
    d. Churchill's manic behaviors were often a liability to him as a leader.
    Answer: d　　　　　　LO: 6; factual　　　　　　page: 172

28. A study by Richards et al. (1988) found people with bipolar or cyclothymic disorders are _____ creative _____ people with no history of these disorders.
    a. more; than
    b. less; than
    c. equally; as
    d. rarely; as
    Answer: a　　　　　　LO: 6; factual　　　　　　page: 174

29. Which of the following is *false* about the role of genetics in mood disorders?
    a. Family history studies have found that the first-degree relatives of people with bipolar disorder are two to three times more likely to have either bipolar or unipolar depression.
    b. Twin studies suggest that the concordance rate of bipolar disorder is 69% among MZ twins and 19% among DZ twins, suggesting heritability.
    c. Family history studies have found that first-degree relatives of people with unipolar depression are more likely than controls to have either bipolar or unipolar depression.
    d. Adoption studies have found that the rate of mood disorders and suicide attempts and completions is significantly higher among the biological relatives of adoptees with a mood disorder than among the adoptive relatives.
    Answer: c　　　　　　LO: 7; factual　　　　　　page: 175

30. Which of the following neurotransmitters **has not been** implicated in mood disorders?
    a. norepinephrine
    b. serotonin
    c. dopamine
    d. acetylcholine
    Answer: d　　　　　　LO: 8; factual　　　　　　page: 177

Mood Disorders

31. Which of the following is *true* about the role of neurotransmitters in mood disorders?
    a. Several studies that have compared people with mood disorders to people without them have found consistent differences between these groups on their levels of monoamine byproducts.
    b. Depressive people with prominent aggressive and suicidal impulses have been found to have low levels of acetylcholine compared to controls.
    c. Several studies suggest that people with major depression have too few receptors for the monoamines, whereas people with bipolar depression have an excess of these receptors.
    d. People with bipolar disorder have monoamine receptors that undergo poorly timed changes in sensitivity, which are correlated with mood changes.
    Answer: d   LO: 8; factual   pages: 177-178

32. The part of the neuroendocrine system that is hyperactive in people with depression is the:
    a. cerebral cortex.
    b. hypothalamic-pituitary-adrenal axis.
    c. limbic system.
    d. nondominant brain hemisphere.
    Answer: b   LO: 9; factual   page: 179

33. Which of the following is *true* about neurophysiological abnormalities in depression?
    a. People who are depressed have more slow-wave sleep and less REM sleep.
    b. Neuroimaging (CT and MRI) studies have shown that depressed people have atrophy in the cerebral cortex, whereas people with bipolar disorder have an enlarged cerebral cortex.
    c. People with severe major depression have increased metabolism in the frontal cerebrum and overactivation of the right hemisphere.
    d. People with severe bipolar disorder have atrophy or deterioration in the cerebellum.
    Answer: d   LO: 9; factual   page: 179

34. Currently, the most common biological treatment for bipolar disorder is:
    a. electroconvulsive shock therapy.
    b. anticonvulsant drugs.
    c. lithium.
    d. exposure to bright lights.
    Answer: c   LO: 9; factual   page: 181

Chapter 5

35. Which of the following is *false* about lithium?
    a. Lithium is more effective at reducing the symptoms of mania than the symptoms of depression.
    b. Most people who take lithium do so only during (or just prior to) a manic episode in order to limit the drug's side effects.
    c. There are enormous differences between people in the rate at which their bodies absorb lithium, which makes a proper dosage difficult to ascertain.
    d. Lithium's side effects include cognitive symptoms, such as difficulties with attention and concentration, in addition to abdominal pain, nausea, and kidney dysfunction.
    Answer: b   LO: 10; factual   pages: 181-182

36. Which of the following is a common reason for people with bipolar disorder stop taking their lithium?
    a. They are cured of the disorder.
    b. They miss their symptoms of mania.
    c. They forget.
    d. They believe they have better insight into their needs than their doctors do.
    Answer: b   LO: 10; factual   page: 182

37. One way to reduce the rate at which patients stop taking their lithium is by:
    a. combining drug treatment with cognitive-behavioral therapy.
    b. reducing the dosage so the side effects are lessened.
    c. combining the drug treatment with psychoanalytic therapy.
    d. giving clear instructions and going over them with the patient and the patient's parents, spouse, or significant other.
    Answer: a   LO: 10; factual   page: 182

38. Which of the following types of drugs for depression and mania has the fewest number of side effects?
    a. anticonvulsants
    b. selective serotonin reuptake inhibitors
    c. monoamine oxidase inhibitors
    d. tricyclic antidepressants
    Answer: b   LO: 11; factual   page: 183-185

39. Doctors often do not prescribe _____ to treat patients who might be suicidal because of the potential for fatality in overdose.
    a. lithium
    b. tricyclic antidepressants
    c. MAO inhibitors
    d. tricyclic antidepressants
    Answer: d   LO: 11; factual   pages: 183-184

Mood Disorders

40. Doctors prescribe _____ carefully because of their propensity to interact with a large number of everyday products, such as cheese, chocolate, or cold medicines.
    a. anticonvulsants
    b. SSRIs
    c. calcium channel blockers
    d. MAO inhibitors
    Answer: d   LO: 11; factual   pages: 183-184

41. _____ is an effective treatment for patients with severe depression and is thought to work by _____.
    a. Electroconvulsive therapy; resetting circadian rhythms
    b. Light therapy; resetting circadian rhythms
    c. Electroconvulsive therapy; stimulating the hypothalamus
    d. Electroconvulsive therapy; causing an acute release of monamines
    Answer: c   LO: 12; conceptual   page: 185

42. One of the most controversial therapies for depression is:
    a. electroconvulsive therapy.
    b. lithium.
    c. light therapy.
    d. use of SSRIs.
    Answer: a   LO: 12; factual   page: 185

43. One of the major complaints about the side effects of ECT has been:
    a. loss of sexual desire.
    b. loss of appetite.
    c. loss of memory.
    d. hypersensitivity to light.
    Answer: c   LO: 12; factual   page: 185

44. Exposure to bright lights is used for treating:
    a. Bipolar I Disorder.
    b. Bipolar II Disorder.
    c. catatonic depression.
    d. seasonal affective disorder.
    Answer: d   LO: 13; factual   page: 186

Chapter 5

45. Light therapy, which is used to treat depression with seasonal onset, is thought to work by:
    a. resetting diurnal rhythms.
    b. resetting circadian rhythms.
    c. causing an acute release of monoamines.
    d. stimulating the hypothalamus.
    Answer: b   LO: 13; factual   page: 186

46. The hypothesis that depression results from frequent or chronic exposure to uncontrollable negative events is known as the _____ theory of depression.
    a. learned helplessness
    b. cognitive distortion
    c. psychodynamic
    d. reformulated learned helplessness
    Answer: a   LO: 14; conceptual   page: 187

47. _____ theories suggest that life stress leads to depression because it creates a reduction in positive reinforcers in the person's life.
    a. Cognitive
    b. Behavioral
    c. Psychodynamic
    d. Humanistic
    Answer: b   LO: 14; conceptual   page: 187

48. Depressed people tend to have _____ chronic life stressors than nondepressed people.
    a. more
    b. fewer
    c. the same number of
    d. different
    Answer: a   LO: 14; factual   page: 187

49. Bruce is having problems with his wife. As a result, in order to avoid conflict, he stops communicating with her. When she pressures him to talk to her about their problems (which Bruce believes never seem to get resolved even if they do talk), he becomes increasingly silent and withdraws into himself. Their communication worsens, he withdraws further, and he becomes depressed. According to the behavioral perspective, Bruce probably:
    a. is attempting to overcome rejection.
    b. is frustrated with not being able to get his point across.
    c. may begin to talk when his wife stops yelling at him.
    d. is purposely upsetting his wife in order to punish her.
    Answer: a   LO: 14; applied   page: 187

-108-

Mood Disorders

50. With respect to Beck's (1967) cognitive distortion theory:
    a. the depressed person is generally accurate in terms of their perspective on the world, the future, and the self.
    b. the depressed person is completely aware of his or her negative views.
    c. the depressed person's errors in thinking perpetuate a negative view of the world, the future, and the self.
    d. the depressed person feels there is no way out of his or her negative situations.
    Answer: c   LO: 15; conceptual   page: 188

51. The theory proposed to explain how cognitive factors influence whether a person becomes helpless and depressed following a negative event is the _____ theory.
    a. learned helplessness
    b. reformulated learned helplessness
    c. causal attribution
    d. cognitive distortion
    Answer: b   LO: 16; conceptual   page: 188

52. Which of the following is an example of the "mental filter" error in thinking?
    a. "If I don't get an A on this test, I'll be a failure."
    b. "I can't believe I missed five questions out of 100. What an idiot I am."
    c. "I feel dumb, so I must be dumb."
    d. "I should be a better person than I really am."
    Answer: b   LO: 15; conceptual   page: 189

53. Which of the following is *false* about the role of causal attributions in depression?
    a. A pessimistic attributional style is one that is internal-stable-global.
    b. Pessimistic causal attributions may lead to depression but only when coupled with negative life events.
    c. As the severity of one's depression increases, one's tendency to make pessimistic causal attributions increases as well.
    d. Depressed people make pessimistic causal attributions and have negative automatic thoughts even when they are not depressed.
    Answer: d   LO: 15; conceptual   page: 189

54. Which of the following *is not* a characteristic of causal attributions as they relate to determining whether a person develops learned helplessness deficits?
    a. internal or external factors
    b. stable or unstable factors
    c. global or specific factors
    d. situational or environmental factors
    Answer: d   LO: 16; conceptual   pages: 189-190

Chapter 5

55. Metalsky, Halberstadt, and Abramson (1987) hypothesized that students who tended to attribute negative events to internal, stable, and global causes would be more likely to show depressive symptoms if they did poorly on an exam than students who attributed negative events to external, unstable, and specific causes. The most significant predictors of students' level of depression after the exam was students':
   a. use of internal attributions.
   b. exam score.
   c. level of depression before the exam.
   d. attributional style.
   Answer: b   LO: 16; factual   pages: 189-190

56. When researchers have compared depressed people with nondepressed people, they have found that:
   a. depressed people are more accurate in their judgments about how much control they have over situations.
   b. nondepressed people are more accurate in their judgments about how much control they have over situations.
   c. when it comes to "luck," depressed people are more accurate in their judgments about how much control they have, but nondepressed people are more accurate in other situations.
   d. both depressed and nondepressed judge their amount of control at a rate no greater than "chance."
   Answer: a   LO: 15; conceptual   page: 191

57. From the research on depressive realism, psychologists are finding:
   a. negative thinking appears to lead to depression.
   b. inaccurate perceptions about the one's self-efficacy lead to depression.
   c. accurate, realistic thinking keeps people from being depressed.
   d. hope and optimism are important factors in keeping people from being depressed.
   Answer: d   LO: 15; conceptual   page: 191

58. According to Aaron Beck (1979), negative thoughts:
   a. appear only when a person is depressed.
   b. are present when a person is depressed or happy.
   c. are latent in people prone to depression when they are not depressed.
   d. are latent in all people, whether or not they are prone to depression.
   Answer: c   LO: 16; conceptual   page: 191

Mood Disorders

59. Research on causal attributions and the reformulated learned helplessness theory has found:
    a. a pessimistic attributional style will lead to depression when coupled with negative life events.
    b. a pessimistic attributional style will lead to depression whether coupled with negative or positive life events.
    c. an optimistic attributional style will lead to depression when coupled with negative life events.
    d. an optimistic attributional style will lead to depression if it is coupled with unexpected life events.
    Answer: a   LO: 16; conceptual   pages: 191-192

60. Which of the following can accurately be said about modern psychodynamic theories?
    a. Their focus on psychosexual concerns is overemphasized and detracts from their ability to provide an effective framework for treating depressives.
    b. Their focus on the depressive's patterns of interpersonal relationships have led to an effective therapy for depression.
    c. There is insufficient empirical evidence to support their effective use with people who suffer from depression.
    d. The only research on these theories is cross-sectional; thus, we do not know what are the causes and what are the symptoms of depression.
    Answer: b   LO: 17; conceptual   page: 192

61. Which of the following aspects of Freud's theory of depression have *not* been supported by empirical evidence?
    a. The self-blame and feelings of guilt evident in depression result from introjection of hostility.
    b. People with depression are self-critical and believe they must be perfect.
    c. The parents of depressed people are remembered as cold and neglectful, demanding perfection and complete devotion from the child in exchange for their love.
    d. People who become depressed are dependent on others and have low self-esteem.
    Answer: a   LO: 17; factual, conceptual   pages: 192-193

62. A major problem with accepting Freud's theory of depression is that:
    a. there is no empirical support for these theories and, therefore, no scientific basis that it is a valid theory.
    b. there are no longitudinal studies to support these theories, so we can't tell if early life experiences led to the depression.
    c. most of the research is cross-sectional so we don't know if the characteristics are symptoms or causes of the depression.
    d. Freud's theories do not lend themselves to empirical research; thus, they cannot be accepted scientifically.
    Answer: c   LO: 17; factual, conceptual   page: 194

Chapter 5

63. Which of the following *is not* a goal of cognitive-behavioral therapy for depression?
    a. to change negative, hopeless patterns of thinking described by the cognitive models of depression
    b. to help depressed people solve concrete problems in their lives
    c. to help depressed people understand the early roots and underlying causes of their depression
    d. to help depressed people develop skills for being more effective in their world
    Answer: c   LO: 18; conceptual   page: 194

64. Which of the following *is not* one of the steps a cognitive-behavioral therapist will use?
    a. help the client discover the negative automatic thoughts the client habitually uses, and their link to the client's depression
    b. help the client challenge negative thoughts
    c. help the client develop new skills to help the client cope better his or her life
    d. help the client understand the client's unconscious processes that lead to the client's depression
    Answer: d   LO: 19; conceptual   page: 194

65. Which of the following is a question that a cognitive behavioral therapist might be expected to ask a depressed client?
    a. "Why don't you look at this differently?"
    b. "What can you do if this worst possible situation occurs?"
    c. "Do you know that you're wrong in the way that you're looking at this?"
    d. "Why are you always so depressed?"
    Answer: b   LO: 19; applied   page: 195

66. The therapist in our text asked, "How do you know you will never get into medical school if you fail this exam?" Which cognitive-behavioral step was the therapist taking?
    a. helping the client discover his or her negative automatic thoughts and understand their link to the client's depression
    b. helping the client challenge his or her negative thoughts
    c. helping the client confront his or her worst fears
    d. helping the client learn new skills he or she might need for coping better in life
    Answer: b   LO: 19; applied   page: 195

67. A form of therapy that grew out of the psychodynamic approach but is more structured and short term is _____ therapy.
    a. cognitive-behavioral
    b. psychoanalytic
    c. interpersonal
    d. humanistic
    Answer: c   LO: 18; factual   page: 198

Mood Disorders

68. Which of the following *is not* something that typically is part of interpersonal therapy?
    a. focus on problems in a client's interpersonal relationships
    b. explore current and past relationships
    c. help the client make decisions about changes he or she wants to make in current relationships
    d. help the client change negative ways of interpreting relationships
    Answer: d   LO: 19; conceptual   page: 198-199

69. A therapist who specifically addresses issues of a depressed patient's grief for loss of a loved one, interpersonal role disputes, role transitions, and deficits in a client's relational skills is most likely a(n) _____ therapist.
    a. psychodynamic
    b. cognitive-behavioral
    c. behavioral
    d. interpersonal
    Answer: d   LO: 18; conceptual   page: 198-199

70. Which of the following is a correct statement about interpersonal therapy?
    a. Interpersonal therapy has a short-term focus.
    b. Interpersonal therapy is not appropriate for treatment of children.
    c. Interpersonal therapy is not appropriate for treatment of older adults.
    d. Interpersonal therapy can be used successfully in individual therapy but does not work well in group therapy.
    Answer: a   LO: 18; factual   page: 198

71. Researchers of therapy outcome effectiveness were surprised to see significant improvement among the pill placebo group. They suggest the effectiveness of the placebo treatment resulted from:
    a. the depressed patients' belief that they were actually receiving medication for their symptoms, and that belief caused the symptoms to abate.
    b. the depressed patients' desire to please the researchers, which caused them not only to act less depressed, but to believe they were less depressed.
    c. the depressed patients interacting with a warm and caring professional, even though no specific type of therapy is being delivered.
    d. None of the above is correct. The placebo treatment was not effective.
    Answer: c   LO: 20; factual   page: 199

Chapter 5

72. A number of studies that have compared psychosocial and drug therapies to assess their effectiveness for treating mildly depressed patients have found _____ to be a particularly important predictor of recovery.
    a. the specific type of therapy used
    b. the relationship between the patient and therapist
    c. length of time in treatment
    d. the patient's intellectual level
    Answer: b   LO: 20; factual, conceptual   pages: 198-199

73. Which of the following statements about the effectiveness of treatments for depression is *false*?
    a. Cognitive therapy, interpersonal therapy, and imipramine work about equally well for treating patients who are depressed (but not severely depressed).
    b. Maintenance doses of therapy that combine psychosocial and drug therapies are no more effective than drug therapy alone for preventing relapse.
    c. Pill placebo treatments can also significantly improve depression but are not effective at preventing relapse.
    d. Drug therapy may be a more effective treatment for the severely depressed because it works faster than cognitive or interpersonal therapy.
    Answer: b   LO: 20; factual   pages: 199-200

74. The research on therapy outcome effectiveness in depression demonstrates that:
    a. drug therapies are consistently more effective than psychosocial therapies.
    b. cognitive-behavioral therapies are overall the most effective.
    c. interpersonal therapies are overall the most effective.
    d. clients have a choice in treatments since all three of these seem equally effective for most people.
    Answer: d   LO: 20; factual   page: 200

75. According to research, which of the following statements about gender differences in depression is *true*?
    a. Women have a higher rate of depression-linked neurobiological abnormalities compared to men.
    b. Women are more likely to experience depression during menopause than at any other time in their lives.
    c. Women have frequent increases in their levels of depression during the premenstrual phase, which are not merely exacerbations of major depression or dysthymia.
    d. Depression with postpartum onset is often linked to severe stress, such as a lack of social support.
    Answer: d   LO: 21; factual   pages: 201-203

Mood Disorders

76. With regard to women's menstrual cycles and depression, recent research has found that:
    a. there is a direct link between the phase of a woman's menstrual cycle and her mood such that women become more depressed immediately before menstruation.
    b. women who become increasingly depressed during their menstrual cycle have a history of frequent major depressive episodes unconnected to their menstrual cycle.
    c. there is a direct link between the phase of a woman's menstrual cycle and her mood, but it is only found in women between the ages of 15 and 35.
    d. there is a no direct link between a woman's menstrual cycle and her mood, but there is a link with her hormones, which is directly linked to post partum depression.
    Answer: b   LO: 21; factual   page: 202

77. Due to the disagreement among mental health professionals about the connection between women's menstrual cycles and depression, the American Psychiatric Association:
    a. chose not to include it in DSM-IV.
    b. gave it a tentative Axis I diagnosis of premenstrual dysphoric disorder.
    c. included diagnostic criteria for premenstrual dysphoric disorder in the appendix.
    d. included the diagnostic criteria for the disorder under sex and gender disorders.
    Answer: c   LO: 21; factual   page: 202

78. According to recent research (Angold & Wortham, 1993), the increase in depression for girls during early adolescence is tied primarily to their:
    a. hormonal changes.
    b. self-esteem.
    c. late maturing.
    d. biochemical abnormalities.
    Answer: b   LO: 22; factual   page: 202

79. Nolen-Hoeksema's (1990) research found that women's _____ may be one of the contributors to women's greater rates of serious depression.
    a. active coping
    b. passive ruminative style of coping
    c. tendency to distract themselves
    d. attempts to problem solve
    Answer: b   LO: 22; factual   page: 203

Chapter 5

80. Psychologists who propose a social explanation for women's depression would conclude that the most determining factor in a woman becoming depressed is:
    a. a passive, traditional personality that puts her at risk for depression.
    b. social expectations that women are emotional and, therefore, at risk for depression.
    c. social acceptability for women to express their emotions and thus more often than men to acknowledge being depressed.
    d. conforming to the traditional sex-role for women that limits their opportunities.
    Answer: d   LO: 22; conceptual   page: 204

81. Proponents of social explanations for women's depressions are likely to assert that traditional marriages are:
    a. good for men, but not for women.
    b. good for women, but not for men.
    c. good for both men and women.
    d. not good for men or women.
    Answer: a   LO: 22; factual   page: 204

82. The most compelling social explanation for women's higher rates of depression is that:
    a. women's hormonal changes put them at high risk for emotional upheaval, which often leads to depression.
    b. women social status puts them at high risk for physical and sexual abuse, which often leads to depression.
    c. women's passive traditional role puts them at high risk for developing low self-esteem, which often leads to depression.
    d. the limitations put on a woman's ability to succeed in a male-dominated world often leads to depression.
    Answer: b   LO: 22; factual, conceptual   page: 204

83. Most studies of rape estimate ___ % of women will be raped at some point in their lifetimes.
    a. less than 5
    b. between 5 and 10
    c. between 14 and 25
    d. more than 25
    Answer: c   LO: 22; factual   page: 204

84. In a study by Straus & Gelles (1990), approximately _____ percent of women reported they had been physically assaulted by their husbands in the previous year.
    a. 11
    b. 13
    c. 18
    d. 20
    Answer: b   LO: 22; factual   page: 204

Mood Disorders

85. Which of the following is *true* about suicide?
    a. More women than men are parasuicidal.
    b. When legislation limits access to guns, people find other ways to kill themselves, and suicide rates do not decrease.
    c. "Egoistic suicide" is Durkheim's term to describe suicide committed by people who experience severe disorientation due to a large change in their relationship to society.
    d. Having a high education level and being from an Eastern culture are highly associated with suicide risk.

    Answer: a   LO: 23; factual, conceptual   pages: 204-207

86. Hendin's (1995) research on suicide in the elderly population has found that:
    a. there has been a 50% increase in suicide rates among the elderly over the last few decades.
    b. when they attempt suicide, they are more successful at it than younger people are.
    c. most older people who attempt suicide do not really intend to die.
    d. only a few of the elderly who attempt suicide actually have a history of psychological problems.

    Answer: b   LO: 23; factual   page: 205

87. In a study by Kellerman and Reay (1986) on deaths by gun in homes of families who owned guns, _____% of the deaths within the home were of family members, whether by suicide, homicide (one family member killing another), or accident.
    a. .5
    b. 25
    c. 37
    d. 98

    Answer: d   LO: 23; factual   page: 206

88. Tony feels alienated from society, withdraws completely from social interaction, and sees himself as being alone in an unsupportive world. Seeing no other way out, Tony commits suicide. Using Durkheim's (1897) criteria, this is _____ suicide.
    a. egoistic
    b. anomic
    c. altruistic
    d. schizoid

    Answer: a   LO: 23; applied   page: 206

Chapter 5

89. People with bipolar disorder:
    a. rarely attempt suicide in the manic state because they are feeling euphoric and elated.
    b. often attempt suicide in the manic state because they are agitated, in despair over their illness, or concerned about oncoming depression.
    c. are more likely to attempt suicide in a depressive phase than in the manic phase.
    d. rarely attempt suicide, but if they do, they are more successful than other segments of the population.
    Answer: b   LO: 23; factual   page: 207

90. Which of the following was a finding of Hendin's (1995) research on suicide?
    a. Persons who feel great rage are more likely to express that rage by harming others than by harming themselves.
    b. Teenagers who are enraged at their parents but cannot express their rage may attempt suicide to punish their parents.
    c. War veterans are less likely than others to attempt suicide because they are able to justify killing in terms of needing to destroy the enemy.
    d. People who attempt suicide tend to be extremely flexible and have considered suicide as the best solution to their problems.
    Answer: b   LO: 23; conceptual   page: 208

91. Which of the following is *true* concerning the connection between suicide and schizophrenia?
    a. Schizophrenics are more likely to commit suicide when they are hallucinating than when they are lucid.
    b. Young educated males who relapse frequently into psychosis are the most likely to commit suicide.
    c. Older educated females with a long history of schizophrenia are the most likely to commit suicide.
    d. While 10% of schizophrenics attempt suicide, only 5% are successful at it.
    Answer: b   LO: 23; factual   page: 208

92. Studies looking for a link between suicide and biological factors found which of the following when they performed post-mortem studies of the brains of people who committed suicide?
    a. high levels of dopamine
    b. low levels of dopamine
    c. low levels of serotonin
    d. high levels of serotonin
    Answer: c   LO: 23; factual   page: 209

Mood Disorders

93. Nolen-Hoeksema, in the text, suggests that:
    a. people have the right to die whenever they choose, even if they are not terminally ill.
    b. preventing suicide is appropriate because many people who attempt suicide are not making a rational or permanent choice.
    c. preventing a person from committing suicide is inappropriate because persons who attempts suicide will keep trying until they are successful.
    d. life is so precious and so fragile, that we should live it to the fullest and make every possible attempt to prevent someone from committing suicide.
    Answer: b   LO: 24; conceptual   page: 209

94. The most important thing to do if you suspect a friend or family member is suicidal is to:
    a. try to joke them out of it.
    b. ignore it, because if they are not, you don't want to put the idea into their head.
    c. get help from mental health professionals as quickly as possible.
    d. tell them to stop thinking about it and show them how wonderful life really is.
    Answer: c   LO: 24; factual, conceptual   page: 209

95. In the case presented of Elaine, the 21-year-old college senior, which of the following would be a focus of cognitive therapists with respect to her problem?
    a. Elaine's role dispute with her parents
    b. a fundamental deficit in social skills
    c. her problems with role transitions
    d. her belief that she needs to please her family, no matter the cost
    Answer: d   LO: 18; applied   page: 213

96. The text gives a case study of a 21-year-old college student, Elaine, who is trying to decide what to do once she graduates. The conflicts between what she wants and what her parents want her to do have caused her to exhibit symptoms of depression. What would an interpersonal therapist focus on in treating Elaine?
    a. her faulty assumption that she has to please her family even if it's not what she wants to do
    b. her negative schema that she is a selfish person for her to want to move to the East Coast when her parents want her on the West Coast
    c. her role dispute with her parents and possibly a conflict over role transitions from college student to working person
    d. her false belief that she will be a horrible person if she moves to the East Coast, as she wishes, rather than to the West Coast, as her parents prefer
    Answer: c   LO: 18; applied   page: 213

Chapter 5

Essay Questions

97. Aisha has been referred to you by the CEO of the company where she works in high-level management. She is a 25-year-old African-American woman who has been rapidly rising in job level and responsibility since she began working for the company 3 years ago. She is the widowed mother of two little girls, and has been their sole support since her husband died 4 years ago. For over 2 years now, she has been plagued with what she believed to be Chronic Fatigue Syndrome, but her physician has not found any physical signs of that disorder. She can remember no periods of time during the past 2 years when she has had a great deal of energy, but the problem seems to be getting worse and is affecting her ability to concentrate and make decisions in both her professional and personal life. She also complains of insomnia and feelings of hopelessness. In the interview, she tells you that when she was a child, her mother was hospitalized for depression. What is your diagnosis, and how did you determine that diagnosis? Specifically, what symptoms support your diagnosis as opposed to a different diagnosis?

The disorder described here is dysthymic disorder. The student should discuss the process of differential diagnosis and how she or he arrived at his or her conclusion by (1) considering the symptoms suggesting dysthymia (pervasive depression most of the time for at least 2 years, and at least two of the following: poor appetite/overeating, insomnia/hypersomnia, low energy or fatigue, low self-esteem, poor concentration/difficulty making decisions, and feeling of hopelessness, without evidence of major depressive episodes or bipolar disorder, and a family history for depression); and (2) eliminating all forms of major depression in terms of severity and disruption of daily functioning, as well as additional criteria (e.g., anhedonia, agitation, inappropriate feelings of guilt, and suicidal thoughts), and any form of bipolar disorder (she has indicated no times when mania would appear to be present).

98. Aisha has been referred to you by the CEO of the company where she works in high-level management. She is a 25-year-old African-American woman who has been rapidly rising in job level and responsibility since she began working for the company 3 years ago. She is the widowed mother of two little girls and has been their sole support since her husband died 4 years ago. For over 2 years now, she has been plagued with what she believed to be Chronic Fatigue Syndrome, but her physician has not found any physical signs of that disorder. She can remember no periods of time during the past 2 years when she has had a great deal of energy, but the problem seems to be getting worse and is affecting her ability to concentrate and make decisions in both her professional and personal life. She also complains of insomnia and feelings of hopelessness. In the interview, she tells you that when she was a child, her mother was hospitalized for depression. What diagnosis would you make, and how would you go about treating her for her problem? Explain your reasons for choosing this method of treating her as opposed to some other method, and explain any concerns you might have about the treatment you do suggest.

Diagnosis of dysthymia, for reasons given previously. Whichever treatment option the students choose, they should discuss the effectiveness versus the side effects of each, particularly with respect to drug therapy; the most conservative in terms of side effects and often the fastest would be the SSRIs. ECT would be extreme for dysthymia, and light therapy is not indicated since it is for SAD. Students should compare and contrast the techniques and effectiveness of cognitive-behavioral therapy and interpersonal therapy, which have both been shown to be highly effective for treatment and relapse prevention.

99. From the perspective of the biological, behavioral, cognitive, and psychodynamic theories, discuss what it is that causes a person to become depressed. What evidence supports or questions the soundness of each theory.

The student should include in the biological perspective the role that genetics, monoamines, and the neuroendocrine system play in depression; behavioral theories should address learned helplessness and operant conditioning (the role of reinforcement); cognitive theories should include either Beck's cognitive distortions theory or the reformulated learned helplessness theory; and psychodynamic theory should discuss Freud's introjected hostility theory. The research support for and limitations of each of these theories should be addressed.

100. Describe the gender differences that are found in the research concerning unipolar depression. How do the biological, personality, and social perspectives explain these differences. Based on what is known about development of depression and the vulnerability of women for developing depression, what intervention would you design to prevent depression from occurring?

In terms of biological explanations, despite its popularity, hormonal fluctuation has not been well-supported because of contradictory findings and flaws in methodology. Personality theories address lack of assertiveness and women's ruminative coping style. Social explanations address women's status in society that leads to higher rates of physical and sexual abuse, limitations for personal growth, and also discusses how the traditional passive feminine role sets women up for low self-esteem and limited opportunities. In terms of prevention, the student should take what has been found in the research and design an intervention/prevention strategy.

Chapter 5

101. Your friend John is a junior in college. He has been acting very strange lately. He has been withdrawing from his usual active, out-going self and has been moody and uncommunicative. You finally confront him one day and ask him what's going on, and he tells you that he's thinking about killing himself. His dad has a gun "hidden" in the hallway closet, and John has been thinking about "swallowing" it, something he learned from seeing the movie *Scent of a Woman*. What factors do you see here that were raised in the chapter, and what is the best course of action for you to take?

The student should discuss gender and age issues as they relate to suicide rates, as well as the evidence suggesting that family-owned handguns increase the risk of suicide. Sociological theories of suicide might be discussed; psychological theories (including cognitive, affective, and biological factors and demographics) should be included in terms of who is at high risk for suicide. The fact that suicide is not usually a rational choice and that most people who attempt suicide but do not complete it do not try again is important in terms of how critical it is to intervene. The best course of action is to take it seriously and get help from mental health professionals immediately.

Chapter 6 The Schizophrenias

1. Which of the following is *not* typical of people with schizophrenia?
    a. loss of touch with reality
    b. almost a complete inability to communicate clearly
    c. peculiar speech patterns that may be difficult to understand
    d. inability to care for oneself
    Answer: b LO: 1; factual page: 216

2. Beliefs that have little grounding in reality are called:
    a. hallucinations.
    b. primary symptoms.
    c. loss of reality.
    d. delusions.
    Answer: d LO: 2; factual page: 216

3. Hallucinations are:
    a. unreal perceptual experiences.
    b. false beliefs.
    c. odd ways of thinking.
    d. schizophrenic language.
    Answer: a LO: 2; factual page: 216

4. The person first credited with deriving the most comprehensive and accurate description of schizophrenia is:
    a. Sigmund Freud.
    b. Emil Kraepelin.
    c. Eugen Bleuler.
    d. Carl Jung.
    Answer: b LO: 1; factual page: 216

5. Kraepelin's label for what is now called schizophrenia was:
    a. schizophrenia.
    b. dementia praecox.
    c. multiple personalities.
    d. split personality.
    Answer: b LO: 1; factual page: 216

Chapter 6

6. The label schizophrenia reflects a belief that:
    a. parts of the personality split apart from each other.
    b. the person with the disorder has a frenetic personality.
    c. there is a splitting of the person's personal beliefs from social norms.
    d. there is a splitting of mental associations, thoughts, and emotions.
    Answer: d   LO: 1; conceptual   page: 216

7. Which of the following is *not* a symptom of schizophrenia?
    a. delusions
    b. hallucinations
    c. disorganized thought and speech
    d. sociopathic behavior
    Answer: d   LO: 2; factual   page: 216

8. Which of the following is the most accurate statement concerning delusions?
    a. Delusions are ideas that the individual believes are true, and there is some evidence that they may actually be true.
    b. Delusions are voices that a schizophrenic hears, telling the schizophrenic to perform certain self-destructive behaviors.
    c. Delusions are ideas that the individual believes are true that are highly unlikely and sometimes totally impossible.
    d. Delusions are dreams that seem so real that the schizophrenic believes them to be real.
    Answer: c   LO: 2; conceptual   page: 217

9. How do the "typical" self-deceptions that most people hold differ from schizophrenic delusions?
    a. While self-deceptions are typically implausible, people other than the person believing them will agree with the person that they could actually happen.
    b. Although people who tend to use self-deceptions may be preoccupied by them, they nonetheless are able to get things done in their lives, such as hold a job.
    c. People holding self-deceptions are as likely as schizophrenics to acknowledge that their beliefs are wrong, but they don't let them interfere with their relationships.
    d. People holding self-deceptions do not view the arguments against their beliefs as part of a conspiracy to silence them.
    Answer: d   LO: 2; conceptual   page: 217

The Schizophrenias

10. The most common type of delusions are:
    a. persecutory delusions.
    b. delusions of reference.
    c. delusions of grandeur.
    d. thought insertion.
    Answer: a   LO: 2; factual   page: 217

11. One day Mr. Abbott walked into a law office and asked for help. He believed that the CIA had a device planted in one of his teeth several years ago, and they were monitoring his thoughts and trying to control his behavior by planting ideas that were not his own in his head. He also believed that others could hear his thoughts, even though he never spoke them out loud. Mr. Abbott appears to have
    a. persecutory delusions and delusions of being controlled.
    b. thought insertion and thought broadcasting.
    c. persecutory delusions and thought broadcasting.
    d. delusions of being controlled and thought broadcasting.
    Answer: b   LO: 2; applied   page: 218

12. Milton Rokeach (1964), a personality and social psychologist, interviewed three men who were institutionalized at Ypsilanti State Mental Hospital in Michigan. Each of these men believed he was Jesus Christ, and each believed the other two were imposters since there can be only one Jesus. This is an example of:
    a. delusions of guilt or sin.
    b. persecutory delusions.
    c. grandiose delusions.
    d. thought insertion.
    Answer: c   LO: 2; applied   page: 218-219

13. Which of the following is true?
    a. Although there are many different types of delusions, it is rare that a schizophrenic would experience more than one type of delusion.
    b. Although a schizophrenic may experience more than one type of delusion, ordinarily he or she experiences only one type at a time.
    c. It is most common for schizophrenics who have delusions to experience two simultaneously.
    d. It is extremely common for schizophrenics who have delusions to have several of them occurring at the same time.
    Answer: d   LO: 2; factual   page: 217-219

Chapter 6

14. In the case study presented in the text of David Zelt, which delusions did he experience?
    a. grandiose, persecutory, reference, and thought control
    b. grandiose, persecutory, reference, and thought insertion
    c. persecutory, being controlled, thought broadcasting, and thought insertion
    d. persecutory, reference, being controlled, and thought insertion
    Answer: a   LO: 2; applied   page: 218-219

15. In the case study presented in the text of David Zelt, his belief that he had discovered the source of telepathy is which type of delusion?
    a. thought broadcasting
    b. persecutory delusion
    c. delusion of reference
    d. grandiose delusion
    Answer: d   LO: 2; applied   page: 219

16. In the case study presented in the text of David Zelt, his belief that the other scientists were talking about him and he could read their minds is which type of delusion?
    a. thought broadcasting
    b. delusion of reference
    c. persecutory delusion
    d. grandiose delusion
    Answer: b   LO: 2; applied   page: 219

17. A study by Chapman, Edell, and Chapman (1980) found that _____ mentally healthy college students reported sometimes hearing voices.
    a. almost no
    b. 5 percent
    c. 15 percent
    d. 20 percent
    Answer: c   LO: 2; factual   page: 219

18. In a study by Chapman, Edell, and Chapman (1980), _____ mentally healthy college students believed they had transmitted thoughts into other people's heads at some time.
    a. no
    b. 3 percent
    c. 6 percent
    d. 9 percent
    Answer: c   LO: 2; factual   page: 219

The Schizophrenias

19. Chapman, Edell, and Chapman's (1980) study of college students who reported hearing voices found these students were unlikely to be diagnosed as schizophrenic because:
    a. college students develop their abilities to perceive things that others might not, so this is not considered unusual.
    b. most of the students who reported these occurrences were taking classes in variations of consciousness and had become hypersensitive.
    c. they were already in a sample of students who were being studied for the schizophrenic symptoms they were exhibiting.
    d. these experiences were occasional and brief, and tended to occur when the students were tired, stressed, or under the influence of alcohol or drugs.
    Answer: d   LO: 2; factual   page: 219

20. The most common type of hallucinations are:
    a. visual.
    b. auditory.
    c. gustatory.
    d. visual and auditory occurring with about equal frequency.
    Answer: b   LO: 2; factual   pages: 219-220

21. The second most common type of hallucinations are:
    a. visual.
    b. auditory.
    c. gustatory.
    d. tactile.
    Answer: a   LO: 2; factual   page: 220

22. Delusions and hallucinations differ across cultures predominantly in:
    a. whether they are auditory, visual, or gustatory.
    b. their general theme, such as persecution and grandiosity.
    c. their specific content, such as whether they involve the CIA or a tribal priest.
    d. the degree to which they debilitate an individual.
    Answer: c   LO: 2; factual   page: 220

23. Vera told her coworkers that she speaks with dead relatives. Since Vera comes from a culture where such beliefs are common, it is most likely that she is:
    a. schizophrenic because she is having persistent hallucinations.
    b. most likely normal but may be suffering from a disorder in which she is highly suggestible to mass hysteria.
    c. probably highly suggestible and suffering from hysteria but should be watched to be sure it does not develop into schizophrenia.
    d. probably normal because belief in spirits are common in her culture.
    Answer: d   LO: 2; applied   pages: 220-224

Chapter 6

24. The cognitive disorganization that is characteristic of schizophrenia is called:
    a. disorganized thoughts.
    b. formal thought disorder.
    c. thought disarray.
    d. loose thinking.
    Answer: b   LO: 3; factual   page: 221

25. Speech that is so disorganized as to render it unintelligible to the listener is called:
    a. clang associations.
    b. formal thought disorder.
    c. word salad.
    d. alogia.
    Answer: c   LO: 3; factual   page: 221

26. When asked about his twin brother, Milton responded: "Hilton is Milton, a twin, a sin, both kin within, from mother to brother, too sad, too bad, too rad, a fad, you cad, go away, Jose." This type of speech is called:
    a. word salad.
    b. neologisms.
    c. alogia.
    d. clang associations.
    Answer: d   LO: 3; applied   page: 221

27. A proposed explanation for the disorganized thinking and speech in schizophrenia supported by evidence with the Continuous Performance Test (CPT) is that schizophrenics:
    a. are too unresponsive to the environment to know that they are not communicating effectively and may proceed to speak while thinking they are coherent.
    b. may be busy "talking" to a visual or auditory hallucination and are thus unable to communicate effectively.
    c. often withdraw from others, get overinvolved with their own thoughts, and lose the ability to organize and present their thoughts to other people.
    d. cannot effectively deploy and control their attention.
    Answer: d   LO: 3; conceptual   page: 222

The Schizophrenias

28. When comparing attentional processes of schizophrenics and normals (using the Continuous Performance Test, CPT), Erlenmeyer-Kimling and Cornblatt (1987) and Nuechterlein (1989) found that:
    a. in the acute phase of the disorder, schizophrenics perform more poorly on the CPT than normals but perform as well as normal controls when their symptoms are in remission.
    b. schizophrenics perform more poorly on the CPT than normal controls in the acute phase and when their symptoms are in remission.
    c. schizophrenics perform more poorly on the CPT than normal controls, but their children and siblings perform about as well as relatives of normal controls.
    d. because of their disorganized manner of thinking, schizophrenics remember better if their rehearsal of stimuli in the CPT are interrupted by a distraction.
    Answer: b　　　　LO: 3; factual, conceptual　　　　page: 222

29. Erlenmeyer-Kimling et al. (1989) suspect attentional problems in the children of schizophrenics:
    a. may overwhelm these children's ability to cope with the everyday stresses of life.
    b. cause those who are very young to have behavioral problems, but the social problems do not surface until middle or late childhood.
    c. are caused by the chaotic environment incident to living with a schizophrenic parent and can be overcome by providing a more stable environment.
    d. may be a marker for vulnerability to schizophrenia but do not necessarily lead to developing the disorder later in life.
    Answer: a　　　　LO: 3; factual; conceptual　　　　page: 222

30. One reason presented in the text that people are often frightened of schizophrenics is that:
    a. they have a higher incidence of committing violent crimes.
    b. the media stereotypes that depict schizophrenics as dangerous.
    c. their behavior is disorganized.
    d. we cannot communicate with them effectively.
    Answer: c　　　　LO: 3; factual, conceptual　　　　page: 223

31. The term used for schizophrenics who exhibit an extreme lack of responsiveness to the outside world is:
    a. disorganized.
    b. catatonic.
    c. dissociated.
    d. withdrawn.
    Answer: b　　　　LO: 3; factual　　　　page: 223

Chapter 6

32. Which of the following most closely describes catatonic behavior?
    a. Jim, who stands in a bizarre position in the corner of a room for hours without moving a muscle.
    b. Janice, who races madly about in an agitated state and cannot be subdued without restraint or medication.
    c. Both are exhibiting catatonic behavior.
    d. Neither is exhibiting catatonic behavior.
    Answer: c   LO: 3; applied   page: 223

33. Type I symptoms in schizophrenia represent:
    a. the presence of salient experiences (e.g., hallucinations).
    b. deficits in certain domains (affect).
    c. abnormal brain structures.
    d. abnormal brain chemistry.
    Answer: a   LO: 4; factual   pages: 223-224

34. Type II symptoms in schizophrenia represent:
    a. the presence of salient experiences (e.g., hallucinations).
    b. deficits in certain domains (affect).
    c. abnormal brain structures.
    d. abnormal brain chemistry.
    Answer: b   LO: 4; factual   page: 224

35. The severe reduction in or absence of emotional responses to the environment often observed in schizophrenics are called:
    a. emotional deficit.
    b. affective flattening.
    c. emotional blunting.
    d. alogia.
    Answer: b   LO: 4; factual   page: 224

36. June has been hospitalized for 7 months with catatonic schizophrenia. She has just been told by her psychiatrist that her mother, whom she loved deeply, died in a car accident. When told this, June remains impassive, and responds to the news by saying, in a monotone voice, "Oh. Mom died." This would demonstrate:
    a. avolition.
    b. anhedonia.
    c. affective flattening.
    d. prodromal symptoms.
    Answer: c   LO: 4; applied   page: 224

The Schizophrenias

37. Avolition is a _____ symptom of schizophrenia and is marked by _____.
    a. positive; wild excitement and agitation for no apparent reason
    b. negative; an inability to persist at common goal-directed activities
    c. negative; a deficit in both the quantity of speech and the quality of its expression.
    d. positive; a prefrontal cortex that is smaller and less active than in people without schizophrenia.
    Answer: b   LO: 4; factual, conceptual   page: 224

38. Which of the following is *not* a common form of alogia, as discussed in the text that is common to schizophrenics?
    a. reduction in speaking
    b. not initiating speech with others
    c. answering questions in brief, empty replies
    d. echoing or repeating what another person said
    Answer: d   LO: 4; factual, conceptual   page: 224

39. Research by Andreason et al. (1990) has found that:
    a. negative symptoms are more responsive to medication than positive symptoms.
    b. persons with many negative symptoms typically have higher levels of education but a poorer prognosis than persons with primarily positive symptoms.
    c. negative symptoms seem less bizarre than positive symptoms but are a primary cause of problems schizophrenics have in functioning in society.
    d. medications are more effective in overcoming flat affect, alogia, and avolition than they are in reducing hallucinations, delusions, and thought disturbances.
    Answer: c   LO: 4; factual, conceptual   page: 224

40. Positive and negative symptoms of schizophrenia:
    a. are rarely seen in the acute phase of the disorder.
    b. are most prominent in the chronic phase of the disorder.
    c. manifest themselves during the acute phase of the disorder.
    d. are evident in both the acute phase of the disorder and in remission.
    Answer: c   LO: 5; conceptual   page: 224

41. Prodromal symptoms of schizophrenia are most evident:
    a. during the acute phase of the disorder.
    b. when the disorder is in remission.
    c. after the schizophrenic comes out of the acute phase.
    d. prior to onset of the acute phase.
    Answer: d   LO: 5; factual, conceptual   page: 224

Chapter 6

42. Residual symptoms of schizophrenia are most evident:
    a. during the acute phase of the disorder.
    b. when the disorder is in remission.
    c. after the schizophrenic comes out of the acute phase.
    d. prior to onset of the acute phase.
    Answer: c   LO: 5; factual, conceptual   page: 224

43. The form of schizophrenia that is characterized by prominent delusions and hallucinations that involves themes of persecution and grandiosity is _____ schizophrenia.
    a. paranoid
    b. disorganized
    c. catatonic
    d. residual
    Answer: a   LO: 5; conceptual   page: 225

44. Tesha experiences delusions of being controlled by a neighbor's television remote control. She visits the neighbor and demands that he hand over his remote, which he refuses to do, calling her "crazy." She takes this as further evidence of a plot against her life organized by the entire neighborhood. Tesha is most likely experiencing:
    a. self-deception.
    b. undifferentiated schizophrenia.
    c. paranoid schizophrenia.
    d. disorganized (hebephrenic) schizophrenia.
    Answer: c   LO: 5; applied   page: 225

45. People with paranoid schizophrenia, as compared with other forms of schizophrenia:
    a. exhibit the most obvious, extreme, and disorganized symptoms.
    b. often do not exhibit disorganized behavior but may be lucid and articulate.
    c. exhibit different, yet equally disorganized, symptoms.
    d. can be differentiated only in terms of the positive and negative symptoms.
    Answer: b   LO: 5; conceptual   page: 226

46. The prognosis for people with paranoid schizophrenia is _____ the prognosis for people with other types of schizophrenia.
    a. better than
    b. the same as
    c. worse than
    d. more difficult to ascertain than
    Answer: a   LO: 5; factual   page: 226

47. Episodes of psychosis in paranoid schizophrenia are often:
    a. insidious and difficult to predict.
    b. interrupted by only brief periods of symptom remission.
    c. more extreme and pronounced than other types of schizophrenia.
    d. triggered by stress.
    Answer: d   LO: 5; factual   page: 226

48. Our text described a young woman who responded to news that her mother was hospitalized for a serious illness by stating, "Mama's sick. (giggle) Sicky, sicky, sicky. (giggle) I flipped off a doctor once, did you know that. Flip. I wanta wear my blue dress tomorrow. Dress mess. (giggle)" This describes which type of schizophrenia?
    a. paranoid
    b. catatonic
    c. disorganized
    d. undifferentiated
    Answer: c   LO: 5; applied   page: 226

49. Disorganized schizophrenia tends to have:
    a. an early onset and be resistant to treatment.
    b. an early onset and be responsive to treatment.
    c. a late onset and be resistant to treatment.
    d. a late onset and be responsive to treatment.
    Answer: a   LO: 5; factual   page: 226

50. Which of the following is *false* about catatonic schizophrenia?
    a. It has some of the most distinct features of all types of schizophrenia.
    b. Catatonic schizophrenics' behaviors suggest extreme unresponsiveness to their environment.
    c. It is one of the most commonly seen forms of schizophrenia.
    d. This type of schizophrenia has not been well researched.
    Answer: c   LO: 5; factual   pages: 226-227

51. Which of the following is *not* a typical symptom of catatonic schizophrenia?
    a. remaining motionless for long periods of time (catatonic stupor)
    b. excessive, purposeless, excited motor activity (catatonic excitement)
    c. repeating the words spoken by another person (echolalia)
    d. rapidly speaking words that make little sense in context (word salad)
    Answer: d   LO: 5; conceptual   pages: 226-227

Chapter 6

52. In undifferentiated schizophrenia:
    a. the symptoms are similar to disorganized schizophrenia but less extreme.
    b. there is an early onset of the disorder; it is chronic and resistant to treatment.
    c. the symptoms are less extreme than those for paranoid schizophrenia.
    d. there is a late onset, the symptoms are chronic, and it responds well to therapy.
    Answer: b   LO: 5; factual, conceptual   page: 227

53. Which of the following people would receive a diagnosis of residual schizophrenia?
    a. James, who has suffered from several episodes of avolition and formal thought disorder, but who now experiences only auditory hallucinations.
    b. Kathy, who has suffered two acute episodes of schizophrenia involving delusions and hallucinations, but who now experiences only mild hallucinates and affective flattening.
    c. Harold, who has suffered from alogia and affective flattening for years, but who now experiences only formal thought disorder.
    d. Jake, who has suffered from at least one episode of acute positive symptoms of schizophrenia, but who now experiences only visual hallucinations and loosening of associations.
    Answer: b   LO: 5; applied   page: 227

54. The highly variable prevalence estimates of schizophrenia across cultures are mostly due to:
    a. language barriers between the assessors and the individuals in the population of interest.
    b. the fact that negative symptoms are more difficult to detect than positive ones.
    c. cultural norms that set relative standards for what counts as schizophrenic behavior.
    d. Prevalence estimates are not variable, they are extremely consistent across cultures.
    Answer: d   LO: 6; factual, conceptual   page: 227

55. Which group is most likely to be misdiagnosed with schizophrenia when they are actually suffering from mood disorders?
    a. European Americans
    b. Native Americans
    c. African Americans
    d. Asian Americans
    Answer: c   LO: 6; factual   page: 227

The Schizophrenias

56. A study by Escobar (1993) found that, despite statistically significant differences in prevalence of schizophrenia across ethnic groups, these differences largely disappeared when _____ was controlled for.
    a. education
    b. socioeconomic status
    c. marital status
    d. parental education
    Answer: b   LO: 6; factual   page: 227

57. Which of the following is *not* a difference between males and females with schizophrenia?
    a. Men are more likely to display negative symptoms of schizophrenia than women.
    b. Women are more likely to have a later age of onset when they develop schizophrenia.
    c. The mesolimbic system in men tends to contain more dopamine than it does in women.
    d. Men are more likely to develop alcohol and substance abuse problems when they have schizophrenia.
    Answer: c   LO: 6; factual   pages: 227-228

58. Women who develop schizophrenia are more likely than men to have:
    a. failed or dropped out of school.
    b. had inadequate social skills early in life.
    c. been single.
    d. married and had children.
    Answer: d   LO: 6; factual   pages: 227-228

59. Studies in the chapter suggest a person's risk for schizophrenia is increased by the person's:
    a. degree of genetic relatedness to someone with schizophrenia and the severity of the schizophrenic relative's disorder.
    b. degree of genetic relatedness to someone with schizophrenia and being exposed to illogical thought, mood swings, and deficits as a result of being raised by schizophrenic parents.
    c. having been reared by schizophrenic parents and the severity of the parents' disorder.
    d. having been raised by schizophrenic parents and general level of life stress.
    Answer: a   LO: 6; factual   page: 229

60. Which of the following is *not* one of the biological theories of schizophrenia discussed in the text?
    a. genetic transmission
    b. structural and functional abnormalities in the brain
    c. insufficient levels of the neurotransmitter serotonin
    d. excess levels of the neurotransmitter dopamine
    Answer: d   LO: 6; factual   pages: 228-234

Chapter 6

61. Which of the following children is at highest risk for developing schizophrenia? One with:
    a. two biological parents and a monozygotic (MZ) twin who are schizophrenic.
    b. two adoptive parents and a monozygotic (MZ) twin who are schizophrenic.
    c. biological parents and a dizygotic (DZ) twin who are schizophrenic.
    d. one biological parent and a dizygotic (DZ) twin who are schizophrenic.
    Answer: a   LO: 6; factual   page: 230

62. Manuel goes to the student health services to check out his mental health status, he advises the therapist there that his cousin Sal was hospitalized for schizophrenia a few years ago, when they were in high school, and Sal has been on medication ever since. Manuel is worried that he, too, may be at risk for developing schizophrenia. What are his chances?
    a. about 1%
    b. about 2%
    c. about 13%
    d. about 50%
    Answer: b   LO: 6; factual, applied   page: 230

63. The concordance rate for schizophrenia in twins:
    a. ranges from 50 to 91 % for monozygotic (MZ) twins, regardless of whether the schizophrenia is mild or severe.
    b. differs significant for monozygotic (MZ) twins, depending on whether the schizophrenia is mild or severe.
    c. is close to 100% for monozygotic (MZ) twins, thus demonstrating the powerful genetic component in this disorder.
    d. is stronger for monozygotic (MZ) twins than for dizygotic (DZ) twins, thus demonstrating the powerful environmental components interacting with genetics.
    Answer: b   LO: 6; factual   page: 230

64. Which of the following is *false* about the structural and functional brain abnormalities associated with some cases of schizophrenia?
    a. Ventricular enlargement resulting from brain atrophy could lead to different manifestations of schizophrenia, depending on which brain areas have shrunken.
    b. Women are more likely than men to show ventricular enlargement, though men tend to have more negative symptoms of schizophrenia.
    c. In some cases, an abnormal brain connection is found that is not present in people without schizophrenia.
    d. The structural deficits could be caused by viral infections.
    Answer: b   LO: 7; factual   pages: 231-232

The Schizophrenias

65. Which statement best describes the involvement of the prefrontal cortex in schizophrenia?
    a. Evidence of a smaller prefrontal cortex is a consistent diagnostic criterion of schizophrenia.
    b. A smaller prefrontal cortex is common in people exhibiting the positive symptoms of schizophrenia.
    c. People with an enlarged prefrontal cortex are most likely to exhibit deficits in language, emotional expression, planning, and social interactions.
    d. It is more common for people with predominantly negative symptoms of schizophrenia to have a less active prefrontal cortex.
    Answer: d   LO: 7; factual   page: 231

66. Which statement is *true* about the relationship between ventricular enlargement and schizophrenia?
    a. Schizophrenics with ventricular enlargement tend to have a poor premorbid history.
    b. Schizophrenics with ventricular enlargement have fewer symptoms, and those symptoms are milder, than schizophrenics with smaller ventricles.
    c. Schizophrenics with ventricular enlargement are more responsive to medication, suggesting a positive interaction between the deformity and certain drugs.
    d. Ventricular enlargement is greater among female schizophrenics than among male schizophrenics.
    Answer: a   LO: 7; factual   pages: 231-232

67. Evidence against a genetic cause for low prefrontal activity and ventricular enlargement is found in:
    a. studies of monozygotic twins who are discordant for schizophrenia.
    b. studies of dizygotic twins who are concordant for schizophrenia.
    c. studies of monozygotic twins who are concordant for schizophrenia.
    d. adoption studies.
    Answer: a   LO: 7; factual, conceptual   pages: 231-232

68. Which of the following *was not* evidence supporting the original dopamine theory of schizophrenia?
    a. Drugs that reduce the functional level of dopamine in the brain tend to reduce to symptoms of schizophrenia.
    b. Drugs that increase the functional level of dopamine in the brain, such as amphetamines, tend to decrease the psychotic symptoms of schizophrenia.
    c. Autopsy and PET scan studies showed more neuronal receptors for dopamine and sometimes higher levels of dopamine in some areas of the brains of schizophrenics.
    d. Levels of HVA (homovanillic acid, a byproduct of dopamine) tend to be higher in the blood and cerebrospinal fluid of people with more severe symptoms of schizophrenia than in schizophrenics with milder symptoms.
    Answer: b   LO: 8; factual   page: 233

Chapter 6

69. Recent research on the dopamine theory suggests:
    a. the original theory was too simplistic in terms of understanding schizophrenia.
    b. the original theory was too complex in terms of understanding schizophrenia.
    c. the original theory is incorrect; new research indicates that dopamine is not involved in schizophrenia.
    d. the original theory is accurate in its implication and description of how dopamine is involved in schizophrenia.
    Answer: a   LO: 8; factual, conceptual   pages: 233-234

70. A drug recently found to be one of the most effective drugs for schizophrenia is:
    a. L-DOPA.
    b. Thorazine (chlorpromazine).
    c. Xanax (alprazolam).
    d. Clozaril (clozapine).
    Answer: d   LO: 8; factual   page: 233-234

71. The revised dopamine theory of schizophrenia suggests that:
    a. high dopamine activity in the mesolimbic system accounts for the positive symptoms.
    b. high dopamine activity in the temporal region accounts for positive the symptoms.
    c. low dopamine activity in the prefrontal area accounts for positive the symptoms.
    d. low dopamine activity in the hypothalamus accounts for the negative symptoms.
    Answer: a   LO: 8; factual   page: 233-234

72. Negative psychosocial factors, such as stress and certain types of family functioning:
    a. can trigger episodes of schizophrenia even in persons without an existing predisposition to the disorder.
    b. can cause schizophrenia only if chronic life stress and poor family functioning are both present together.
    c. will not affect the severity of a schizophrenic person's symptoms if the schizophrenic is on proper doses of medication.
    d. cause a relapse in those who already have the disorder.
    Answer: d   LO: 9; conceptual   page: 234

73. The term *nervous breakdown*, as discussed in the text, refers to:
    a. a psychotic break, which is the development of schizophrenia.
    b. a complete break from normal social interactions and ability to function.
    c. development of severe depression or an anxiety disorder.
    d. Any or all of the above could be true.
    Answer: c   LO: 9; conceptual   page: 235

The Schizophrenias

74. According to the text, the social selection explanation of schizophrenia suggests:
    a. the burdens of living in an impoverished inner-city neighborhood and having low status occupations are so extraordinarily stressful that these factors can selectively lead to schizophrenia.
    b. the symptoms of schizophrenia interfere with a person's ability to finish school and hold a job; thus, they tend to "drift" below the social class of their family of origin.
    c. the stress of everyday living is so overwhelming for persons who are genetically vulnerable that, in order to escape social expectations, these persons develop schizophrenia.
    d. that some persons who live in high-risk situations, such as impoverished inner-city neighborhoods with high unemployment and low education, are highly resistant to these stressors and are able to select themselves out and remain emotionally healthy.
    Answer: b   LO: 9; conceptual   page: 235

75. As described by Fromm-Reichman (1948) and Arieti (1955), the schizophrenogenic mother is one who was:
    a. overprotective and allows no boundaries between herself and her children.
    b. overcontrolling and does not allow her children to make decisions for themselves.
    c. dominant and cold, and rejected her children.
    d. authoritarian and demanded total obedience from her children.
    Answer: c   LO: 9; factual, conceptual   page: 236

76. When Mrs. Hardin came to visit her son, Daniel, he greeted her with a handshake. She asked, "What's the matter, don't you love me? Give me a hug." When he complied and gave her a hug, his mother became rigid and pushed him away. These mixed messages were a part of Daniel's daily life as a child. The pattern of behavior exhibited by Mrs. Hardin is called:
    a. schizophrenogenic.
    b. a double bind.
    c. a double blind.
    d. crazy-making.
    Answer: b   LO: 9; applied   page: 236

77. Research on deviant patterns of communication demonstrates that:
    a. they are typical of how people in families communicate with each other.
    b. they have no long-term effects on children from nonschizophrenic families.
    c. they have no long-term effects on children at risk for developing schizophrenia.
    d. high levels of communication can have detrimental effects on children at risk for developing schizophrenia.
    Answer: b   LO: 9; conceptual   pages: 236-237

Chapter 6

78. Which statement best describes "expressed emotion," as characterized by researchers?
    a. Families that routinely express their emotions create an environment that facilitates relapse by creating stress for the schizophrenic family member, who cannot deal with the constant emotion that appears to the exclusion of rational, reasonable interactions.
    b. Families that express, rather than inhibit or suppress, their emotions actively model maladaptive behavior patterns that the schizophrenic picks up through observation; he or she then feels no restrictions upon expressing delusional beliefs and describing hallucinations.
    c. Families in which the members are overinvolved with each other, who express self-sacrificing attitudes toward the schizophrenic member but also appear cold, resentful, and rejecting create an atmosphere that puts the schizophrenic family member at a greater risk for relapse.
    d. Families that are high in expressed emotion tend to show abnormally high levels of affection and concern for one another, yet they show the schizophrenic family member practically no warmth or concern at all.
    Answer: c   LO: 9; conceptual   pages: 236-237

79. Cross-cultural studies addressing the role of families and family communication patterns in schizophrenia have found that families of schizophrenics:
    a. in the United States, Europe, Mexico, and India tend to score higher on measures of expressed emotion than families of nonschizophrenics.
    b. in the United States and Europe tend to score lower on measures of expressed emotion than those in Mexico and India.
    c. in the United Stats, Europe, Mexico, and India tend to score lower on measures of expressed emotion than families of nonschizophrenics.
    d. in the United States and Europe tend to score higher on measures of expressed emotion than those in Mexico and India.
    Answer: d   LO: 9; factual   page: 237

80. The best evidence implicating family expressed emotion on relapse in schizophrenic patients is:
    a. the difficulty therapists have in bringing about changes in entrenched communication patterns.
    b. the foreseeable outcome that persons who lack motivation and demonstrate blunted affect will elicit more negative expressed emotion from family members.
    c. that the observed family patterns actually result from instead of cause the symptoms exhibited by the schizophrenic.
    d. that interventions that reduce family expressed emotion tend to reduce relapse rate in schizophrenic family members.
    Answer: d   LO: 9; factual   pages: 236-237

The Schizophrenias

81. A treatment for schizophrenia used early in this century, that caused the patient to go into a coma was:
    a. insulin therapy.
    b. shock therapy.
    c. prefrontal lobotomy.
    d. psychosurgery.
    Answer: a   LO: 10; factual   page: 238

82. Electroconvulsive therapy has been found to have:
    a. little effect on the symptoms of schizophrenia.
    b. dramatic effects on the symptoms of schizophrenia.
    c. similar long-term results as phenothiazines on treating schizophrenia.
    d. detrimental side effects for schizophrenics.
    Answer: a   LO: 10; factual   page: 238

83. The most common treatment for schizophrenia during the first half of this century was:
    a. drug therapy.
    b. custodial care.
    c. insulin therapy.
    d. shock therapy.
    Answer: b   LO: 10; factual   page: 238

84. The use of phenothiazines for treating schizophrenia emerged from:
    a. extending the research on insulin therapy.
    b. the newly discovered tranquilizer, thalidomide.
    c. the discovery of antihistamines.
    d. long years of research in trying to find an effective drug for schizophrenia.
    Answer: c   LO: 10; factual   page: 238

85. Which of the following is *true* of the drug Thorazine (chlorpromazine)?
    a. It affects more neurotransmitters than dopamine alone, which is one reason it is thought to help reduce negative as well as positive symptoms of schizophrenia.
    b. It binds to different dopamine receptors than other neuroleptic drugs and, consequently, has fewer side effects than most drug treatments for schizophrenia.
    c. It helps schizophrenic people control the positive symptoms of their disorder by blocking the D_1 and D_2 receptors for dopamine.
    d. It should only be taken when a relapse is expected or when symptoms are particularly bothersome; otherwise, neurological side effects can occur.
    Answer: c   LO: 10; factual   page: 238

Chapter 6

86. A movement disorder marked by persistent, involuntary movements of the face and mouth is called _____ and occurs as a result of _____.
    a. akinesia; neuroleptic drug treatment for schizophrenia
    b. akathesis; phenothiazine drug treatment for schizophrenia
    c. tardive dyskinesia; clozapine drug treatment for schizophrenia
    d. tardive dyskinesia; phenothiazine drug treatment for schizophrenia
    Answer: d   LO: 10; factual   page: 239

87. A common side effect of neuroleptic drugs involves slowed motor activities, a monotonous voice, and an expressionless face. This side effect is called:
    a. akathesis.
    b. akinesia.
    c. tardive dyskinesia.
    d. agranulocytosis.
    Answer: b   LO: 10; factual   page: 239

88. Which of the following is a potential side effect of Clozaril (clozapine)?
    a. agranulocytosis protect immune function
    b. tardive dyskinesia
    c. akinesia
    d. Tests so far been found to have no serious side effects for Clozaril (clozapine).
    Answer: a   LO: 10; factual   page: 239

89. Which of the following is *true* concerning cross-cultural studies of the research on neuroleptics?
    a. They are relatively consistent across cultures.
    b. They have been found to be useful in the United States and European countries but not in other countries.
    c. Dosage may need to be modified for patients of Asian descent.
    d. Dosage may need to be increased for patients of Hispanic descent.
    Answer: c   LO: 10; factual   page: 239

90. As a social worker, you are assisting a schizophrenic person in learning how to initiate and maintain conversations with others, gather needed information from doctors, and remain persistent. To accomplish this, you are taking the person with you to the doctor's office and around town to demonstrate directly how to accomplish these tasks. The type of intervention you are performing is:
    a. cognitive intervention.
    b. social intervention.
    c. humanistic intervention.
    d. behavioral intervention.
    Answer: d   LO: 11; applied   pages: 240-241

The Schizophrenias

91. Research that evaluates the effectiveness of psychosocial interventions has shown that psychosocial interventions are:
    a. very costly and are not practical for a managed-care health system.
    b. effective but only when they involve the schizophrenic's entire family.
    c. effective, but schizophrenic people tend to lose the gains that they make during the intervention over time, which means they must be ongoing.
    d. best delivered in a cognitive-behavioral format, with time-limited numbers of sessions.
    Answer: c   LO: 11; factual   pages: 240-241

92. Group therapy for schizophrenics has:
    a. not been particularly useful, since one of the major symptoms of schizophrenia is social withdrawal; thus, the patient is not able to interact with others.
    b. been useful by providing a forum where the patient can express frustrations of making others understand the disorder and their fears of relapse.
    c. not been useful in terms of providing feedback on problem areas, since schizophrenics have such a distorted view of reality.
    d. been useful for allowing schizophrenics to vent their angry feelings toward their schizophrenogenic mothers as the root of their problems.
    Answer: b   LO: 11; conceptual   page: 241

93. Which of the following is *not* a skill that schizophrenics need to develop?
    a. understanding how their medications work, why maintenance drug therapy is used, and the benefits of medication
    b. identifying personal warning signs of symptom relapse and monitoring them with assistance of others
    c. identifying people upon whom the schizophrenic can become dependent to carry out tasks of daily living
    d. learning effective verbal and nonverbal listening techniques to promote effective conversational skills
    Answer: c   LO: 11; conceptual   page: 242

94. In a study by Hogarty et al. (1986, 1991), which of the following forms of intervention had the most effective and longest-lasting results?
    a. medication only
    b. medication plus social skills training for the schizophrenic
    c. medication plus family-oriented therapy
    d. social skills training for the schizophrenic plus family-oriented therapy.
    Answer: c   LO: 11; factual   page: 243

Chapter 6

95. You are a religious healer in a developing country. If you are treating a schizophrenic person according to your traditional method, which involves a series of rituals designed to transform the meanings of the symptoms for the schizophrenic person, your treatment method would fall under the _____ according to Karno and Jenkins (1993).
    a. social support model
    b. mystical model
    c. persuasive model
    d. structural model
    Answer: c   LO: 11; applied   page: 244

96. The model that states there are interrelated levels, such as the body, emotion, and cognition, or the person, society, and culture, and symptoms arise when that integration is lost would be the _____ model.
    a. social support
    b. structural
    c. clinical
    d. persuasive
    Answer: b   LO: 11; conceptual   pages: 244-245

97. The model of treating schizophrenia that is described by anthropologists and cultural psychologists suggesting that rituals can transform the meaning of symptoms for the patient is the _____ model.
    a. social support
    b. mystical
    c. clinical
    d. persuasive
    Answer: d   LO: 11; conceptual   pages: 244-245

98. The model of treating schizophrenia that is described by anthropologists and cultural psychologists suggesting that it is the faith that the patient puts in the traditional healer to provide a cure for his or her symptoms that relieves the symptoms is the _____ model.
    a. social support
    b. structural
    c. clinical
    d. persuasive
    Answer: c   LO: 11; conceptual   pages: 244-245

The Schizophrenias

99. Which of the following is *false* of the prognosis for people with schizophrenia?
    a. Schizophrenic people commit suicide at a rate of about 10%.
    b. Between 50 and 80 percent of schizophrenic people who are hospitalized once for an episode will be rehospitalized at a later point in their lives for another episode.
    c. Schizophrenic people have a lower life expectancy than people without it by about 10 years.
    d. Schizophrenia tends to become worse with age, which means that more older schizophrenics end up in nursing homes or group homes.
    Answer: d   LO: 12; factual   page: 245

100. From which of the following types of schizophrenic people would you expect the best prognosis?
    a. A woman who reports that she first noticed her symptoms at age 20, who has catatonic schizophrenia, and who is a resident of western Europe.
    b. A man who reports that he first noticed his symptoms at age 45, who has paranoid schizophrenia, and who is a U.S. citizen.
    c. A woman who reports that she first noticed her symptoms at age 40, who has paranoid schizophrenia, and who is a citizen of India.
    d. A man who reports that he first noticed his symptoms at age 25, who has undifferentiated schizophrenia, and who is a citizen of South Korea.
    Answer: c   LO: 12; applied   pages: 245-247

101. Prognosis of schizophrenia is better with:
    a. broader, closer family networks and lower measures of expressed emotion.
    b. broader, closer family networks and higher measures of expressed emotion.
    c. smaller family networks and lower measures of expressed emotion.
    d. smaller family networks and higher measures of expressed emotion.
    Answer: a   LO: 12; conceptual   page: 246

102. Which of the following may explain gender differences with respect to schizophrenia?
    a. Women have a better prognosis than men because they tend to develop the disorder later.
    b. Women have a worse prognosis than men because their estrogen levels would promote an excess of dopamine.
    c. Men have a better prognosis than women because their greater dependence on the left hemisphere keeps them more grounded in logic and reality.
    d. There are no consistent research findings that suggest either men or women have a better prognosis when it comes to schizophrenia.
    Answer: a   LO: 12; factual   pages: 246-247

Chapter 6

Essay Questions

103. You have gotten into a discussion of abnormal psychology with a friend of yours, and the friend says, "I know all about those 'schizos.' They are the people with split personalities." Describe how you would explain the history and derivation of the term *schizophrenia* to your friend, and discuss why it is not synonymous with the notion of "split personalities." Be sure to provide specific characteristics of schizophrenia to support your answer.

    The student should discuss how the term involves not a splintering off of different personalities, but a splitting of the person from reality and among the schizophrenic's psychological capacities (e.g., thought, emotion, attention, behavior). Kraepelin's initial role in categorizing schizophrenic behaviors is in order, as well as examples of positive and negative cognitive, social, affective, and behavioral symptoms.

104. You have recently been told by one of your friends that one of your favorite high school teachers has been diagnosed as schizophrenic. You ask your friend what type of schizophrenia, but your friend doesn't know. In order to determine which type it is, you need to explain each of them to this friend. State how you would name, describe, and differentiate the five different types of schizophrenia so you could figure out which type your former teacher has.

    The student should be able to list paranoid, catatonic, disorganized, undifferentiated, and residual, and give the general classes of symptoms, and then differentiate among them by noting: the characteristic symptoms and diagnostic criteria in terms of degree of both positive and negative symptoms; the specific age of onset and prognosis that is typical with each; and the degree to which and how each responds to medication.

105. You have been asked to give a speech in your speech class on schizophrenia. Since you know that most of the other students in the class are biology majors, you decide to "improve their education" by describing the biological theories of schizophrenia. State how you would explain these theories, and provide evidence that supports and limits each of these theories.

    The student should be able to discuss genetics (twin studies, family studies, and adoption studies); structural abnormalities (frontal cortex and ventricles); and excessive dopamine (simple and complex mediating factors, and responsiveness to drugs). Evidence and limitations of each should be presented.

106. Lucy is a 25-year-old Hispanic woman who comes to you for help. She is hearing voices that tell her she is evil and does not deserve to live. She sees the spirit of a dead aunt whom she always feared as a child, and she believes that this aunt has cursed her. What diagnosis would you give her, what do you feel her prognosis is for recovery, and how would you suggest she be treated?

The Schizophrenias

The student needs to consider the schizophrenic symptoms in the context of Lucy's belief system. An assessment would have to be made of her cultural ties. If a belief in spirits and spirit possession is common among her family and community, it would be appropriate for the student to discuss bringing in a *currandero* to perform a healing ritual--the student should describe the type of ritual that might be expected. If, however, Lucy's family and friends do not subscribe to a belief in spirits, then the student would have to look at the positive symptoms of hallucinations and delusions and go from there. In terms of prognosis, her age, gender, and cultural background would be relevant issues to discuss.

107. While medications have been a modern "miracle" in terms of reducing many symptoms of schizophrenia, they are not a cure. Discuss the various medications that are currently used, which forms of schizophrenia they are used to treat, the symptoms they do modify, the symptoms they do not change, and the side effects of each of the medications that might be used. Then discuss the type of treatment that has been found to be the most effective not only in terms of symptom reduction, but also with regard to long-term effectiveness.

Explain the mechanism of neuroleptic drugs in reducing positive symptoms, such as delusions and hallucinations, by blocking dopamine receptors and reducing its quantity, but they do not eliminate negative symptoms, such as lack of social skills; the student must address the negative side effects of akinesia, akathesis, and tardive dyskinesia (the student should explain the characteristics of each). Then explain how clozapine blocks a different dopamine receptor (D_4), reduces both positive and negative symptoms, and has fewer side effects, although the side effect it has (potentially destroying the immune system) can be lethal. The most effective long-term treatment has been a combination of drug therapy and family therapy (social skills training has been useful, but is more useful in conjunction with family therapy). To maintain long-term effectiveness, treatment should be ongoing.

108. As the only psychology major in your Diversity class, you have been asked to relate issues of diversity to the class. Explain how you would discuss the role of age, gender, and culture in onset and prognosis of schizophrenia.

The earlier the onset, the more insidious and severe the disorder; although it is a chronic and debilitating disorder, predicting lower life expectancy and a 10% suicide rate, its impact is reduced with age. Men are more likely than women to experience negative symptoms, and women have a later age of onset than men and better levels of functioning prior to and between acute episodes. The later the age of onset, the better the prognosis. Third World countries have extended family networks to care for the schizophrenic, which greatly improves prognosis.

Chapter 7   Dissociative and Somatoform Disorders

1. An extreme mechanism the mind uses to escape traumatic, painful situations or emotions is:
   a. withdrawal.
   b. escapism.
   c. dissociation.
   d. splitting.
   Answer: c   LO: 1; conceptual   page: 254

2. Which of the following statements is *true* concerning dissociation?
   a. Dissociative experiences are extremely common.
   b. A student who, during exam week, feels his soul floating above his body should be sufficiently concerned about this experience to pursue therapy.
   c. There has been consistent scientific interest in dissociation over the past few centuries.
   d. Freud was the first modern mental health practitioner to address issues of dissociation.
   Answer: a   LO: 1; factual, conceptual   page: 254

3. Freud became fascinated with _____ that arose out of dissociative processes.
   a. hysterical symptoms
   b. glove anesthesia
   c. functional paralysis
   d. neurological inconsistencies
   Answer: a   LO: 1; factual, conceptual   page: 254

4. Freud's studies of patients with severe dissociative experiences contributed to his theory of the mind and the role of _____ in psychopathology.
   a. early childhood experiences
   b. repression
   c. ego strength
   d. neurological factors
   Answer: b   LO: 1; factual, conceptual   page: 254

5. French neurologist, Pierre Janet, viewed dissociation as:
   a. a simple form of dealing with stress, such as daydreaming or being creative.
   b. a process whereby systems of ideas are split off from consciousness, and there is no way to access them, although they have a major impact on our behavior.
   c. a process whereby systems of ideas are split off from consciousness but are available to consciousness through dreams and hypnosis.
   d. a way to rid oneself of unacceptable urges, thoughts, or behaviors that one wishes not to acknowledge.
   Answer: c   LO: 1; factual, conceptual   page: 254

Dissociative and Somatoform Disorders

6. Hilda states she cannot feel anything in her left hand. She has been to many doctors, including three neurologists, and none of them can find any physiological basis for this problem. Most likely Hilda is suffering from:
   a. a psychosomatic illness.
   b. glove anesthesia.
   c. hysterical neurosis.
   d. physiological paralysis.
   Answer: b   LO: 1; applied   page: 254

7. In Hilgard's (1977, 1986) experiments with the "hidden observer," the _____ mode consists of the plans, desires, and voluntary actions of which we are aware, and the _____ mode, in which we can register and store information about which we are unaware.
   a. conscious; unconscious
   b. aware; unaware
   c. open; closed
   d. active; receptive
   Answer: d   LO: 1; factual, conceptual   page: 255

8. Studies on the "hidden observer" have found that:
   a. subjects could be cued to remember pain they had been instructed not to feel while they were under hypnosis, but surgical patients could not recall any events that occurred while they were under anesthetic.
   b. subjects could be cued to remember pain they had been instructed not to feel while they were under hypnosis, and surgical patients could recall events that occurred while they were under anesthetic.
   c. the memories of both subjects under hypnosis and surgical patients under anesthesia were vague and relatively dissociated from the actual events that occurred.
   d. people have a basic tendency to avoid integrating voluntary and involuntary components of consciousness when they are in pain.
   Answer: b   LO: 1; factual, conceptual   page: 255

9. A fundamental lesson we may learn from Hilgard's (1977, 1986) research on the "hidden observer" is:
   a. there is much we do not know about the unconscious mind and how it works.
   b. the active, voluntary component of consciousness is more powerful than the receptive, recording mode.
   c. we are highly suggestible under altered states, such as hypnosis and anesthesia, and must be vigilant to protect ourselves at such times.
   d. people who develop dissociative disorders may have chronic disruptions in integrating the active and receptive modes of consciousness.
   Answer: d   LO: 1; conceptual   page: 255

Chapter 7

10. Which of the following is common to all of the dissociative disorders?
    a. separate personalities in the same individual that may or may not be aware of each other
    b. a sense of feeling detached from one's mental state or body
    c. frequent experiences in which different aspects of a person's self are split off from each other
    d. moving away and assuming a new identity with no memory for the previous identity
    Answer: c   LO: 2; conceptual   page: 255

11. The disorder in which a person develops more than one distinct personality is:
    a. dissociative identity disorder.
    b. dissociative fugue.
    c. dissociative amnesia.
    d. depersonalization disorder.
    Answer: a   LO: 2; factual   page: 256

12. The most common type of "alter" found in dissociative identity disorder is the:
    a. child.
    b. persecutor.
    c. helper.
    d. host.
    Answer: a   LO: 2; factual   page: 257

13. Which statement is *false* about the "persecutor personality"?
    a. It may engage in dangerous behavior, such as overdosing on medication, then leave the host personality to suffer the consequences.
    b. It believes that it can harm the host (or other alters) without harming itself.
    c. Its primary goal is to get back at the host's abusive parent by inflicting potentially fatal harm.
    d. It inflicts pain or punishment on the other personalities by engaging in self-mutilative behaviors, such as self-burning.
    Answer: c   LO: 2; factual, conceptual   page: 257

14. The "helper personality" in dissociative identity disorder has the function of:
    a. protecting the host, but harming the other personalities by engaging in self-mutilating and other dangerous behavior.
    b. serving as the victim of the trauma.
    c. acting as a "big brother" or "big sister" to protect the host personality from trauma.
    d. offering advice to other personalities or performing functions that the host personality is unable to perform.
    Answer: d   LO: 2; factual, conceptual   page: 258

Dissociative and Somatoform Disorders

15. Which of the following is typical of persons with dissociative identity disorder (DID)?
    a. They have complete amnesia for specific times and people in their lives.
    b. None of the personalities knows what any of the others are doing.
    c. The host is aware of other personalities, but many alters are unaware of each other.
    d. They have rigidly controlled, stable emotions.
    Answer: a   LO: 2; conceptual   page: 258

16. Which statement is *true* about why diagnoses of dissociative identity disorder (DID) and schizophrenia are confounded?
    a. People with both disorders exhibit flat affect and illogical associations, which makes a differential diagnosis difficult.
    b. People with schizophrenia experience such intense delusions of being someone else that they begin to act so differently (exhibiting a different voice or physical appearance) that they are misdiagnosed with DID.
    c. People with both disorders often hear voices, which makes a differential diagnosis difficult.
    d. People with both disorders experience visual hallucinations, which makes a differential diagnosis difficult.
    Answer: c   LO: 3; conceptual   page: 258

17. Which of the following is *true* about the comorbidity of dissociative identity disorder (DID) with other disorders?
    a. DID is usually the first diagnosis a person receives, and other diagnoses, if any, are subordinate to that primary diagnosis.
    b. There is usually not a problem of differential diagnosis between schizophrenia and DID because the voices are perceived to come from "outside" for the schizophrenic and from "inside" with DID.
    c. There is rarely an issue of comorbidity since DID is so all-encompassing that symptoms of any other disorders would be absorbed within that diagnosis.
    d. The majority of persons diagnosed with DID also are diagnosed with serious depression or anxiety as well as a personality disorder.
    Answer: d   LO: 3; factual   page: 258

18. Which statement is *true* about gender differences in dissociative identity disorder (DID)?
    a. Though an equal number of adult males and females are diagnosed with DID, there are more female children diagnosed than male children.
    b. Women with DID are more likely to be convicted of crimes, whereas men with DID are more likely to have substance abuse and alcohol addictions.
    c. Women with DID engage in more suicidal behavior than men with DID.
    d. Men are more likely to develop persecutor alter personalities, whereas women are more likely to develop child alters or helper personalities.
    Answer: c   LO: 3; factual   page: 259

Chapter 7

19. Which of the following is *true* about the diagnosis of dissociative identity disorder (DID)?
    a. DID has been a common diagnosis, affecting approximately 1% of the population since it was first included in the DSM in 1917.
    b. DID is diagnosed more frequently in Asian countries, such as India and Japan, than it is in Europe and the United States.
    c. The majority of persons diagnosed with DID are adult women.
    d. There has been a decrease in diagnosis of DID since publication of DSM-IV in 1980 due to the concern about personalities being "planted" by therapists.
    Answer: c   LO: 3; factual   page: 259

20. A plausible reason that Hispanics may not be diagnosed with dissociative identity disorder (DID) as often as other groups in the United States is that:
    a. mental illness is considered to be a stigma among Hispanics; thus, they tend to cover up or make excuses about bizarre behaviors.
    b. it is likely that what may otherwise be diagnosed as DID is misdiagnosed as *ataque de nervios*, a more socially acceptable stress reaction.
    c. Hispanics have such large and supportive extended families that the children do not generally experience the types of trauma that may lead to DID.
    d. genetically Hispanics are not predisposed to DID, and a person who is traumatized in early childhood will develop other disorders, such as substance abuse.
    Answer: b   LO: 3; factual, conceptual   pages: 259-260

21. A major criticism of categorizing dissociative identity disorder (DID) as a diagnosable disorder comes from the belief that:
    a. the disorder is artificially created by therapists in suggestible clients.
    b. there are insufficient data to allow for creating such a diagnostic category.
    c. because it is primarily an American female disorder and rarely applies to other individuals, it does not belong in the DSM.
    d. it gets overused by criminal defendants who try to get out on an insanity plea.
    Answer: a   LO: 4; factual, conceptual   page: 261

22. Which is *false* about Spanos et al.'s (1985) research on hypnotic suggestion?
    a. Most subjects in the experimental group, who were hypnotized to connect with a "hidden part" of themselves, displayed symptoms of DID.
    b. Most subjects in the experimental group, who were hypnotized to connect with a "hidden part" of themselves, assumed a different name for their "separate part."
    c. Subjects in the experimental group who connected with a "hidden part" of themselves, scored differently on standardized personality tests when role playing a murderer under hypnotic suggestion.
    d. Subjects in the experimental group who connected with a "hidden part" of themselves maintained their hypnotically induced "alter" for a long period of time.
    Answer: d   LO: 4; factual   page: 261

Dissociative and Somatoform Disorders

23. The most common underlying factor for developing dissociative identity disorder (DID) is:
    a. chronic physical and/or sexual abuse over an extended period during childhood.
    b. a child with low intelligence but high creativity.
    c. one abusive parent and one overprotective parent during childhood.
    d. a biological predisposition to the disorder.
    Answer: a   LO: 5; factual   page: 262

24. Which of the following is *not* typical of individuals who develop dissociative identity disorder (DID)?
    a. chronic sexual and/or physical abuse during childhood
    b. being highly suggestible
    c. ineffective defenses against trauma
    d. using the personalities as a way to cope with life
    Answer: c   LO: 5; factual, conceptual   page: 262

25. According to the text, the goal of treatment for dissociative identity disorder (DID) is to:
    a. have the various alters communicating with each other.
    b. integrate the alters into one coherent personality.
    c. eliminate the alters so the host personality can function effectively.
    d. help the client understand that each alter is a part of the whole person.
    Answer: b   LO: 5; factual, conceptual   page: 262

26. Which of the following is *not* typically a part of treating a person with dissociative identity disorder (DID)?
    a. identifying the functions or roles of each personality
    b. helping alters confront and work through the traumas leading to their creation
    c. negotiating with the alters to fuse into one personality
    d. eliminating each alter as its role becomes known and no longer needed
    Answer: d   LO: 5; factual, conceptual   page: 262

27. Thomas, a 39-year-old single man, has abruptly left behind his home and belongings to move across the country. When found at his new residence, he has difficulty remembering the events that preceded his arrival and cannot remember important facts about himself. The most likely diagnosis for Thomas is:
    a. dissociative fugue.
    b. depersonalization disorder.
    c. retrograde amnesia.
    d. anterograde amnesia.
    Answer: c   LO: 8; factual, conceptual   pages: 263-264

Chapter 7

28. According to the chapter, a factor that predisposes people to both dissociative identity disorder and dissociative fugue is having:
    a. a genetic history of either disorder.
    b. a highly suggestible personality.
    c. depression in childhood.
    d. a previous history of amnesia.
    Answer: b   LO: 6; factual   page: 264

29. The major differential diagnostic characteristic of dissociative fugue involves:
    a. loss of memory.
    b. cycling between identities.
    c. travel.
    d. dissociating.
    Answer: c   LO: 6; factual   page: 264

30. Which of the following is *false* about dissociative fugue?
    a. A person may experience repeated fugue states or only a single episode.
    b. Fugue states may last for as little as a few days or as long as several years.
    c. Persons experiencing dissociative fugue has total amnesia for their prior identity.
    d. Once a person recovers from the fugue state, he or she will be able to remember what happened during the dissociative state.
    Answer: d   LO: 6; factual, conceptual   page: 264

31. The precipitating factor in dissociative fugue is typically:
    a. chronic stress.
    b. post-traumatic stress disorder.
    c. early childhood abuse.
    d. anger that cannot be openly expressed.
    Answer: a   LO: 7; factual   page: 264

32. The major difference between dissociative fugue and dissociative amnesia is:
    a. that amnesia has an organic base, and fugue has a psychogenic base.
    b. in fugue, the person's entire identity is forgotten; in amnesia, there are merely large gaps in memory about themselves.
    c. in amnesia, the person travels great distances to get away from stress; in fugue, they often remain where they are.
    d. in fugue, old memories are forgotten; in amnesia, there is an inability to remember new information.
    Answer: b   LO: 8; factual, conceptual   pages: 264-265

Dissociative and Somatoform Disorders

33. Which of the following statements is *true*?
    a. Organic amnesia is typically anterograde; psychogenic amnesia is typically retrograde.
    b. Organic amnesia is typically retrograde; psychogenic amnesia is typically anterograde.
    c. People with long-term organic retrograde amnesia typically lose the ability to recall personal information and lose their sense of identity, but they retain general information.
    d. People with long-term psychogenic retrograde amnesia typically lose the ability to recall general and personal information, but retain a sense of personal identity.
    Answer: a LO: 8; conceptual page: 265

34. Which of the following is *true* about psychogenic amnesia?
    a. It is often caused by biological as well as psychological factors.
    b. It generally involves anterograde amnesia, thus causing an inability to learn new information since the onset of the amnesia.
    c. It can involve retrograde amnesia, meaning the amnesic person is unable to remember events from the past.
    d. The amnesic person usually has retrograde amnesia for both personal and general information.
    Answer: c LO: 8; factual page: 265

35. Which of the following is *true* about organic amnesia?
    a. It is often caused by psychological as well as biological factors.
    b. It rarely involves retrograde amnesia.
    c. It often involves anterograde amnesia.
    d. If an amnesic has retrograde amnesia, it will often be only for personal information, not for general information.
    Answer: c LO: 8; factual page: 265

36. Ed, who is 60 years old, has been asked by his employer to retire early. He has been making serious mistakes, either because he is drunk on the job or forgets important information (or both). He thinks he holds his liquor well, but others are seeing the toll it has taken, particularly in terms of his memory loss. It is likely that Ed has:
    a. dissociative fugue.
    b. organic anterograde amnesia.
    c. Munchausen's syndrome.
    d. Korsakoff's syndrome.
    Answer: d LO: 8; applied page: 266

Chapter 7

37. Korsakoff's syndrome is caused in part by _____ and is a form of _____ amnesia.
    a. head injury; organic anterograde
    b. severe alcohol abuse; psychogenic retrograde
    c. surgery; psychogenic anterograde
    d. severe alcohol abuse; organic retrograde
    Answer: d   LO: 8; factual   page: 266

38. Which of the following is *false* concerning psychogenic amnesias?
    a. They may result from the use of dissociation as a defense against intolerable memories or stressors.
    b. They may be for specific events that occurred when a person was in such a high state of arousal that he or she did not encode information during the event and thus cannot retrieve the information.
    c. Information about the event may be stored at the time of the event but is associated with such a high state of arousal of painful emotions that the person cannot access the emotion-laden information.
    d. Amnesias for specific periods of time around trauma as well as for one's entire past are relatively common.
    Answer: d   LO: 9; factual   pages: 265-266

39. Which statement is *false* about the connection between amnesia and criminal activity?
    a. True amnesias can occur in conjunction with the commission of a crime.
    b. Amnesia is most often seen in arson cases, with approximately 25% of persons arrested for arson claiming to have amnesia for the crime.
    c. A person may have amnesia for committing a crime due to a head injury incurred during the commission of the crime.
    d. Crimes committed while the person is under the influence of alcohol or other drugs can cause amnesia for the period of intoxication.
    Answer: b   LO: 9; factual   pages: 266-267

40. With respect to amnesia for a homicide, which of the following is most likely?
    a. The victim had first assaulted the killer causing the killer to dissociate into a state of rage.
    b. The killer was in a psychotic state at the time of the homicide.
    c. The victim was closely related to the killer, who was in a state of high emotional arousal at the time of the crime.
    d. It is relatively easy to determine whether the amnesia is true or fake by putting the killer under hypnosis.
    Answer: c   LO: 9; factual   page: 266

Dissociative and Somatoform Disorders

41. Janet, a junior in college majoring in physics, has been under a great deal of stress. Recently, she has had a strange sensation that she is outside of her body, watching herself. These experiences are becoming increasingly more frequent and are beginning to interfere with her work. It is likely that she has:
    a. dissociative identity disorder.
    b. depersonalization disorder.
    c. dissociative fugue.
    d. dissociative amnesia.
    Answer: b   LO: 10; applied   page: 267

42. In treating a client with a dissociative disorder, a therapist is probably most likely to:
    a. prescribe antianxiety medications and use relaxation techniques to reduce the client's stress.
    b. help the client explore past experiences and develop a more integrated sense of self.
    c. confront the client with his or her distorted beliefs and provide a supportive atmosphere for changing them.
    d. help the client identify his or her distorted beliefs and integrate them into a more complete sense of self.
    Answer: b   LO: 10; conceptual   page: 267

43. A prospective soldier reporting for a medical examination prior to his possible conscription for the Persian Gulf War who experiences tremendous pain in several areas of his body, but whose symptoms cannot be detected by medical tests, is likely suffering from _____. However, if he fakes his symptoms and does not truly experience them, then his condition would be called _____.
    a. psychosomatic disorder; somatoform disorder
    b. somatoform disorder; factitious disorder
    c. malingering; psychosomatic disorder
    d. somatoform disorder; malingering
    Answer: d   LO: 11; applied   pages: 267-268

44. The major difference between somatoform disorders and psychosomatic disorders is that:
    a. there is a detectable physical problem with somatoform disorders, but not with psychosomatic disorders.
    b. there is a detectable physical problem with psychosomatic disorders, but not with somatoform disorders.
    c. with somatoform disorders the person is really suffering, whereas in psychosomatic disorders the person is faking the ailment.
    d. There is no difference between the two--they are synonyms for each other.
    Answer: b   LO: 11; conceptual   page: 268

Chapter 7

45. Harvey went for his induction physical and complained of chronic stomach pains that he said he had had for years. He was precise about where the pains were, when they occurred (he stated they even occurred in his sleep), and the intensity never seemed to ease up. A review of his medical records revealed no previous stomach problems. We might assume Harvey:
    a. is malingering.
    b. has from a somatoform disorder.
    c. has a factitious disorder.
    d. has a psychosomatic illness.
    Answer: a   LO: 11; applied   page: 268

46. Cindy is a quiet, passive young lady who often goes unnoticed, even by people close to her. One day she doubles over in pain that cannot be controlled by heat, ice packs, or any medications. Concerned about her well being, her parents call 911. An ambulance arrives and she is taken to the hospital, where a handsome young doctor treats her. For the moment, at least, her symptoms abate. Cindy is suffering from:
    a. dissociative disorder.
    b. somatoform disorder.
    c. factitious disorder.
    d. psychosomatic disorder.
    Answer: c   LO: 11; applied   page: 268

47. The relationship between somatoform disorders and dissociative disorders is that:
    a. many theorists believe they result from repression of painful memories or emotions.
    b. they both involve a separating of parts of the personality.
    c. they are equally as difficult to treat.
    d. they produce similar types of symptoms by persons who have these disorders.
    Answer: a   LO: 11; conceptual   page: 268

48. Which of the following is *not* a distinct type of somatoform disorder?
    a. conversion disorder
    b. somatization and pain disorder
    c. hypochondriasis
    d. anorexia nervosa
    Answer: d   LO: 11; factual   page: 268

49. Of the four somatoform disorders, only _____ is not characterized by the experience of one or more physical symptoms.
    a. body dysmorphic disorder
    b. depersonalization disorder
    c. hypochondriasis
    d. conversion disorder
    Answer: a   LO: 11; factual   page: 268

Dissociative and Somatoform Disorders

50. One reason that people with conversion disorder can be difficult to treat is:
    a. *ataque de nervios.*
    b. *la belle indifference.*
    c. that while they often admit to having a psychological problem, they will not make the connection between psychological and physical factors.
    d. that their physical symptoms can be detected with medical tests, which makes it difficult to convince them that the root of the problem is psychological, not physical.
    Answer: b   LO: 11; factual, conceptual   page: 271

51. People with _____ actually perceive they have physical symptoms, whereas people with _____ only worry about experiencing symptoms or having a certain disorder.
    a. somatization disorder; hypochondriasis
    b. pain disorder; malingering
    c. hypochondriasis; factitious disorder
    d. conversion disorder; somatization disorder
    Answer: a   LO: 11; factual, conceptual   pages: 271-274

52. The disorder in which a person loses functioning in some part of their body is:
    a. malingering.
    b. hypochondriasis.
    c. conversion disorder.
    d. factitious disorder.
    Answer: c   LO: 11; factual   page: 269

53. Which of the following is *true* about conversion disorder?
    a. A person with conversion disorder is likely to have more than one symptom at a time.
    b. A person can have repeated episodes of conversion disorder involving different parts of the body.
    c. The symptoms occur gradually until the person suddenly loses the ability to control a specific party of the body.
    d. People with conversion disorder are deeply disturbed by their inability to use the affected body part.
    Answer: b   LO: 12; factual, conceptual   page: 269

54. An apparent lack of concern about losing functioning in some part of a person's body is referred to as:
    a. *ataque de nervios.*
    b. anhedonia.
    c. anesthetic indifference.
    d. *la belle indifference.*
    Answer: d   LO: 12; factual, conceptual   page: 269

Chapter 7

55. The previous term for conversion disorders were:
    a. conversion hysterias.
    b. hysterical anesthesia.
    c. phantom limb.
    d. conversion anesthesia.
    Answer: a   LO: 12; factual   page: 269

56. According to the ancient Greeks, conversion disorders were experienced only by:
    a. women and were caused by a dislodged, wandering uterus.
    b. women and were caused by unexpressed rage over their status.
    c. men and were caused by a dislodged, wandering prostate gland.
    d. men and resulted from fear of being forced to go to war.
    Answer: a   LO: 12; factual   page: 269

57. Current knowledge about conversion disorders states that they are:
    a. diagnosed more often in women than in men, since it is more likely that a uterus can become dislodged than a prostate gland.
    b. diagnosed more often in women than in men but are unrelated to internal organs.
    c. diagnosed as often in men as in women and result largely from stress.
    d. diagnosed more often in men than in women.
    Answer: b   LO: 12; factual   page: 269

58. In the famous case of Anna O. (Bertha Pappenheim), the patient was plagued with ongoing bouts of:
    a. hypochondriasis.
    b. dissociative disorder.
    c. conversion disorder.
    d. factitious disorder.
    Answer: c   LO: 12; factual   pages: 269-270

59. Which of the following is *true* about conversion disorders?
    a. Early psychoanalytic theorists believed the symptoms arose from a woman's unfulfilled desires for sexual gratification and children.
    b. They were extremely common among women during World War I and World War II, apparently because men were off at war.
    c. They were extremely rare among both men and women during World War I and World War II.
    d. They were more common in Victorian Europe than they are today in Europe or the United States.
    Answer: d   LO: 13; factual, conceptual   pages: 269-270

Dissociative and Somatoform Disorders

60. According to the text, people with _____ have higher rates of _____.
    a. dissociative disorder; schizophrenia
    b. conversion disorder and somatization disorder; depression, anxiety, antisocial personality disorder, and alcohol abuse
    c. hypochondriasis and pain disorder; dissociative identity disorder
    d. body dysmorphic disorder; obsessive-compulsive disorder
    Answer: b   LO: 13; factual   page: 270

61. Anderson, Yaenik, and Ross (1993) found that _____ may be common among sexual abuse survivors.
    a. conversion disorder
    b. hypochondriasis
    c. factitious disorder
    d. malingering
    Answer: a   LO: 13; factual   page: 270

62. Conversion disorder may serve the purpose of:
    a. getting attention.
    b. avoiding unpleasant memories or events.
    c. getting sympathy.
    d. creating arousal.
    Answer: b   LO: 13; conceptual   page: 270

63. _____ treatment believes that recovery from conversion disorder is prompted by the patient drawing the connection between the traumatizing event and the symptom.
    a. Psychoanalytic
    b. Cognitive
    c. Behavioral
    d. Cognitive-behavioral
    Answer: a   LO: 14; conceptual   page: 271

64. Behavioral treatments of conversion disorder focus on:
    a. exaggerating the trauma by flooding so the client sees she is now safe from harm.
    b. relieving the client's anxiety around the initial traumatizing event.
    c. encouraging the client to shout out her anger.
    d. showing the client how her symptoms are connected with the trauma they symbolize.
    Answer: b   LO: 14; conceptual   page: 271

Chapter 7

65. Samuel has been diagnosed by his psychiatrist as having conversion disorder. We might expect that it will be difficult to treat Samuel because people with conversion disorder typically:
   a. enjoy the attention they are getting.
   b. lack the insight necessary to see the connection between their disorder and their emotional pain.
   c. have trauma that is so deep that as soon as one symptom is relieved another arises.
   d. do not believe anything is wrong.
   Answer: d   LO: 14; applied   page: 271

66. Which of the following is *true* about individuals who suffer from somatization disorder?
   a. They have a long history of seeking medical attention for complaints about physical symptoms affecting different areas of their bodies, although no physical cause has been found for these complaints.
   b. They have a long history of seeking medical attention for complaints about physical symptoms affecting different areas of their bodies and have been found reinforced by finding physical causes for these complaints.
   c. Typically, they complain about only one problem at a time, but when that problem is resolved, they immediately move on to another.
   d. They are extremely specific yet understated about their physical complaints and often seek surgery to relieve them.
   Answer: a   LO: 15; conceptual   page: 271

67. _____ is a subset of somatization disorder, in which _____.
   a. Conversion disorder; one pain continues to be replaced by another
   b. Pain disorder; people complain only of chronic pain
   c. Hysterical conversion; a specific part of the body is found to have neurological damage.
   d. Somatoform disorder; people complain only of chronic pain
   Answer: b   LO: 15; factual, conceptual   page: 271

68. In _____ the person actually experiences physical symptoms and seeks help for them, whereas in _____ the person may just worry about having a disorder.
   a. somatization disorder; pain disorder
   b. hypochondriasis; factitious disorder
   c. psychosomatic illness; somatization disorder
   d. somatization disorder; hypochondriasis
   Answer: d   LO: 15; factual, conceptual   page: 271

Dissociative and Somatoform Disorders

69. The difference between somatization and conversion disorders is that:
    a. in somatization, the loss of functioning of a body part is part of a broader spectrum of symptoms that apparently have psychological causes.
    b. in somatization disorder the individual rarely complains about their physical symptoms.
    c. conversion disorder generally is part of a broader spectrum of symptoms that apparently have psychological causes.
    d. somatization is the older name for the disorder, which was changed to conversion disorder with the publication of DSM-IV.
    Answer: a   LO: 15; factual, conceptual   pages: 271-272

70. People with somatization or pain disorder:
    a. constantly express their feelings of anxiety and depression.
    b. tend to experience their distress through physical symptoms or mask it in alcohol abuse or antisocial behavior.
    c. are more often male than female.
    d. are more often middle-aged adults than older adults or young children.
    Answer: b   LO: 15, 16; factual, conceptual   page: 271

71. Which groups are most likely to experience somatization disorder?
    a. Caucasians and Asians
    b. Caucasians and Hispanics
    c. Hispanics and Asians
    d. They are all equally likely to express distress in physical complaints.
    Answer: c   LO: 16; factual   page: 272

72. Which of the following groups are most likely to have somatization disorder?
    a. Hispanics, Asians, and middle-aged adults.
    b. men, young children, and Hispanics.
    c. women, middle-aged adults, and Asians.
    d. Asians, Hispanics, and young children.
    Answer: d   LO: 16; factual   page: 272

73. A critical concern in distinguishing somatization disorder from organic disorders is that:
    a. people who complain of physical symptoms that cannot be substantiated often have medical histories with many actual physical disorders.
    b. there are physical disorders that we cannot yet adequately detect.
    c. if these individuals do not get help for their psychological disorders, they may exacerbate into more serious emotional problems.
    d. if these individuals do not get help for their psychological disorders, they may exacerbate into actual, serious medical problems.
    Answer: b   LO: 16; factual, conceptual   page: 272

Chapter 7

74. A disorder that is commonly confused with somatization disorder is:
    a. *ataque de nervios*.
    b. Korsakoff's syndrome.
    c. chronic fatigue syndrome.
    d. conversion disorder.
    Answer: c   LO: 16; factual   page: 272

75. In a study by Manu et al. (1989) of 100 adults complaining of chronic fatigue syndrome, how many met the criteria of somatization disorder?
    a. 1
    b. 5
    c. 15
    d. 20
    Answer: c   LO: 16; factual   page: 273

76. Family history studies of somatization and pain disorders have found:
    a. there is no support for genetic transmission but a great deal of evidence for environmental causes.
    b. parents who are somatizers tend to overprotect their children.
    c. children of parents who are somatizers have an increased vulnerability to a wide range of psychological problems.
    d. people who are somatizers are more likely to be from alcoholic families.
    Answer: c   LO: 17; factual   page: 273

77. Which of the following is *not* an explanation of somatization disorder?
    a. Persons with these disorders tend to experience bodily sensations as more intense than other people, they pay more attention to physical symptoms, and they tend to catastrophize these symptoms.
    b. Somatization disorder may be part of post-traumatic stress disorder (PTSD).
    c. Individuals with somatization disorder may have been neglected as children, and as children, they learned that the only way to receive care and attention was to be ill.
    d. Several genes have been identified that interact with each other to create a hypersensitivity to infectious diseases that currently are undetectable.
    Answer: d   LO: 17; factual, conceptual   page: 273

78. The female relatives of people with somatization disorder have higher rates of _____. The male relatives have higher rates of _____.
    a. alcohol abuse and depression; antisocial personality disorder and anxiety
    b. pain disorder; anxiety
    c. depression and anxiety; alcohol abuse and antisocial personality disorder
    d. depression and antisocial personality disorder; alcohol abuse and anxiety
    Answer: c   LO: 17; factual   page: 273

Dissociative and Somatoform Disorders

79. Which of the following does *not* belong in the cognitive theory of somatization?
    a. People with these disorders tend to experience bodily sensations as more intense than other people.
    b. People with this disorder were often neglected as children and got attention only by being sick.
    c. People with this disorder pay more attention to physical symptoms than other people do.
    d. People with this disorder tend to catastrophize their symptoms.
    Answer: b   LO: 17; factual, conceptual   page: 273

80. Tula's physician referred her to a psychologist because of recurrent somatization symptoms. Which technique would *not* be appropriate for treating Tula?
    a. teaching her to express negative feelings or memories and to understand the relationship between her emotions and her physical symptoms.
    b. helping her learn to interpret her physical symptoms appropriately, and to avoid catastrophizing physical symptoms.
    c. working within her belief system and using her belief in the spirits' power to produce physical pain to understand how that has caused her to neglect the care of her body.
    d. confronting her with how the somatization is hurting not only her, but also other people in her life.
    Answer: d   LO: 18; applied   pages: 273-274

81. Hypochondriasis resembles somatization disorder in that:
    a. people with both disorders often do not believe that their problems are caused by psychological factors and are thus difficult to treat.
    b. people with both disorders actually experience physical symptoms.
    c. both disorders tend to be accompanied by *la belle indifference*.
    d. both disorders tend to run in families.
    Answer: d   LO: 19; factual, conceptual   page: 274

82. Conversion disorder resembles somatization disorder in that:
    a. both disorders tend to be accompanied by *la belle indifference*.
    b. both disorders tend to run in families.
    c. people with both disorders often do not believe that their problems are caused by psychological factors and are thus difficult to treat.
    d. people with both disorders often develop them in conjunction with post-traumatic stress disorder.
    Answer: d   LO: 19; factual, conceptual   pages: 271-272

Chapter 7

83. Which of the following body parts is *not* one of the most frequently focused on by people with body dysmorphic disorder?
   a. knees
   b. face and head
   c. arms and legs
   d. sexual body parts
   Answer: a   LO: 20; factual   page: 275

84. According to Phillips (1991), case studies of some people with body dysmorphic disorder indicate that:
   a. their preoccupation with the notion that their body parts are deformed are so extreme as to indicate that these individuals may, in fact, suffer a form of schizophrenia.
   b. their belief that some part of their body is deformed can be so severe and bizarre as to be considered delusional.
   c. at times these individuals show no concern at all for their bodies, while at other times they are so obsessed that psychologists are beginning to see a connection with DID.
   d. these individuals have such a distorted image of their bodies that researchers are now coming to suspect there is some connection with anorexia nervosa.
   Answer: b   LO: 20; factual, conceptual   page: 275

85. Which of the following is most likely to seek treatment for body dysmorphic disorder?
   a. Joan, a single female who has waited 6 years to get treatment.
   b. Beverly, a married woman whose husband has prodded her for over a year to get treatment.
   c. Ben, a single male who has considered marriage for approximately 1 year but is concerned that his fiancée will not marry him unless he is treated.
   d. Angelica, a single female who has had ten plastic surgeries by the time she seeks treatment.
   Answer: a   LO: 20; applied   page: 276

86. While American researchers and clinicians have tended to ignore _____, they have been accused of overemphasizing _____.
   a. conversion disorder; depersonalization disorder
   b. body dysmorphic disorder; dissociative fugue
   c. dissociative amnesia; dissociative identity disorder
   d. body dysmorphic disorder; dissociative identity disorder
   Answer: d   LO: 4; 20; factual   page: 276

Dissociative and Somatoform Disorders

87. If Selena is typical of other people with body dysmorphic disorder, we would expect that she:
    a. also suffers from depression and anxiety.
    b. has antisocial personality disorder.
    c. has severe levels of depression or anxiety.
    d. has merely an exaggerated concern for her body.
    Answer: c   LO: 21; applied   page: 276

88. Phillips (1991) has suggested that body dysmorphic disorder may be a form of:
    a. dissociative disorder.
    b. obsessive-compulsive disorder.
    c. anxiety disorder.
    d. personality disorder.
    Answer: b   LO: 21; factual   page: 271

89. Which treatment is *not* mentioned in the text for body dysmorphic disorder?
    a. psychoanalytic therapy focused on helping the client gain insight into the real concerns behind her obsession with her body part(s)
    b. use of Xanax (alprazolam) to reduce the symptoms of anxiety that accompany this disorder
    c. behavioral therapy employing systematic desensitization to help the client stop engaging in compulsive behaviors around her body part and to reduce the client's anxiety about her body part
    d. use of selective serotonin reuptake inhibitors (SSRIs) to reduce the obsessional thoughts and compulsive behaviors in persons with this disorder.
    Answer: b   LO: 22; factual, conceptual   page: 271

90. Truddi has been diagnosed with dissociative identity disorder. Each of her 92 alters has different heart rates, blood pressure, handwriting, and even allergies. This is an excellent example of the age-old philosophical debate involving:
    a. mind-body interaction.
    b. nature versus nurture.
    c. genetics versus environment.
    d. vulnerability to stress.
    Answer: a   LO: 2; applied   page: 277

91. Since we all somatize our distress to some extent, somatization disorder is actually a matter of:
    a. intent.
    b. exaggeration.
    c. internalization.
    d. understatement.
    Answer: b   LO: 18; conceptual   page: 277

Chapter 7

92. The text suggests that what differentiates a person who develops somatization disorder from persons who don't is a matter of:
    a. ineffective coping techniques that lead to body breakdown.
    b. reduced ability to distinguish between what is going on in their mind from what is going on in their bodies.
    c. what is socially acceptable in terms of expressing anger and sadness.
    d. a choice of whether to somatize or internalize.
    Answer: b LO: 18; conceptual page: 277

93. Mariette's 8-month-old baby has been hospitalized three times for mysterious stomach problems. Previously, Mariette had another baby who had died from gastrointestinal problems. Both babies appeared to be completely healthy when they were born. The hospital staff put up cameras to observe Mariette when she comes to visit her baby, and they have now learned that she creates these illnesses in her children, which the hospital psychiatrist determined is to get attention for themselves. This tragic disorder is called:
    a. factitious disorder.
    b. malingering by proxy.
    c. factitious disorder by proxy.
    d. body-dysmorphic disorder by proxy.
    Answer: c LO: 11; applied page: 279

94. Which of the following is *not* a reason it may take a long time for authorities to intervene in factitious disorder by proxy?
    a. Parents with this disorder may be very adept at hiding what they are doing to their children.
    b. Authorities must be extremely cautious about accusing a parents of causing harm to their children because of the repercussions to the child and the family.
    c. Parents with this disorder appear to be extremely loving and protective, drawing praise for their dedicated nursing.
    d. Case workers for Departments of Children Services are so overloaded and underappreciated that they often let these cases "slip through the cracks."
    Answer: d LO: 11; factual, conceptual page: 279

95. Which of the following disorders has aroused controversy due to its possible creation by means of hypnosis and therapist suggestion?
    a. dissociative fugue
    b. factitious disorder
    c. depersonalization disorder
    d. dissociative identity disorder
    Answer: d LO: 4; factual, conceptual page: 261

Dissociative and Somatoform Disorders

96. Richard has been accused of murdering an intruder who broke into his house, but the last thing he remembers is falling asleep on the couch while drinking a few beers and watching the evening news. When the police question him, he claims to have no memory of the event. Which term would *not* appropriately describe his condition?
    a. organic retrograde amnesia
    b. psychogenic retrograde amnesia
    c. malingering
    d. splitting
    Answer: d   LO: 8; applied   page: 264-268

Essay Questions

97. You have been asked to present at talk to your local Hospital Volunteers of America Group. They have asked you to help them understand the different forms of dissociative disorders. They have asked that you begin by listing and describing the four basic forms of dissociative disorder. Then, you will need to expand on this by discussing the elements of each, how they develop, how they are similar, and how they differ from each other. Advise them how would you go about making a differential diagnosis? What treatment techniques would you use for each of these disorders?

The student should describe the specific characteristics of dissociative identity disorder (DID), dissociative fugue, dissociative amnesia (anterograde and retrograde), and depersonalization disorder, and address the part that amnesia and the fragmenting of aspects of the personality play in each of them, and then go on to discuss how they are different from each other. The student should also discuss the role of early trauma and excessive levels of stress as they relate to these disorders. The various drug therapies that are or are not effective and the appropriate psychosocial therapies for each disorder need to be addressed--with respect to DID, the student might want to look at whether "integration" of the personalities is optimal goal, or whether getting them to communicate with each other is more (or less) appropriate. A nice touch would be if a student added a cross-cultural perspective by discussing whether an Hispanic client might be diagnosed with DID or *ataque de nervios*.

Chapter 7

98. The topics of repressed memory and false memory syndrome have been receiving a lot of attention from researchers, clinicians, and the media, not to mention the courts. Discuss how each of these relates to dissociative identity disorder, then present the evidence supporting and disputing each side. Finally, address the ethical issues relevant to this debate.

First the student must explain what repressed memories are and how they help a person to survive; then the issue of a client's vulnerability to suggestion, whether or not under hypnosis. The student should connect the issue of repressed memory to DID and talk about how it has been used and abused in criminal cases (particularly homicide)--what exactly are the conditions under which a traumatic event will be repressed? The genetic evidence for dissociation should be debated here, as well as any empirical evidence discussed. There are clear ethical issues involving abuse of authority with respect to therapist/client relationship and disruption of family relations IF the memories are planted but need for working through the issues and achieving closure if the memories are real.

99. Your favorite uncle has suddenly lost his memory. You know from your Abnormal Psychology class that amnesia can have a variety of causes. In an attempt to understand your uncle's problem, discuss three causes of organic amnesia and three causes of psychogenic amnesia. What types of information are typically lost and retained in both organic and psychogenic amnesia?

Organic: biological factors of disease, drugs, accidents; Psychogenic: defense against intolerable memories, failure to encode due to a high state of arousal at the time of the event, failure to retrieve due to association with a high state of arousal from painful emotions. Discuss anterograde and retrograde amnesia, and which is most likely to be exhibited depending on whether the amnesia is organic or psychogenic.

100. Between 25 to 45% of people arrested for homicide claim to have amnesia for the killing. What are three ways in which they could experience true amnesia for the event? If they are fabricating their amnesia, what is one way that one of these three "real ways" of experiencing amnesia could be ruled out?

Here the issues of psychogenic amnesia involving repression of intolerable memories and the failure to encode or retrieve due to high arousal, as well as organic amnesia due to an accident such as falling on the head during the crime, may account for the amnesia. In terms of assessing whether the person is faking, Spanos' research on the "Bianchi" effect should be discussed with respect to inducing DID but can be countered with Ross, Norton, and Fraser's concerns about failure to have long-term effects.

Dissociative and Somatoform Disorders

101. Imagine that one of your friends is complaining to you about having terrible stomach pains, but this friend says the doctors can't find anything physically wrong. You suspect this might be a somatoform disorder of some type, but you have to think through all you know about these disorders so you can try to help your friend. Explain the various types of somatoform disorders, including their symptoms and differential diagnoses. How do these differ from psychosomatic illnesses? Consider the possible causes of these disorders, including gender and cultural factors. What types of treatment have been effective for each of these disorders? How will this information help your friend?

Here the student should explain what somatoform disorders are and should discuss conversion (including the telling symptom of *la belle indifference*), somatization and pain disorders, hypochondriasis, and body dysmorphic disorder. Factitious disorder by proxy would be a bonus to discuss. The concept of depersonalization is relevant, and the differentiation from psychosomatic illnesses in that the latter actually have a physical problem. A discussion of how some of these disorders may actually exist as physical problems that we cannot yet (do not have sufficiently sophisticated tests) detect, as has been an issue with chronic fatigue syndrome, would be a nice inclusion here. The student should discuss how females are more apt to somatize than males (who tend to turn to alcohol, other drugs, and aggression), and that Western cultures are less likely than others to exhibit somatic symptoms--and the reasons given for these differences. The appropriateness of using drugs for each of these should be discussed, as well as psychoanalytic, but the focus would be on the cognitive-behavioral treatments (watch out for challenging clients beliefs here). Finally, the student should indicate how the information presented here can help the friend.

Chapter 8   Personality Disorders

1. All of the ways of acting, thinking, believing, and feeling that makes an individual unique are called:
   a. personality.
   b. personality traits.
   c. individuality.
   d. disposition.
   Answer: a   LO: 1; conceptual   page: 282

2. A complex pattern of behavior, thought, and feeling that is stable across time and across many situations is called:
   a. personality.
   b. personality trait.
   c. individuality.
   d. individuality trait.
   Answer: b   LO: 1; conceptual   page: 282

3. A personality disorder is:
   a. a long-standing pattern of behavior, thoughts, and feeling that are highly maladaptive for an individual or for people around that individual.
   b. a mental illness that causes an individual to act in a way that is not consistent with his or her usual pattern of behavior.
   c. a mental illness that causes an individual to act in a way that is not consistent with how other people would like the individual to act.
   d. a social judgment that determines an individual's behavior is inconsistent with societal norms.
   Answer: a   LO: 1; conceptual   page: 282

4. Which of the following is *false* concerning personality disorders?
   a. For a diagnosis of personality disorder, the patterns of behavior must have been present continuously from adolescence or early adulthood into adulthood.
   b. DSM-IV calls special attention to personality disorders by placing them on Axis II.
   c. Typically, an individual diagnosed with a personality disorder will not have an Axis I (acute) diagnosis.
   d. People with personality disorders do not typically seek treatment for the personality disorder.
   Answer: c   LO: 1; factual, conceptual   page: 282

Personality Disorders

5. The personality disorders that contain some of the features of schizophrenia or paranoid psychotic disorder, without the psychosis, are:
   a. Cluster A: odd or eccentric behaviors and thinking.
   b. Cluster B: dramatic, erratic, and emotional behavior and interpersonal relationships.
   c. Cluster C: anxious and fearful emotions, and chronic self-doubt, leading to maladaptive behaviors.
   d. Cluster D: personality disorders not otherwise specified ("NOS").
   Answer: a   LO: 2; factual   page: 283

6. The personality disorders that describe persons who tend to be manipulative, volatile, and uncaring in social relationships and prone to impulsive behaviors are:
   a. Cluster A: odd or eccentric behaviors and thinking.
   b. Cluster B: dramatic, erratic, and emotional behavior and interpersonal relationships.
   c. Cluster C: anxious and fearful emotions, and chronic self-doubt, leading to maladaptive behaviors.
   d. Cluster D: personality disorders not otherwise specified ("NOS").
   Answer: b   LO: 2; factual   page: 283

7. Which of the following is *not* an issue of controversy with respect to classifying personality disorders as diagnosable categories in DSM-IV?
   a. Each disorder is described as if it represents something qualitatively different from a "normal" personality, but there is evidence that most of these disorders are merely extreme versions of "normal" personality traits.
   b. There is much overlap in diagnostic criteria of the personality disorders, so most people who are diagnosed with one disorder meet the criteria for at least one other.
   c. There is a great deal of research on these disorders but much of it is conflicting with respect to judging which specific diagnosis (or diagnoses) a person should receive.
   d. Diagnosing a personality disorder often requires information that may be difficult for a therapist to get, such as stability of the individual's behavior since childhood.
   Answer: c   LO: 3; factual, conceptual   pages: 282-283

8. Which of the following is *true* concerning the odd-eccentric personality disorders?
   a. The behaviors in this group are so odd as to be considered beyond the edge of "reality."
   b. Many researchers consider this group of disorders to be part of the "schizophrenia spectrum."
   c. Although closely resembling schizophrenic behaviors, these are actually quite different disorders.
   d. Researchers have been unsuccessful in their attempts to find a genetic link between these disorders and schizophrenia.
   Answer: b   LO: 4; conceptual   page: 283

Chapter 8

9. Sherman's wife demanded that he see a therapist because his constant, pervasive, unwarranted mistrust of others was causing her great distress. He finally agreed, even though he believed she was trying to find a reason to "dump" him. It is most likely that Sherman has which personality disorder?
    a. paranoid personality disorder
    b. schizotypal personality disorder
    c. schizoid personality disorder
    d. borderline personality disorder
    Answer: a   LO: 5; applied   page: 283

10. Sam trusts no one. He learned that from his father, who constantly interfered with the boy's relationships with others, saying, "Sam, you're better than they are and they know it. They're jealous of you. They'll try to harm you. You can't trust them." Sam tried hard to win his father's love, but every time he made a mistake or didn't know the answer to a question his father asked, the young boy would be ridiculed and criticized. Sam now believes everyone is out to get him, that his wife is cheating on him, and everything anyone says by way of denial is further confirmation of its truth. Sam probably has:
    a. schizoid personality disorder.
    b. schizotypal personality disorder.
    c. paranoid personality disorder.
    d. borderline personality disorder.
    Answer: c   LO: 5; applied   page: 283-284

11. Which of the following is *true* concerning paranoid personality disorder?
    a. It affects somewhere between 1 to 2% of the population.
    b. Males are twice as likely as females to be diagnosed with the disorder.
    c. There is an increased risk for depression, anxiety disorders, substance abuse, and psychotic episodes concomitant with this disorder.
    d. There is a good prognosis for the disorder because under stress the symptoms intensify and the individual is likely to receive treatment.
    Answer: c   LO: 5; factual, conceptual   page: 284

12. According to psychodynamic theorists, people with paranoid personality disorder are riddle with hostile feelings that they:
    a. repress and displace.
    b. rationalize and project.
    c. intellectualize and deny.
    d. deny and project.
    Answer: d   LO: 5; factual, conceptual   page: 284

Personality Disorders

13. The parents of people with paranoid personality disorder:
    a. are critical and intolerant of any weakness, but also emphasize to their child that he or she is "special" and "different" from others.
    b. are harsh and inconsistent, and alternate between being neglectful and being hostile and violent toward their children.
    c. derive pleasure from their child's dependence on them in early life, do not encourage the child to develop a separate sense of self, and punish the child's attempts at individuation.
    d. are overcontrolling and punitive when their child makes mistakes but do not praise or reward their child when he or she does well.
    Answer: a   LO: 5; factual, conceptual   page: 284

14. Which of the following would be expected to be most effective in terms of treating a person with paranoid personality disorder?
    a. challenging their distorted perceptions of reality
    b. being calm, respectful, and straightforward
    c. establishing a warm, personal relationship
    d. interpreting the client's beliefs in a more positive light
    Answer: b   LO: 6; factual, conceptual   pages: 285-286

15. Which of the following is *not* something that a cognitive therapist would do in attempting to treat someone with paranoid personality disorder?
    a. examine the "worst possible case scenario"
    b. increase the client's sense of self-efficacy for dealing with difficult situations
    c. help the client reframe the situation into a less threatening scenario
    d. help the client see that his or her perceptions are distorted
    Answer: d   LO: 6; applied   pages: 285-286

16. A person who is described as "aloof, reclusive, and detached," who shows little emotion in interpersonal interactions, and views relationships with others as "unrewarding, messy, and intrusive," would most likely be diagnosed with which personality disorder?
    a. paranoid
    b. schizophrenic
    c. schizoid
    d. schizotypal
    Answer: c   LO: 7; applied   page: 286

Chapter 8

17. Harlin is about the most dull, uninteresting, humorless person you ever met. It's no wonder you aren't friends with him, even though he's your next-door neighbor. In fact, he is so aloof and reclusive that you hardly ever see him, and you never see anyone visiting him. He rarely responds to your "Good mornings" or "Hellos," and you gave up trying to tell him jokes years ago; the guy obviously has no sense of humor at all. If Harlin were diagnosed with a personality disorder, it would be:
a. paranoid.
b. schizophrenic.
c. schizoid.
d. schizotypal.
Answer: c LO: 7; applied page: 286-287

18. Which of the following is *true* about schizoid personality disorder?
a. It is a relatively common disorder, with about 2.5% of the adult population manifesting it at some point in their lives.
b. Among people seeking treatment for the disorder, there are slightly more men than women with this disorder.
c. Schizoids are able to function in society, especially if they have jobs that do not require much interpersonal interactions.
d. There is a clear link between schizoid personality disorder and schizophrenia.
Answer: c LO: 7; factual page: 287

19. Which of the following is *true* concerning development of schizoid personality disorder?
a. Behavioral theorists believe this is learned behavior that develops out of severely disturbed mother-child relationships in which the child never learns to give or receive love and thus come to view relationships as dangerous.
b. Cognitive theorists see schizoid persons as hypersensitive to cues that produce emotions, and their behavior of withdrawal is in response to being overwhelmed by emotionally charged environmental stimuli.
c. Psychoanalytic theorists focus on the severely disturbed father-child relationships, where the child learns that the people around him or her cannot be trusted.
d. Cognitive theorists believe in part that the schizoid person is unresponsive to cues that produce emotions.
Answer: d LO: 7; factual, conceptual page:

Personality Disorders

20. According to cognitive theories, people with schizoid personality disorder:
    a. have low self-regard and are led to reject other people and social interactions due to a fear of being rejected themselves.
    b. have beliefs that other people are malevolent and deceptive, combined with a lack of self-confidence about being able to defend themselves against others, leading them to be suspicious and to reject others before they themselves are rejected.
    c. develops out of severely disturbed mother-child relationships, in which the child never learns to give or receive love.
    d. have cognitive styles that are impoverished and unresponsive to cues that produce emotions.
    Answer: d LO: 7; factual, conceptual page: 287

21. With respect to treating schizoid personality disorder:
    a. psychoanalytic treatments focus on recreating the mother-child relationship and helping the individual gain insight into how that affects current problems in dealing with the individual's social environment.
    b. cognitive treatments are aimed at helping the client understand his or her distorted perceptions so they can be reworked into healthy attitudes that will help the client build relationships.
    c. psychoanalytic and cognitive treatments focus on increasing the person's awareness of his or her feelings and his or her social skills and social contacts.
    d. psychoanalytic and cognitive treatments refrain from use of group therapy because they offer the opportunity to model group members' behavior, which is something therapists do not want to occur in this disorder.
    Answer: c LO: 8; factual, conceptual pages: 287-288

22. Which of the following is *not* a cognitive anomaly exhibited by people with schizotypal personality disorder?
    a. dissociative states
    b. illusions and ideas of reference
    c. odd beliefs and magical thinking
    d. paranoia or suspiciousness
    Answer: a LO: 9; factual page: 288

23. Which of the following is *not* a way in which schizotypal personality disorder resembles schizophrenia?
    a. Both schizophrenics and schizotypals have difficulty initiating, sustaining, and controlling their attention on cognitive tasks.
    b. Both schizophrenics and schizotypals have enlarged ventricles.
    c. Both schizophrenics and schizotypals experience hallucinations and delusions.
    d. Both schizophrenics and schizotypals have odd or inappropriate emotional responses.
    Answer: c LO: 9; factual, conceptual page: 288

Chapter 8

24. The distinguishing characteristic of schizotypal personality disorder is:
    a. their oddities in cognition.
    b. the overriding paranoia they exhibit.
    c. their social reclusiveness.
    d. their pervasive lack of trust.
    Answer: a   LO: 9; factual, conceptual   page: 288

25. Many of us, as we lie in bed and look up at the ceiling, see faces, or people, or animals, but we know they are not real. The schizotypal sees them and believes them to be real. This is an example of the cognitive oddity called:
    a. magical thinking.
    b. illusions.
    c. hallucinations.
    d. delusions.
    Answer: b   LO: 9; factual, conceptual   page: 288

26. Which of the following is *true* concerning schizotypal personality disorder?
    a. It is a relatively rare disorder, with a lifetime prevalence rate of less than 1%.
    b. It is diagnosed approximately three times as much in males as in females.
    c. Although schizotypals are at increased risk for schizophrenia, they are at decreased risk for depression and anxiety disorders.
    d. It is arguably overdiagnosed in people of color because culturally-bound beliefs are often misinterpreted.
    Answer: d   LO: 9; factual, conceptual   page: 289

27. Which of the following is *false* about the biological bases of schizotypal personality disorder?
    a. Family history studies, adoption studies, and twin studies indicate that it is at least to some degree genetically transmitted.
    b. It is often considered to be a mild form of schizophrenia that is transmitted through similar genetic mechanisms as schizophrenia.
    c. As with schizophrenic, people with schizotypal personality disorder tend to have high levels of platelet monamine oxidase, and low levels of homovanillic acid, both of which are related to dopamine production.
    d. Patients with schizotypal personality disorder show increases in ventricular regions of the brain that are similar to those of schizophrenic patients.
    Answer: c   LO: 9; factual   page: 289

Personality Disorders

28. Which of the following is *true* about the biopsychosocial factors of schizotypal personality disorder?
    a. Persons with schizotypal personality disorder show problems in their ability to sustain attention on cognitive tasks, but not in involuntary control of attention.
    b. Family history studies, adoption studies, and twin studies suggest that schizotypal personality disorder is much more common in the first-degree relatives of people with schizophrenia than in the relatives of other psychiatric groups or healthy control groups.
    c. The psychoanalytic researchers believe that this disorder is created by a schizoprenogenic mother who constantly gives the child mixed, contradictory messages that place the child in a double bind or no-win situation.
    d. The cognitive researchers believe that parents of the schizotypal were overcontrolling and punitive when their child made mistakes, but did not praise or reward the child when he or she did well.
    Answer: b   LO: 9; factual, conceptual   page: 289

29. Which of the following is *not* one of the treatments that has been found to be effective for schizotypal personality disorder?
    a. use of neuroleptic drugs to reduce psychoticlike symptoms
    b. helping the client increase social contact and learn socially appropriate behaviors through social skills training
    c. use of aversive therapies, such as shocking the client each time he or she expresses a bizarre thought, and teaching the client to monitor his or her thoughts so they can be examined and disregarded
    d. teaching them to look for objective evidence in the environment for their thoughts and to learn to disregard their bizarre thoughts
    Answer: c   LO: 10; factual   page: 290

30. Which two Cluster B personality disorders (dramatic-emotional) are most well researched?
    a. antisocial; borderline
    b. borderline; narcissistic
    c. narcissistic; histrionic
    d. antisocial; narcissistic
    Answer: a   LO: 11; factual   page: 290

31. The most striking gender difference among the personality disorders appears in _____ personality disorder: men are five times more likely to be diagnosed with it than females.
    a. schizotypal
    b. antisocial
    c. paranoid
    d. narcissistic
    Answer: b   LO: 11; factual   page: 292

Chapter 8

32. Which of the following is *false* about antisocial personality disorder?
    a. The disorder has been recognized for over two hundred years.
    b. People with this disorder can be extremely charming, gracious, and cheerful.
    c. People with this disorder often become successful businesspeople and professionals.
    d. People with this disorder tend to avoid risk because they are concerned with their own well-being
    Answer: d   LO: 11; factual, conceptual   pages: 291-292

33. Which statement about antisocial personality disorder has been most strongly substantiated?
    a. People with antisocial personality disorder are highly intelligent.
    b. The tendency to engage in antisocial behaviors tends to begin in childhood and is one of the most stable personality characteristics.
    c. People with antisocial personality disorder are able to inhibit their impulsive behaviors when it suits their purposes.
    d. People with antisocial personality disorder engage in impulsive and dangerous acts in order to increase their low levels of arousability.
    Answer: b   LO: 11; factual, conceptual   pages: 292-293

34. At age 23, Andrea crashed her thirteenth car into a tree with such force that it killed her. There was no evidence that she was drunk, although she began drinking when she was 12. She never finished high school, and during her lifetime the longest she held a job was a month. She "stole" her friend's boyfriend and married him. A year later they had a daughter, whom she lost in a custody battle with the child's father when they got divorced, because the daughter was barefoot and dirty and there was no food or furniture in the apartment when the social worker came to visit. She made commitments to her friends and family that she consistently failed to follow through on because "something else came up." If Andrea had sought treatment for her problem, the diagnosis would probably be:
    a. dependent personality disorder.
    b. narcissistic personality disorder.
    c. substance abuse.
    d. antisocial personality disorder.
    Answer: d   LO: 11; applied   pages: 290-294

35. Which of the following is *not* one of the reasons given in the text to explain how antisocial behavior tends to diminish as people become older?
    a. It may be due to biological maturation.
    b. Many people with the disorder are in jail or otherwise constrained from acting out their antisocial tendencies.
    c. It may be due to psychological maturation.
    d. Because antisocials engage in such high-risk behaviors, many of them die before they reach old age.
    Answer: d   LO: 11; factual, conceptual   pages: 292-293

Personality Disorders

36. Which of the following is correct about studies addressing a genetic influence on antisocial behaviors?
    a. Twin studies find that the concordance rate for criminal behaviors is nearly 80% in monozygotic (MZ) twins, compared with 50% or lower in dizygotic (DZ) twins.
    b. Adoption studies find that the criminal records of adopted sons are more similar to the records of their biological fathers than their adoptive fathers.
    c. Family history studies show that first- and second-degree relatives of people with this disorder show increased rates of the disorder, as well as increased rates of alcoholism but not necessarily increased criminal activity.
    d. Twin studies show that the concordance rate for low serotonin levels is nearly 55% in monozygotic (MZ) twins, compared with 23% in dizygotic (DZ) twins.
    Answer: b   LO: 11; factual   pages: 293-294

37. Research on social and personality factors that contribute to antisocial behavior has found that children with antisocial tendencies:
    a. come from homes in which they have experienced harsh and inconsistent parenting.
    b. have parents who are hostile, cruel, domineering, and controlling.
    c. have parents who are neglecting and rejecting, and leave the children to grow up by themselves.
    d. come from homes where children are allowed to do as they wish, with no limits on their behavior, and no disciplinary boundaries set.
    Answer: a   LO: 11; factual   page: 294

38. In terms of curing antisocial personality disorder:
    a. there have been excellent results with the drug lithium.
    b. they are so resistant to treatment that there is little hope that any person with this disorder will ever be cured.
    c. many theorists believe that the only successful cure for this disorder is age.
    d. a combination of lithium and SSRIs currently looks like the most successful treatment for the disorder.
    Answer: c   LO: 12; factual   page: 294

39. Among people with borderline and antisocial personality disorders, low levels of serotonin have been linked to:
    a. paranoia.
    b. shyness.
    c. dissociative states.
    d. impulsivity.
    Answer: d   LO: 11, 13; factual   page: 297

Childhood Disorders

5. Which child is *least likely* to develop a psychological disorder?
   a. Terry, a 5-year-old boy who lives in the projects with his single mother, who has always had a happy, outgoing personality.
   b. Kenny, a grumpy 5-year-old boy who lives with his parents in an exclusive neighborhood.
   c. Sarah, a shy 6-year-old girl who has become socially withdrawn since being sexually molested by her mother's boyfriend.
   d. Cindy, a very active 3-year-old whose mother died in childbirth and whose father is a rich, but alcoholic professional.
   Answer: a   LO: 1; applied   page: 319

6. Which of the following is *not* one of the factors listed in the text that developmental psychopathologists consider with respect to its impact on the symptoms of childhood psychopathology?
   a. level of cognitive development
   b. level of social development
   c. level of emotional development
   d. level of behavioral development
   Answer: d   LO: 1; conceptual   page: 319

7. The behavior disorders include:
   a. attention deficit disorder, oppositional defiant disorder, and conduct disorder.
   b. separation anxiety and childhood depression.
   c. autism and mental retardation.
   d. enuresis and encopresis.
   Answer: a   LO: 1; factual   page: 320

8. A child whose behavior involves hyperactivity has:
   a. a behavior disorder.
   b. an emotional disorder.
   c. a developmental disorder.
   d. a habit disorder.
   Answer: a   LO: 1; factual   page: 320

9. Which of the following statements about attention deficit/hyperactivity disorder (ADHD) is *false*?
   a. ADHD is a common precursor to conduct disorder.
   b. ADHD continues into adolescence for two-thirds of children.
   c. Many adults with a history of underachievement and poor relationships have been found to have had ADHD as children but were not diagnosed.
   d. ADHD children typically perform below their intellectual capabilities.
   Answer: c   LO: 1; factual   page: 320-321

Chapter 11

6. The least common sexual disorder is:
   a. sexual dysfunction.
   b. paraphilia.
   c. vaginismus.
   d. transsexualism.
   Answer: d   LO: 1; factual   page: 386

7. The sexual dysfunctions are:
   a. a set of disorders in which people have trouble engaging in and enjoying sexual interchanges with other people.
   b. deviant behaviors that are typically kept hidden for fear that the person with the disorder may be arrested.
   c. physical disorders that affect a person's ability to engage in sexual intercourse with another person.
   d. psychological disorders that inhibit a person's ability to engage in sexual intercourse with another person.
   Answer: a   LO: 1; factual, conceptual   page: 386

8. The physiological change occurring with penile erection and vaginal lubrication is known as _____ and first occurs during the _____ phase of the sexual response cycle.
   a. myotonia; desire
   b. vasocongestion; plateau
   c. engorgement; desire
   d. vasocongestion; excitement
   Answer: d   LO: 1; factual   page: 387

9. Which of the following *is not* one of the phases of the sexual response cycle?
   a. foreplay
   b. arousal
   c. orgasm
   d. plateau
   Answer: a   LO: 1; factual   page: 387

10. Sandy and Chris are engaging in sexual intercourse. The phases of the sexual response cycle they would normally be expected to experience are:
    a. foreplay, excitement, and orgasm.
    b. desire, excitement, plateau, orgasm, and resolution.
    c. stimulation, arousal, orgasm, and resolution.
    d. stimulation, plateau, orgasm, and completion.
    Answer: b   LO: 1; applied   page: 387

Chapter 8

40. A person who exhibits out-of-control emotions that cannot be soothed, a hypersensitivity to abandonment, a tendency to cling too tightly to other people, and a history of self-injurious behavior would be diagnosed with _____ personality disorder.
    a. dependent
    b. borderline
    c. obsessive-compulsive
    d. histrionic
    Answer: b   LO: 13; factual, conceptual   pages: 295-296

41. Eileen had a distressing habit of leaning on people physically and emotionally. When friends did not answer their phones, she believed they were purposely avoiding her, and she would go to their homes and bang on their doors. She threw herself on top of her ex-husband's car, screaming and banging on the windshield as he was driving away from an argument she started in the middle of the street. It is likely that Eileen has _____ personality disorder.
    a. narcissistic
    b. dependent
    c. histrionic
    d. borderline
    Answer: d   LO: 13; applied   pages: 295-296

42. A key feature of borderline personality disorder is:
    a. lability.
    b. rigidity.
    c. paranoid.
    d. anxiety.
    Answer: a   LO: 13; factual   page: 295

43. With respect to diagnosing borderline personality:
    a. clinicians have, by and large, been in agreement on the diagnostic characteristics.
    b. the varied list of symptoms reflects the complexity of the disorder.
    c. the varied list of symptoms was designed to simplify differential diagnosis.
    d. because the list of symptoms is so inclusive, they will probably not be diagnosed with another personality disorder.
    Answer: b   LO: 13; factual, conceptual   page: 296

44. People with borderline personality are at greatest risk for suicide:
    a. soon after developing the disorder.
    b. early on in treatment.
    c. a year or two after commencing treatment.
    d. It is not borderlines, but the people with whom they interact who are at high risk for suicide.
    Answer: c   LO: 13; factual   page: 296

Personality Disorders

45. Which of the following would be most likely to be diagnosed with borderline personality disorder?
    a. an African-American woman with an annual income of $11,500
    b. an Hispanic-American man with an annual income of $10,900
    c. a Euro-American man with an annual income of $65,000
    d. a Euro-American woman with an annual income of $11,500
    Answer: a   LO: 13; factual   page: 296

46. Relatives of people with _____ personality disorder have higher rates of schizophrenia than control subjects; relatives of people with _____ personality disorder have higher rates of mood disorders than control subjects.
    a. paranoid; borderline
    b. schizoid; avoidant
    c. schizotypal; paranoid
    d. borderline; dependent
    Answer: a   LO: 5; 13; factual   pages: 284, 296

47. Studies of the effects of serotonin level on mood and psychological disorders suggest that:
    a. low serotonin levels are associated primarily with borderline personality disorder.
    b. low serotonin levels are associated primarily with antisocial personality disorder.
    c. low serotonin levels are linked with impulsive behaviors.
    d. high serotonin levels are linked with mood disorders.
    Answer: c   LO: 13; factual   page: 297

48. Psychoanalysts describe the parents of a borderline personality as having:
    a. been cold and detached with the child, although excessively punitive.
    b. discouraged the child from developing independence and a sense of self.
    c. been hostile, cruel, and demanding regardless of what the child did.
    d. given ambiguous but mixed messages so that whatever the child did was wrong.
    Answer: b   LO: 13; factual, conceptual   page: 297

49. The process through which a borderline sees people as either "all good" or "all bad" is called:
    a. dichotomy.
    b. detaching.
    c. separating.
    d. splitting.
    Answer: d   LO: 13; factual   page: 297

Chapter 8

50. The emotional lability seen in the relationships of persons with borderline personality disorder is due to:
    a. fear of rejection.
    b. splitting.
    c. confusion about reality.
    d. inability to read environmental cues.
    Answer: b   LO: 13; factual   page: 297

51. Millon (1981) suggested that persons with borderline personality disorder have a _____, which he attributes to _____.
    a. fundamental deficit in self-identity; biological, psychological, and sociological factors
    b. problem separating self from other; biological, psychological, and sociological factors
    c. fundamental deficit in self-identity; residual dependence from childhood
    d. problem with internalized anger; psychological factors
    Answer: a   LO: 13; factual, conceptual   page: 297

52. According to Linehan (1987), people with borderline personality disorder:
    a. have a psychologically based deficit in the ability to regulate their emotions.
    b. have impulsive actions that lead to extreme emotional reactions to situations.
    c. have a history of discounting and criticizing the emotional experiences of others.
    d. rely on others to help them cope with difficult situations but lack the self-confidence to ask for help in mature ways.
    Answer: d   LO: 13; factual, conceptual   page: 297

53. Studies addressing the effectiveness of drugs for treating borderline personality disorder:
    a. have found that antidepressants improve many borderlines, but others become worse.
    b. have found serotonin reuptake inhibitor fluoxetine effective in treating depressed mood but not in reducing impulsive behaviors.
    c. have found that antianxiety drugs are effective in reducing impulsive behavior, and SSRIs have been effective in reducing symptoms of depression.
    d. are not yet conclusive about their effectiveness.
    Answer: d   LO: 14; factual   page: 298

54. Which of the following is *not* a focus of psychodynamic treatment for borderline personality disorder?
    a. helping the client clarify feelings
    b. confronting the client with the tendency to split images of self and other
    c. learning to monitor and challenge self-disparaging thoughts and black-and-white thinking about people and situations
    d. interpreting the client's transference relationship with the therapist
    Answer: c   LO: 14; factual   pages: 298-299

Personality Disorders

55. Which of the following is *not* a focus of cognitive treatment for borderline personality disorder?
    a. helping the client learn adaptive skills at solving problems and regulating emotions
    b. correcting dichotomous thinking
    c. interpreting the client's transference relationship with the therapist
    d. learning to monitor and challenge self-disparaging thoughts and black-and-white thinking about people and situations

    Answer: c   LO: 14; factual, conceptual   page: 299

56. Therapists who deal with clients with borderline personality disorder must keep in mind:
    a. the need to challenge the borderline client's way of seeing the world.
    b. the borderline client's tendency either to idealize or totally reject a therapist.
    c. that being totally honest with a borderline may make the client feel rejected.
    d. how trusting and gullible, and thus vulnerable to suggestion, the borderline client is.

    Answer: b   LO: 14; factual, conceptual   page: 299

57. Which of the following statements concerning borderline personality disorder is correct?
    a. Of all the clients a therapist may see with different personality disorders, the borderline is the most gratifying to work with since change can be seen quickly.
    b. Setting limits on a borderline client's behaviors can jeopardize the therapeutic relationship.
    c. Clients with borderline personality disorder are among the most motivated to improve, and thus idealizing their therapist is extremely common.
    d. There is an extremely high drop-out rate of borderline clients from therapy, which is around 60%.

    Answer: d   LO: 14; factual, conceptual   page: 299

58. One important diagnostic difference between the borderline and histrionic personality disorders is that the borderline _____, while the histrionic _____.
    a. always wants to be the center of attention; is often self-effacing in an attempt to win favor from others
    b. is often self-effacing in an attempt to win favor from others; always wants to be the center of attention
    c. clings to other people; screams at other people
    d. sees the world in global terms; sees the world in terms of black-and-white

    Answer: b   LO: 15; conceptual   page: 299

Chapter 8

59. Desiree attempts to get attention by being highly dramatic and overtly seductive. She is seen by others as self-centered and shallow, unable to delay gratification, demanding, and overly dependent. It is likely that Desiree has a _____ personality disorder.
    a. borderline
    b. obsessive-compulsive
    c. dependent
    d. histrionic
    Answer: d   LO: 15; factual, conceptual   page: 299

60. Which of the following is *least* likely to be a characteristic of the histrionic personality disorder?
    a. separated or divorced
    b. increased rate of suicide gestures and threats
    c. resistance to obtaining medical care
    d. female
    Answer: c   LO: 15; factual   page: 299

61. According to family history studies, the family members of the histrionic personality are most likely to have:
    a. borderline personality disorder, antisocial personality disorder, and somatization disorder.
    b. dependent personality disorder, borderline personality disorder, and bipolar disorder.
    c. dependent personality disorder, obsessive-compulsive disorder, and unipolar depression.
    d. obsessive-compulsive disorder, somatization disorder, and unipolar depression.
    Answer: a   LO: 15; factual   page: 300

62. Which of the following is *not* considered by psychodynamic theorists to be at the root of histrionic personality disorder?
    a. deep dependency needs stemming from poor resolution of the anal stage
    b. the need for approval from others
    c. repression of one's own feelings and needs
    d. poor resolution of the oral stage
    Answer: a   LO: 15; factual, conceptual   page: 300

Personality Disorders

63. Cognitive theorists note that people with many disorders suffer from the belief that "I am inadequate and unable to handle life on my own." The difference between the behavior of a person with histrionic personality disorder and the behavior of other people is that:
    a. the person with histrionic personality disorder tries to draw attention to herself by being seductive.
    b. the person with histrionic personality disorder works to get nurtured by other people by seeking their attention and approval.
    c. the person with histrionic personality disorder acts out the behavior by reacting to the world in terms of black-and-white, good-and-evil, "you're either with me or against me."
    d. in most of the other disorders, the belief is seen in terms of mood, not behavior.
    Answer: b   LO: 15; factual, conceptual   page: 300

64. Which of the following is *not* a theory suggested for how histrionic personality disorder develops?
    a. deep dependency needs and repression of emotions stemming from poor resolution of the oral or phallic stage
    b. a deep-seated belief that the histrionic person is inadequate and unable to handle her own life
    c. as a child, the person with histrionic personality disorder was subjected to on-going physical and/or sexual abuse
    d. as a child, the person with histrionic personality disorder had to "do something" (like look pretty) to get her parents' attention and receive praise
    Answer: c   LO: 15; factual, conceptual   page: 300

65. Which of the following is *not* a focus of treating a person with histrionic personality disorder?
    a. use of antianxiety drugs to reduce impulsive and seductive behavior
    b. uncovering the repressed emotions and needs, and teaching the client to express these emotions and needs in more appropriate ways
    c. identifying the histrionic's assumptions that they cannot function on their own
    d. toning down the client's dramatic evaluations of situations by challenging them and suggesting more reasonable evaluations
    Answer: a   LO: 16; factual   pages: 300-301

66. The narcissistic personality disorder appears similar to the _____ personality disorder except that the narcissist _____.
    a. histrionic; relies on his own self-evaluations
    b. borderline; does not use the defense of splitting
    c. histrionic; looks to others for approval
    d. antisocial; is more concerned for the welfare of others
    Answer: a   LO: 17; factual, conceptual   page: 301

Chapter 8

67. Connie dreams of controlling the school district. She displays her accomplishments on her office walls, including the newspaper article in which she was named "Woman of the Year." She rarely does her own work but creates a situation where her secretary, Rose, must do both of their work. Then Connie takes credit for *all* of the work and criticizes Rose if errors are made. One weekend, when no one else was in the office, Connie came in, accessed Rose's files, then put her own name on all the charts Rose had painstakingly prepared over the past two years. Don't make plans to meet her for lunch--if she shows up at all, she'll be anywhere from half an hour to an hour and a half late since she is more important than you are, so she's entitled to be late. From this description, a therapist might diagnosis Connie as having:
    a. antisocial personality disorder.
    b. borderline personality disorder.
    c. histrionic personality disorder.
    d. narcissistic personality disorder.
    Answer: d   LO: 17; applied   page: 301-303

68. Which of the following is *true* about narcissistic personality disorder?
    a. Narcissists can be extremely successful in societies (such as the United States) that reward self-confidence and assertiveness.
    b. Because of their unending need for approval, narcissists generally make good choices.
    c. While narcissists annoy and alienate many people, they are usually able to maintain relatively good relations with the most important people in their lives.
    d. When narcissists seek treatment, it is generally for anxiety disorders.
    Answer: a   LO: 17; factual, conceptual   page: 302

69. Which of the following is *false* about narcissistic personality disorder?
    a. It is a relatively rare diagnosis, with a lifetime prevalence rate of less than 1%.
    b. It is more frequently diagnosed in men than in women.
    c. Because narcissists are self-confident and assertive, they tend to be well-liked by the people who know them.
    d. According to Freud, narcissism is a natural developmental phase for children.
    Answer: c   LO: 17; factual, conceptual   page: 302

70. Which of the following psychodynamic theories was stated by Freud, rather than the later psychodynamic writers?
    a. The narcissist suffers from low self-esteem and feelings of emptiness and pain.
    b. The narcissist was rejected by his parents.
    c. Narcissistic behaviors are reaction formations against the narcissist's problems in self-worth.
    d. A child can fixate in the narcissistic phase if they experience caregivers as untrustworthy and decide they can only rely on themselves.
    Answer: d   LO: 17; factual, conceptual   page: 302

Personality Disorders

71. Which of these is the most likely therapy for a person with narcissistic personality disorder?
    a. psychodynamic therapy that addresses the client's early childhood fixation
    b. drug therapy to reduce the client's anxieties about being judged and rejected
    c. cognitive therapy to help the client develop more sensitivity to the needs of others
    d. humanistic therapy to help the client become more in touch with his or her inner self
    Answer: c   LO: 18; factual, conceptual   page: 303

72. Sarah is so anxious about being criticized that she has taken a job as a night guard at Lonely Hills Cemetery. On those few occasions when she must interact with others, such as her employer, she is so nervous that he might find something wrong with how she does her job, that she is barely able to speak. Sarah most likely is suffering from
    a. dependent personality disorder.
    b. avoidant personality disorder.
    c. obsessive-compulsive personality disorder.
    d. conversion disorder.
    Answer: b   LO: 19; applied   page: 303

73. The text notes the obvious overlap between avoidant personality disorder and:
    a. simple phobia.
    b. social phobia.
    c. agoraphobia.
    d. obsessive-compulsive disorder.
    Answer: b   LO: 19; factual   page: 304

74. The text states the major difference between avoidant personality disorder and social phobia is that with avoidant personality it is the fear of _____ that causes them to avoid social situations.
    a. other people
    b. being expected to perform and being unable to do so
    c. being unable to escape
    d. being criticized and a general sense of inadequacy
    Answer: d   LO: 19, 20; factual, conceptual   page: 304

75. Which of the following is *true* about avoidant personality disorder?
    a. Children who are naturally shy are at high risk for developing this disorder.
    b. Women are more likely than men to have this disorder.
    c. People with this disorder are at high risk for dysthymia, depression, and anxiety.
    d. The major concern of the avoidant person is fear of performing in public.
    Answer: c   LO: 19; factual, conceptual   page: 304

Chapter 8

76. Mallory is seeing a cognitive therapist, who has diagnosed her with avoidant personality disorder. Dr. Kidd suggests that when Mallory was a child, she was:
   a. rejected by her parents.
   b. overprotected by her parents.
   c. her parents made all her decisions for her.
   d. abused by her parents.
   Answer: a   LO: 19; applied   page: 305

77. The therapies that have been most successful for treating avoidant personality disorder are:
   a. cognitive and psychodynamic, which help the client to understand the underlying causes of the disorder and examine ways to become more self-confident.
   b. cognitive and behavioral, which gradually expose the client to social settings, teach social skills, and challenge negative automatic thoughts.
   c. cognitive and drug therapies to help the client reduce the anxiety engendered by social interactions.
   d. behavioral and drug therapies to help the client reduce the anxiety engendered by social interactions.
   Answer: b   LO: 21; factual, conceptual   page: 305

78. People with avoidant personality disorder _____, whereas people with dependent personality disorder _____.
   a. fear social interactions; need social interactions
   b. fear they will be criticized; have a deep need to be care for by others
   c. fear they will be rejected; fear they will be criticized
   d. avoid people who will reject them; avoid people altogether
   Answer: b   LO: 22; factual, conceptual   page: 305

79. A person with dependent personality disorder:
   a. does not initiate new activities.
   b. attempts to make decisions on the basis of what will please someone else.
   c. allow themselves to be exploited and abused rather than lose a relationship.
   d. avoid people out of fear that they will be exploited and abused.
   Answer: c   LO: 22; factual, conceptual   page: 305

80. Epidemiological studies of dependent personality disorder have reported that:
   a. clinicians are more likely to diagnose this disorder than their clients are to indicate they have it in self-report measures.
   b. more women than men are diagnosed with this disorder in clinical settings.
   c. persons with this disorder are at high risk for alcohol and other substance abuse.
   d. the lifetime prevalence rate of this disorder is approximately 3.4%.
   Answer: b   LO: 22; factual   page: 306

Personality Disorders

81. According to the research reported in our text, it is *most likely* that parents of people with dependent personality disorder were:
    a. neglecting-rejecting.
    b. overprotective.
    c. abusive.
    d. exploitative.
    Answer: b   LO: 22, 27; factual   page: 306

82. A person with which of the following personality disorders would be *most likely* to seek therapy?
    a. dependent personality disorder
    b. avoidant personality disorder
    c. narcissistic personality disorder
    d. histrionic personality disorder
    Answer: a   LO: 22; factual   page: 306

83. Which of the following is *should be avoided* when working with a client who has dependent personality disorder?
    a. helping the client gain insight into the early experiences with caregivers that led to the dependent behaviors
    b. reinforcing the client's tendency to depend on the therapist for help in overcoming the client's problems
    c. exposing the client gradually to anxiety provoking situations and teaching assertiveness in such situations
    d. challenging the client's assumptions about the need to rely on others
    Answer: b   LO: 22; conceptual   pages: 306-307

84. Many societies value the person who demonstrates self-control, attention to detail, perseverance, and reliability. The one word that might *most* accurately differentiate a person with those highly valued characteristics from a person with obsessive-compulsive personality disorder is:
    a. affect.
    b. extreme.
    c. rational.
    d. logical.
    Answer: b   LO: 24; factual   page: 307

Chapter 8

85. Which of the following is *not* an appropriate descriptor for a person with obsessive-compulsive personality disorder?
    a. grim and austere
    b. moralistic
    c. lacking spontaneity
    d. persistent
    Answer: d   LO: 24; factual, conceptual   page: 307

86. Which of the following is *true* about obsessive-compulsive personality disorder?
    a. It is more common in women than in men.
    b. Obsessive-compulsive personality disorder has been linked by family history and twin studies to obsessive-compulsive disorder.
    c. There is a relatively high lifetime prevalence of obsessive-compulsive disorder, between 1.7 and 6.4%.
    d. Their perfectionism, workaholism, and obsessions enhance their value as employees.
    Answer: c   LO: 24; factual, conceptual   page: 308

87. According to Theodore Millon (1981), people with _____ personality disorder had parents who were overcontrolling and punitive when their child made mistakes and did not praise or reward their child when he or she did well.
    a. paranoid
    b. dependent
    c. avoidant
    d. obsessive-compulsive
    Answer: d   LO: 24; factual, conceptual   page: 308

88. Which of the following is *not* mentioned in the text as an appropriate treatment for obsessive-compulsive personality disorder?
    a. being given an assignment to change his usual schedule
    b. learning relaxation techniques to overcome anxiety
    c. understanding early childhood events that led to the disorder
    d. challenging automatic negative thoughts
    Answer: c   LO: 24; factual, conceptual   page: 309

89. _____ personality disorder and _____ personality disorder are similar in terms of their concerns about inadequacy to function competently.
    a. Avoidant; borderline
    b. Avoidant; obsessive-compulsive
    c. Obsessive-compulsive; histrionic
    d. Dependent; avoidant
    Answer: b   LO: 24; factual, conceptual   page: 309

Personality Disorders

90. Some researchers argue that some of the DSM-IV personality disorders perpetuate gender bias because they represent extreme negative stereotypes of women's personalities. Identify the set of personality disorders thought to contain this bias.
    a. antisocial; borderline; dependent
    b. borderline; histrionic; dependent; obsessive-compulsive
    c. borderline; histrionic; dependent
    d. antisocial; avoidant; dependent
    Answer: c   LO: 3; factual, conceptual   page: 309

91. Which personality disorder has been argued to represent an extreme negative stereotype of men?
    a. antisocial
    b. schizoid
    c. schizotypal
    d. obsessive-compulsive
    Answer: a   LO: 3; factual, conceptual   pages: 309-310

92. Which of the following contrasting values was noted in the text to reflect the Western views of mental health and may result in bias in diagnosing persons from other cultural backgrounds?
    a. nature versus nurture
    b. collectivism versus individuality
    c. cooperation versus competition
    d. pluralism versus assimilation
    Answer: b   LO: 3; factual   page: 310

93. Psychodynamic theorists believe that _____ personality disorder results from a poor resolution of the _____ stage of psychosexual development.
    a. antisocial; anal
    b. dependent; oral
    c. histrionic; oral
    d. borderline; oral
    Answer: b   LO: 27; factual, conceptual   page: 312

94. Dr. Morf is a psychodynamic therapist. She has diagnosed Harold as having obsessive-compulsive personality disorder and has determined that this disorder results from a poor resolution of the _____ stage.
    a. oral
    b. anal
    c. phallic
    d. genital
    Answer: b   LO: 27; applied   page: 312

Chapter 8

95. Which of the following statements is *true* about the treatments for certain personality disorders?
    a. Cognitive-behavioral therapy has been shown to increase the number of social contacts and enjoyment of social interactions among people with avoidant personality disorder.
    b. Neuroleptic drugs help schizoid clients reduce their odd thinking.
    c. Group therapy may be especially effective for histrionic personality disorder.
    d. Selective serotonin reuptake inhibitors have been shown to reduce obsessions and compulsive behaviors among people with obsessive-compulsive personality disorder.
    Answer: a   LO: 10, 16, 21, 24; factual   page: 305

96. Which of the following is *least likely* to attempt and to complete suicide?
    a. borderline personality disorder
    b. histrionic personality disorder
    c. antisocial personality disorder
    d. narcissistic personality disorder
    Answer: d   LO: 17; factual, conceptual   pages: 292, 296, 300, 303

97. Carrie began to see signs of the various personality disorders in most of the people she knew. Which of the following questions would be *least* helpful to her in deciding if these people really do have the disorders?
    a. What are the situational factors that influence the behavior?
    b. Am I selectively remembering (or forgetting) behaviors?
    c. How interesting are these behaviors to me?
    d. Are these behaviors significantly impairing or causing distress for this person or others involved with this person?
    Answer: c   LO: 3 ; applied   page: 313

Personality Disorders

Essay Questions

98. Imagine that you are a parent and want to ensure that your child will grow up emotionally healthy. Consider the theories presented in this chapter that argue that certain types of parenting practices, and their effects on a growing child, can lead to personality disorders (either directly or in conjunction with genetic factors). Along similar lines, many of the psychotherapies for personality disorders described in this chapter use methods that are similar to certain types of adaptive parenting practices. Select two of the personality disorders and do the following with each: (1) summarize its key features, including its symptoms and any associated disorders or risks that accompany it; (2) describe in detail the type of parenting believed to lead to the disorder (including the theorist whose theory you are describing); and (3) explain how psychotherapy for the disorder focuses on eliminating maladaptive behaviors acquired as a result of the parenting described in (2), and how it attempts to construct adaptive behaviors.

    For each disorder, the student should present the diagnostic criteria that characterize the disorders and differential diagnosis, as well as how the disorders are associated with other similar disorders (such as those found in relatives) and other problems that might result from having the disorder. The various forms of parenting (whether harsh and abusive, neglecting rejecting, overprotective, etc.) should be addressed as relevant to the particular disorders and the theorists connected with that perspective (e.g., Klein and object relations). The student will need to address the cognitive and psychodynamic approaches to understanding the roots of the problem, and the psychodynamic, cognitive, behavioral, and cognitive-behavioral techniques that have been found to be effective, as appropriate.

99. The personality disorders are highly controversial in clinical psychology and psychiatry. What are the reasons for these controversies? Do you think that the DSM-IV personality disorders can be defended against these claims? If so, why? If not, why not? Are there any ways that you can think of to improve the DSM-IV so that its authors are not accused of these claims?

    One major issue here is bias--both gender bias and cultural bias. This should be addressed by the student (many of these disorders stereotype women as dependent, labile, etc., and men as aggressive and ruthless; and they assume a value system based on Western belief systems), as well as the question of whether these are actually sufficiently distinct from normal behavior as to deserve categorization. Then the student should become creative in defending one side or the other and talking about how to improve the system.

Chapter 8

100. Many theorists claim that the personality disorders perpetuate both gender-based and cultural biases. Summarize the arguments and the points made by theorists who hold these views. Do you think that the DSM-IV personality disorders can be defended against these claims? If so, why? If not, why not? Are there any ways that you can think of to improve the DSM-IV so that its authors are not accused of these biases?

    This question would require similar responses as in question 99 without the issue of whether the disorders are sufficiently different to require categorization. The student should present the four arguments concerning gender bias and the two arguments concerning cultural bias presented in the text.

101. The text discusses that one view of the personality disorders is that they are merely exaggerations of normal behaviors; another suggests that at least some of these are milder forms of Axis I disorders. Discuss one personality disorder that supports the former position and a second to support the latter. Include the diagnostic criteria for both personality disorders as well as the Axis I disorder, and include a differential diagnosis for the comparison between the personality disorder and the Axis I disorder. Then present your own position in this debate, supporting your argument with evidence from the text.

    The primary issue here is exactly how different these disorders are from (a) normal behavior, and (b) Axis I disorders. The student should proceed on a continuum from normal to extreme, with the personality order of choice in the middle. One suggestion may be to discuss the relationship between schizotypal personality disorder and schizophrenia. The student then will support his or her argument using evidence from the text

102. It is common for students of abnormal psychology to see signs of many mental disorders in themselves as well as in other people they know. Further, people are more likely to state they have such a disorder when completing a self-report questionnaire than a therapist would do when assessing someone in a clinical setting. Explain the two reasons for this that are discussed in the text. Then pick two personality disorders that you considered as you read the chapter would apply to yourself or someone you know, and (1) state what each disorder is and the diagnostic criteria for those disorders; (2) state why you felt they would apply; (3) discuss the rationale in the chapter for why they probably do not apply. If, after answering this question, you still believe they do apply, what action (if any) do you feel would be appropriate from your own perspective, and how do you think a therapist would work with each of these persons?

    The text suggested that diagnoses for personality disorders are vague and thus leave room for much interpretation, and then it addresses the fundamental attribution error, viz., overattributing behavior to personality traits and underestimating the power of the situation. For each of the two disorders the student chooses, she or he should

Personality Disorders

name the disorder and provide the DSM-IV diagnostic criteria, apply the behaviors in self or others that would be consistent with those in DSM, explain how they differ and the cautions noted in the text about how they probably do not apply--look at situational influences, are certain behaviors being exaggerated while others are being ignored, are these consistent patterns of behavior or only seen occasionally, and do the behaviors cause distress in anyone's life (self or other)? The student should then determine, if these seem to be a diagnosable disorder (a) what the student should do about it and (b) how a therapist would treat each of these disorders.

Chapter 9   Childhood Disorders

1. Although we like to think of childhood as a wonderful, relatively stress-free period, where children are able to enjoy a "carefree existence," the reality is that almost ____% of children and ____% of adolescents suffer from significant emotional or behavioral disorders.
   a. 10; 20
   b. 15; 30
   c. 20; 40
   d. 25; 50
   Answer: c LO: 1; factual page: 318

2. Which of the following is *not* listed in the text as one of the major stressors faced by children in the United States on a daily basis?
   a. lack of education
   b. severe physical abuse
   c. living in poverty
   d. exposure to violence
   Answer: a LO: 1; factual page: 318

3. Which of the following is likely to be a factor in helping children to become sufficiently resilient as to avoid major problems resulting from stress?
   a. financial security
   b. a safe environment
   c. good physical health
   d. a competent adult mentor
   Answer: d LO: 1; factual, conceptual page: 318

4. Most psychological disorders in children result from:
   a. primarily biological factors.
   b. primarily environmental factors.
   c. multiple factors, including biological and environmental.
   d. innate temperament.
   Answer: c LO: 1; factual, conceptual page: 319

Childhood Disorders

5. Which child is *least likely* to develop a psychological disorder?
    a. Terry, a 5-year-old boy who lives in the projects with his single mother, who has always had a happy, outgoing personality.
    b. Kenny, a grumpy 5-year-old boy who lives with his parents in an exclusive neighborhood.
    c. Sarah, a shy 6-year-old girl who has become socially withdrawn since being sexually molested by her mother's boyfriend.
    d. Cindy, a very active 3-year-old whose mother died in childbirth and whose father is a rich, but alcoholic professional.
    Answer: a   LO: 1; applied   page: 319

6. Which of the following is *not* one of the factors listed in the text that developmental psychopathologists consider with respect to its impact on the symptoms of childhood psychopathology?
    a. level of cognitive development
    b. level of social development
    c. level of emotional development
    d. level of behavioral development
    Answer: d   LO: 1; conceptual   page: 319

7. The behavior disorders include:
    a. attention deficit disorder, oppositional defiant disorder, and conduct disorder.
    b. separation anxiety and childhood depression.
    c. autism and mental retardation.
    d. enuresis and encopresis.
    Answer: a   LO: 1; factual   page: 320

8. A child whose behavior involves hyperactivity has:
    a. a behavior disorder.
    b. an emotional disorder.
    c. a developmental disorder.
    d. a habit disorder.
    Answer: a   LO: 1; factual   page: 320

9. Which of the following statements about attention deficit/hyperactivity disorder (ADHD) is *false*?
    a. ADHD is a common precursor to conduct disorder.
    b. ADHD continues into adolescence for two-thirds of children.
    c. Many adults with a history of underachievement and poor relationships have been found to have had ADHD as children but were not diagnosed.
    d. ADHD children typically perform below their intellectual capabilities.
    Answer: c   LO: 1; factual   page: 320-321

Chapter 9

10. Which of the following is a ***true*** statement concerning ADHD?
    a. Approximately 15% of children with ADHD have serious learning disabilities that make it especially difficult for them to concentrate in school and learn.
    b. Children with ADHD tend to select only one or two really close friends and are generally rejected by the remainder of their peers.
    c. Approximately 40% of children with ADHD develop conduct disorders or become juvenile delinquents.
    d. ADHD has become a popular diagnosis for children who are disruptive in school or at home.
    Answer: d LO: 2; factual, conceptual page: 321

11. With respect to the prevalence factors of ADHD, which of the following is ***true***?
    a. Approximately 10% of children in the United States develop ADHD.
    b. Boys are three times more likely than girls to develop ADHD.
    c. ADHD is unique to industrialized cultures.
    d. ADHD is probably underdiagnosed in adulthood.
    Answer: b LO: 2; factual page: 321

12. Which of the following have ***not*** been found to predispose children to ADHD?
    a. premature delivery
    b. having an older mother
    c. maternal nicotine consumption
    d. exposure to high concentrations of lead
    Answer: b LO: 3; factual pages: 322-323

13. Which of the following is ***true*** concerning the neurological findings for ADHD children?
    a. They have been noted to have brain damage.
    b. They have higher cerebral blood flow than other children.
    c. They have a variety of abnormalities in EEG readings.
    d. Most children with some brain injury develop ADHD.
    Answer: c LO: 3; factual page: 322

14. What connection have researchers found between diet and ADHD?
    a. Sugar has been implicated as a major contributor to hyperactive behavior.
    b. High sodium will exacerbate an ADHD child's already high activity level.
    c. Coca Cola is beneficial for children with ADHD because even though the sugar may create more hyperactivity, the caffeine actually calms them down.
    d. In controlled research studies, no connection has been found between diet and ADHD.
    Answer: d LO: 3; factual page: 323

Childhood Disorders

15. Children with ADHD are more likely than children without psychological disturbances to:
    a. come from families with schizophrenic fathers and depressed mothers.
    b. exhibit minimal brain damage.
    c. consume inordinate amounts of sugar.
    d. have fathers with criminal behavior.
    Answer: d   LO: 1; factual   page: 323

16. The drugs *most likely* to reduce the disruptive behavior of hyperactive children are:
    a. antidepressants.
    b. stimulants.
    c. tranquilizers.
    d. anti-anxiety drugs.
    Answer: b   LO: 4; factual   page: 323

17. The controversy surrounding the use of drugs for treating children diagnosed with ADHD concerns:
    a. their highly addictive nature.
    b. the high profits that drug manufacturers make by having the drugs overprescribed.
    c. overdiagnosing the disorder and using drugs to control all disruptive behavior.
    d. whether they are actually effective in controlling the targeted behaviors.
    Answer: c   LO: 4; factual, conceptual   page: 323

18. The most effective long-term treatments for ADHD have been seen with:
    a. use of such stimulant drugs as Ritalin.
    b. extinguishing impulsive behaviors and reinforcing prosocial behaviors.
    c. treating the parents' psychological problems and teaching better parenting skills.
    d. All of the above in combination provide the best long-term treatment.
    Answer: d   LO: 4; factual, conceptual   page: 324

19. The most positive treatment outcomes for ADHD are seen when:
    a. parents are taught to deal with their children so they can take over training the child.
    b. treatment begins early in childhood.
    c. treatment waits until the child is older and has the cognitive ability to learn.
    d. the child is placed on drug therapy.
    Answer: b   LO: 4; factual, conceptual   page: 324

20. A child with a chronic pattern of unconcern for the basic rights of others is diagnosed with:
    a. attention deficit disorder (ADD).
    b. attention deficit/hyperactivity disorder (ADHD).
    c. oppositional defiant disorder (ODD).
    d. conduct disorder.
    Answer: d   LO: 5, 6; factual   page: 324

Chapter 9

21. A child who is argumentative, negative, irritable, and defiant is likely to be diagnosed with:
    a. attention deficit disorder (ADD).
    b. attention deficit/hyperactivity disorder (ADHD).
    c. oppositional defiant disorder (ODD).
    d. conduct disorder.
    Answer: c   LO: 5, 6; factual   page: 324

22. Which statement about conduct disorder and oppositional defiant disorder is *false*?
    a. Conduct disorder begins early in life, during toddler and preschool years, whereas oppositional defiant disorder does not begin until the mid-elementary school years.
    b. The majority of children with conduct disorder have problems into adulthood, such as unstable relationships and impulsive aggression, while most children with oppositional defiant disorder outgrow their symptoms.
    c. Girls with conduct disorder have high rates of criminal activity as adults.
    d. Boys tend to manifest aggression in a physical manner, whereas girls tend to manifest aggression in an indirect and verbal manner.
    Answer: a   LO: 5, 6; factual, conceptual   pages: 326-327

23. Studies that have examined the biology of conduct disorder and aggression have found that many children with the disorder have any or all of the following *except*:
    a. neurological deficits.
    b. a genetic history of antisocial behavior among first-degree relatives.
    c. higher levels of adrenaline.
    d. difficult temperaments as infants.
    Answer: c   LO: 5, 6; factual   page: 327

24. In terms of prevalence factors for oppositional defiant disorder and conduct disorder, which of the following is *false*?
    a. Boys are three times more likely than girls to be diagnosed with both disorders.
    b. The disorders are found more frequently in children in lower socioeconomic classes.
    c. The disorders are found more frequently in children in rural rather than urban settings.
    d. Both boys and girls with these disorders are at risk for severe problems throughout their lives.
    Answer: c   LO: 5, 6; factual, conceptual   page: 327

25. Which of the following is *not* a reason the text states is a possible explanation for higher rates of conduct disorder and oppositional defiant disorder children of low socioeconomic status?
    a. poverty
    b. poor parenting
    c. downward social drift
    d. neurological deficits.
    Answer: d   LO: 5, 6; factual   page: 327

Childhood Disorders

26. Research exploring the connection between neurological disorders and child psychopathology have found evidence that neurological deficits play a:
    a. role in ADHD but not in conduct disorders.
    b. role in both ADHD and conduct disorders.
    c. role in conduct disorders but not in ADHD.
    d. different role in ADHD than they do in conduct disorders.
    Answer: b   LO: 7; factual   pages: 327-328

27. Loeber (1990) suggested that the path to developing conduct disorder begins with:
    a. exposure to neurotoxins and drugs in utero or in preschool years.
    b. poor parenting practices.
    c. difficult socioeconomic conditions.
    d. genetic heritage.
    Answer: a   LO: 7; factual   page: 328

28. As infants, children with conduct disorder were:
    a. relatively nonresponsive to their environments.
    b. shy and reticent.
    c. irritable and demanding.
    d. overactive.
    Answer: c   LO: 7; factual   page: 328

29. Research by Loeber (1990) on conduct disorder found that one of the best predictors of children's conduct disturbances is:
    a. the child's temperament in infancy.
    b. parental supervision.
    c. genetic heritage.
    d. neurological functioning.
    Answer: b   LO: 8; factual, conceptual   page: 329

30. Which of the following is *false* about the parenting practices of parents of children with conduct disorders?
    a. The parents tend to neglect their children and are often absent from the home.
    b. The parents lashes out violently at their children when the youngsters "transgress."
    c. Interactions with their children are characterized by hostility, violence, and ridicule.
    d. Perhaps because they are easier targets, girls receive more severe punishments than boys.
    Answer: d   LO: 8; factual   page: 329

Chapter 9

31. Henry has been a schoolyard bully since he was 8 years old. When he first began starting fights with other kids it was just with his fists, now that he's older he's begun using a knife that he carries around in his pocket. He also uses the knife to scratch the sides of people's cars, and he's been in juvenile hall twice already for petty theft and arson. Most likely he has:
    a. ADD.
    b. ADHD.
    c. oppositional defiant disorder.
    d. conduct disorder.
    Answer: d   LO: 8; applied   pages: 324-330

32. Which of the following is *not* a typical way of thinking of a youngster with conduct disorder?
    a. "Bobby bumped into me. He was trying to get into a fight. I'll get him good after recess."
    b. "My pen was on Miss Marchand's desk. James knew it was my pen, and he took it on purpose. I'll get even with him."
    c. "Becky ignores me whenever I try to talk to her. Maybe if I smile at her or carry her books for her, she'd stop ignoring me."
    d. "Ginger snubbed me. The whole world's against me. But just wait. One day I'll let her know who's superior."
    Answer: c   LO: 8; applied   page: 330

33. Psychosocial therapies for conduct disorder use all of the following steps *except* teaching the child:
    a. how to use aggressive rather than assertive behavior.
    b. to take and care about other people's perspectives.
    c. to use "self-talk" to control impulsive behaviors.
    d. adaptive ways to achieve conflict resolution.
    Answer: a   LO: 9; factual, conceptual   page: 331

34. Jimmy complained to his therapist that Aaron, a boy he can't stand, cut in front of him in the lunch line. The therapist worked with Jimmy on understanding why Aaron might have done this and also on ways to use assertiveness to make his feelings known. What type of technique is the therapist using?
    a. behavior modification
    b. systematic desensitization
    c. problem-solving skills
    d. challenging assumptions
    Answer: c   LO: 9; applied   page: 330

Childhood Disorders

35. The psychosocial therapies for conduct disorder are based on:
    a.   classical conditioning.
    b.   operant conditioning.
    c.   insight learning.
    d.   social learning theory.
    Answer: d   LO: 9; factual, conceptual   page: 331

36. If a child's problem involves excessive shyness and fear, the child has:
    a.   a behavior disorder.
    b.   an emotional disorder.
    c.   a conduct disorder.
    d.   a developmental disorder.
    Answer: b   LO: 10; factual, conceptual   page: 333

37. An emotional disorder that is specific to childhood and not diagnosed for adults is:
    a.   separation anxiety disorder.
    b.   dependency disorder.
    c.   autism.
    d.   ADHD.
    Answer: a   LO: 11; factual   page: 333

38. Children whose parents have _____ are three times more likely to develop separation anxiety disorder than the children of parents without the disorder.
    a.   generalized anxiety disorder
    b.   post-traumatic stress disorder
    c.   social phobia
    d.   panic disorder
    Answer: d   LO: 11; factual   page: 334

39. Three-year-old Tiffany cried inconsolably almost the entire day, from the time her mother dropped her off at day care until her mother picked her up. She might stop for a few moments if "Teacher Mary" distracted her but would resume within a short period of time. Despite cooperation from Tiffany's mother and different interventions, the behavior went on for months until Tiffany had to be removed from the day care center because her behavior so disrupted the other children and the staff. Tiffany appears to have had:
    a.   panic disorder.
    b.   depression.
    c.   separation anxiety.
    d.   oppositional defiant disorder.
    Answer: c   LO: 11; applied   pages: 333-334

Chapter 9

40. Which of the following is *true* about separation anxiety disorder?
    a. It occurs in about 5% of preadolescent children.
    b. It is more common in boys than in girls.
    c. Left untreated, the child will eventually grow out of it.
    d. Children with the disorder tend to have somatic symptoms.
    Answer: d   LO: 11; factual   page: 334

41. The symptoms that children with separation anxiety exhibit when separated from their parents are similar to symptoms seen in adults with:
    a. social phobias.
    b. dependent personality disorder.
    c. panic disorder.
    d. dissociative disorders.
    Answer: c   LO: 11; factual   page: 334

42. Which of the following is *most accurate* concerning the development of separation anxiety?
    a. It often develops following a traumatic event.
    b. The parents of children with separation anxiety tend to be neglecting and rejecting.
    c. The parents of children with separation anxiety tend to use harsh punishment.
    d. The families of children with separation anxiety are disengaged, with extremely loose boundaries.
    Answer: a   LO: 12; factual   page: 334

43. Which of the following components of treatment for separation anxiety disorder *has not been* shown consistently to help children recover from the disorder?
    a. teaching relaxation exercises to children with the disorder
    b. administering imipramine to reduce the symptoms of the disorder
    c. teaching parents to model non-anxious reactions to separation from their child
    d. adding a cognitive component to the therapy by teaching children to use "self-talk"
    Answer: b   LO: 13; factual   pages: 335-336

44. Children over the age of 5 are diagnosed with _____ when they have wet the bed or their clothes at least twice a week for 3 months.
    a. enuresis
    b. encopresis
    c. urinary tract infection
    d. bladder disorder
    Answer: a   LO: 14; factual   page: 336

Childhood Disorders

45. Children over the age of four are diagnosed with _____ when they have defecated into their clothing or onto the floor at least once a month for at least 3 months.
    a. enuresis
    b. encopresis
    c. intestinal infection
    d. bowel disorder
    Answer: b   LO: 14; factual   page: 336

46. Which of the following theories is *not* mentioned in the text as a likely basis of enuresis?
    a. biological
    b. psychodynamic
    c. cognitive
    d. behavioral
    Answer: c   LO: 14; factual   pages: 336-337

47. Research on enuresis indicates that:
    a. about 75% of children with enuresis have a biological relative who had it also.
    b. many of the children with the disorder have enlarged bladders that tend to overfill.
    c. this disorder is considerably less common than encopresis.
    d. if parents can be patient, the disorder will resolve itself by age 5.
    Answer: a   LO: 14; factual   page: 336

48. With respect to prevalence of enuresis:
    a. it is more common in girls.
    b. it is more common in boys.
    c. it is an extremely rare disorder for both boys and girls.
    d. it is more likely to occur in industrialized countries than nonindustrialized societies.
    Answer: b   LO: 14; factual   page: 336

49. The most effective treatment for enuresis is:
    a. patience--waiting for the child to outgrow it.
    b. peer pressure.
    c. the bell-and-pad method.
    d. antidepressant medication.
    Answer: c   LO: 14; factual   page: 337

Chapter 9

50. Eight-year-old Matthew has no friends, although he and his two older brothers have been involved in sports from a young age. Matthew's peers at school want nothing to do with him because they say he "stinks." His parents are strict but warm and loving and clearly enjoy interacting with their sons. Matthew's mother has taken him to doctors who treat him with laxatives and other high fiber remedies, and suggest schedules for feeding and going to the toilet; she has taken him to therapists to look for a psychological reason for the "accidents" he has, both at home and at school, where he defecates in his clothes. Matthew is plagued with:
    a. enuresis.
    b. encopresis.
    c. bowel disorder.
    d. intestinal tract disorder.
    Answer: b LO: 14; applied pages: 336-337

51. When important cognitive, motor, and social skills do not emerge fully in a child, such as not beginning to crawl or walk until many months after most other children, we would suspect that the child has a _____ disorder.
    a. behavioral
    b. emotional
    c. developmental
    d. psychosocial
    Answer: c LO: 15; factual, conceptual page: 337

52. Jenny has trouble holding onto objects, such as drinking glasses, pencils, and crayons. She began crawling and walking a full 10 months after most children and still stumbles a lot when she tries to run. We would suspect that the type of developmental disorder Jenny has is:
    a. an expression disorder.
    b. a motor skills disorder.
    c. a social skills disorder.
    d. a cognitive skills disorder.
    Answer: b LO: 15; applied page: 337

53. The two types of developmental disorder that involve deficits in a wide range of skills are:
    a. motor skills disorder and social skills disorder.
    b. mental retardation and autism.
    c. mental retardation and cognitive skills disorder.
    d. mental retardation and social skills disorder.
    Answer: b LO: 15; factual page: 337

Childhood Disorders

54. Children with significant delays in language development, who can acquire very simple vocational skills with special education, but cannot achieve beyond the second grade in academic skills, and have IQ scores between 35 and 50, are said to have which level of mental retardation?
    a. mild
    b. moderate
    c. severe
    d. profound
    Answer: b   LO: 16; factual, conceptual   page: 338

55. To be diagnosed as mentally retarded, a child must not only score low on an IQ test but must also show significant problems in performing the tasks of daily life on at least two of the following activities:
    a. communication and self-care.
    b. reading and math skills.
    c. home living and math skills.
    d. use of community resources and spatial skills.
    Answer: a   LO: 16; factual   page: 338

56. Most people who are mentally retarded fall into which category of mental retardation?
    a. mild
    b. moderate
    c. severe
    d. profound
    Answer: a   LO: 16; factual   page: 338

57. Charlie is 35 years old, yet he can only speak in sentences of two or three words, and he has a very limited vocabulary. He can use a spoon to feed himself and can button his jacket, but he can't cook and doesn't travel by himself because he gets confused and doesn't know where he is. When his IQ was tested, his score was 32. Charlie would be categorized as:
    a. mildly retarded.
    b. moderately retarded.
    c. severely retarded.
    d. profoundly retarded.
    Answer: c   LO: 16; applied   page: 338

Chapter 9

58. Johnny has a round, flat face and almond-shaped eyes, a small nose, slightly protruding lip and tongue, and short square hands. He is short, slightly obese, and mildly retarded. It is like that Johnny has:
    a. Tay-Sachs disease.
    b. phenylketonuria.
    c. Down syndrome.
    d. autism.
    Answer: c   LO: 16; factual   page: 338

59. Cultural-familial retardation results from _____ factors.
    a. genetic
    b. environmental
    c. genetic and environmental
    d. environmental and sociological
    Answer: c   LO: 16; factual   pages: 338-339

60. Down's syndrome results from:
    a. faulty learning.
    b. a metabolic abnormality.
    c. a deficient neurotransmitter.
    d. a chromosomal abnormality.
    Answer: d   LO: 16; factual   page: 339

61. Which of the following childhood diseases resembles Alzheimer's disease in that both consist of tangles and plaques on neurons in the brain, as well as memory loss and an inability to care for oneself?
    a. phenylketonuria (PKU)
    b. fetal alcohol syndrome
    c. fragile X syndrome
    d. Down syndrome
    Answer: d   LO: 17; factual   page: 339

62. Which of the following genetic dysfunctions is the most common cause of mental retardation?
    a. Tay-Sachs disease
    b. fragile X syndrome
    c. Trisomy 21
    d. phenylketonuria
    Answer: c   LO: 17; factual   page: 339

Childhood Disorders

63. Phenylketonuria (PKU) results from:
    a. behavioral origins.
    b. a metabolic abnormality.
    c. a neurotransmitter deficiency.
    d. a hormonal abnormality.
    Answer: b   LO: 17; factual   page: 339

64. A disease caused by a faulty recessive gene that occurs primarily in Jewish families from eastern Europe and causes a progressive degeneration of the nervous system that leads to mental and physical deterioration that is generally fatal by age 6 is:
    a. phenylketonuria.
    b. Tay-Sachs disease.
    c. Trisomy 21.
    d. fetal alcohol syndrome.
    Answer: b   LO: 18; factual   page: 339

65. All of the following genetic abnormalities lead to severe or profound mental retardation (as opposed to mild or moderate) *except*:
    a. Trisomy 13.
    b. fragile X syndrome.
    c. Trisomy 18.
    d. Trisomy 21.
    Answer: d   LO: 17; factual   pages: 339-340

66. Christopher is severely retarded. He has speech defects and is incapable of establishing or maintaining effective interpersonal interactions. His ears are large and his face is long. He most likely has:
    a. fragile X syndrome.
    b. autism.
    c. Down syndrome.
    d. Trisomy 18.
    Answer: a   LO: 18; applied   pages: 339-340

67. Which of the following will *not* have an effect on the intellectual development of the fetus?
    a. rubella
    b. herpes and syphilis
    c. maternal high blood pressure and diabetes
    d. sudden infant death syndrome (SIDS)
    Answer: d   LO: 18; factual   page: 340

Chapter 9

68. How much alcohol may a pregnant woman consume without endangering her unborn child?
    a. one glass of beer or wine a day
    b. one ounce of hard liquor a day
    c. one glass of beer or wine a week
    d. It is not currently known whether there is *any* safe amount during pregnancy.
    Answer: d　　　　　LO: 18; factual　　　　　　　　　　　page: 340

69. Michael Dorris, an anthropologist, became a single father when he adopted an orphaned Lakota boy named Adam. Adam was a beautiful, loving, and affectionate child, but he was never able to learn from experience. He was easily distractible, had difficulty perceiving social cues, could not follow directions, and was almost uneducable. After years of frustration in trying to overcome Adam's early years of deprivation, Dorris traced his son's beginnings, learned the birth mother had died from alcoholism, and finally realized that his son was retarded due to:
    a. fragile X syndrome.
    b. fetal alcohol syndrome.
    c. autism.
    d. Down syndrome.
    Answer: b　　　　　LO: 18; applied　　　　　　　　　　page: 340

70. Which of the following does *not* increase the risk of premature births?
    a. smoking cigarettes
    b. poor prenatal care
    c. drug abuse
    d. rubella
    Answer: d　　　　　LO: 18; applied　　　　　　　　　　page: 340

71. A primary reason that infants born several week premature are at increased risk for mental retardation is that:
    a. they are more likely to have central nervous system damage.
    b. their respiratory system is not fully developed.
    c. their motor skills are not sufficiently developed to interact with the environment.
    d. their mothers are more likely to be of low intelligence.
    Answer: a　　　　　LO: 18; factual　　　　　　　　　　　page: 340

72. Which of the following is *false* about shaken baby syndrome?
    a. It is caused when a baby is shaken violently.
    b. It can cause bleeding in and around the brain and behind the eyes.
    c. It almost always occurs within a pattern of physical abuse by a parent.
    d. It can lead to seizures, blindness, paralysis, mental retardation, or death.
    Answer: c　　　　　LO: 18; factual　　　　　　　　　　　pages: 340-341

Childhood Disorders

73. Which of the following is *not* a sociocultural factor presented in the text as being associated with mental retardation?
    a. parental mental retardation
    b. poor prenatal care
    c. lack of attention from teachers
    d. high crime rates
    Answer: d   LO: 19; factual   page: 341

74. Which of the following is *true* about the effectiveness of interventions for mental retardation?
    a. Children with intellectual deficits who participate in early intervention programs, such as Head Start, tend to show long-term gains in academic and social skills.
    b. African-American and Latino children with mental retardation are more likely to be institutionalized than Euro-American children.
    c. Studies have shown that retarded children who are mainstreamed into regular classrooms outperform children of the same age who are in special education classes.
    d. African-American children benefit more than Euro-American children from interventions that target children at risk for mental retardation.
    Answer: d   LO: 20; 21; factual   pages: 341-343

75. Which of the following educational strategies has been most effective for training mentally retarded children?
    a. mainstreaming them
    b. placement in special education classes
    c. institutionalization
    d. the research is inconclusive on whether it is best to mainstream these children, institutionalize them, or segregate them into special education classes.
    Answer: d   LO: 20; 21; factual   pages: 341-343

76. As an infant, Robert was diagnosed as moderately mentally retarded. He has had seven major illnesses so far in his short five years of life, which the doctors attribute to his genetic abnormalities. His brother, Ron, and sister, Robin, are both healthy children who do well socially and academically. There is no family history of retardation. What type of retardation does Robert have?
    a. organic
    b. cultural-familial
    c. social
    d. genetic
    Answer: a   LO: 20; applied   pages: 343-346

Chapter 9

77. As an infant, Robert was diagnosed as moderately mentally retarded. He has had seven major illnesses so far in his short five years of life, which the doctors attribute to his genetic abnormalities. His brother, Ron, and sister, Robin, are both healthy children who do well socially and academically. There is no family history of retardation. What is his prognosis for improved functioning?
    a. no possibility of improvement or cure
    b. possibly improvement but no cure
    c. possibly complete cure
    d. It will not be possible to determine this until he has started school.
    Answer: b   LO: 20; applied   pages: 343-346

78. When Sondra entered first grade, Ms. Maxwell noticed the child was having difficulty with learning the alphabet, as well as learning the names of her classmates. When Ms. Maxwell consulted the school psychologist, she found that Sondra's older sister had similar problems. Both girls are in good health, and although they wear the same clothes almost every day, they are always neat and clean. If Sondra has cultural-familial retardation, what is her prognosis for improved functioning?
    a. no possibility of improvement or cure
    b. possibly improvement but no cure
    c. possibly complete cure
    d. It will not be possible to determine this until she has finished first grade.
    Answer: c   LO: 20; applied   page: 339

79. Which of the following is *true* about autism?
    a. Autistic children have deficits in social interactions because they are preoccupied with delusions and hallucinations.
    b. Most autistic children have parents who are poorly educated and are of low socioeconomic status.
    c. Autistic children engage in repetitive behaviors, such as hand-flapping or echolalia, that are similar to some symptoms of schizophrenia.
    d. The majority of autistic children are people with severe deficits in some areas but some special talents in others, known as "idiot savants."
    Answer: c   LO: 22; factual, conceptual   page: 344

80. Which of the following have *not* been found to be associated with the development of autism?
    a. having parents who are cold, distant, and uncaring, which leads a child to retreat to an inward world of fantasies
    b. having a biological relative with autism and thus a greater genetic vulnerability
    c. having fragile X syndrome
    d. having prenatal and birth complications and thus possible neurological damage
    Answer: a   LO: 22; factual   page: 346

Childhood Disorders

81. Which of the following is *not* a symptom of autism?
    a. little reciprocity in social interactions
    b. unattractive physical appearance
    c. delay in or total absence of spoken language
    d. stereotyped and repetitive movements
    Answer: b   LO: 22; factual   pages: 344-345

82. As a baby, Ricky rocked back and forth in his crib for hours on end. The movement was so vigorous that his next door neighbor could hear the crib banging up against their shared bedroom walls. By the time he was 4 years old he was still not toilet trained and his language abilities were limited to repeating exactly what was said to him, although sometimes he would sing jingles he heard from television commercials. When his mother held him, he became rigid and fought to be let go. As his pediatrician, you would diagnose Ricky with:
    a. mental retardation.
    b. oppositional defiant disorder.
    c. autism.
    d. Down syndrome.
    Answer: c   LO: 22; applied   pages: 344-346

83. Whenever Enrique talked, he would repeat the exact words that were said to him. So, if you asked him, "How are you, Enrique?" he would respond, "How are you, Enrique?" This type of language deficit in autistic children is referred to as:
    a. echolalia.
    b. apraxia.
    c. alogia.
    d. mimicking.
    Answer: a   LO: 22; applied   page: 345

84. Which of the following is of major importance to autistic children?
    a. new toys
    b. routines and rituals
    c. being held
    d. communication
    Answer: b   LO: 22; factual, conceptual   page: 345

85. Which of the following is *true* about autism?
    a. The onset is after entry into school.
    b. Somewhere between 10 and 20% of autistic children "grow out" of autism.
    c. A person who "recovers" from autism will be able to lead a completely normal life.
    d. Children who live in poverty are at highest risk for developing autism.
    Answer: b   LO: 23; factual   page: 345

Chapter 9

86. The child's _____ is the ***best predictor*** of the outcome of autism.
    a. ethnicity and socioeconomic status
    b. genetic makeup
    c. family history
    d. IQ and amount of language development
    Answer: d   LO: 23; factual   page: 345

87. The current belief about the etiology of autism focuses primarily on:
    a. parenting (specifically, the "refrigerator mother").
    b. unconscious desires to withdraw from a frightening world.
    c. biological causes.
    d. learned behavior.
    Answer: c   LO: 24; factual   pages: 346-347

88. The biological evidence noted in relation to autism would suggest:
    a. that it is primarily an environmentally determined disorder.
    b. that there are several subtypes of the disorder.
    c. that parenting practices are the most critical element in its development.
    d. that there is currently no support for a biological basis of the disorder.
    Answer: b   LO: 24; factual   page: 346

89. All of the following drugs have been shown to reduce some of the symptoms of autism ***except***:
    a. phenothiazines and stimulants.
    b. selective serotonin reuptake inhibitors.
    c. lithium.
    d. All of these drugs appear to be effective for reducing autistic symptoms.
    Answer: d   LO: 25; factual   page: 347

90. Currently, the most effective treatments for autism revolve around _____ therapies.
    a. behavioral
    b. biological
    c. cognitive
    d. psychoanalytic
    Answer: a   LO: 25; factual   page: 347

Childhood Disorders

91. Studies conducted by Ivar Lovaas (1987) have found that _____ resulted in almost 50% of autistic children achieving normal intellectual and educational functioning by age 7.
    a. intensive use of behavioral techniques of modeling and reinforcement to increase social interactions and reduce inappropriate behaviors
    b. teaching parents to use warmth and affection when interacting with their children
    c. providing institutional care where children's physical needs were looked after on a constant basis
    d. ignoring unacceptable behaviors and reinforcing desired behaviors
    Answer: a   LO: 25; factual   page: 347

92. Which of the following disorders is a child *least likely* to "grow out of"?
    a. enuresis
    b. encopresis
    c. autism
    d. separation anxiety disorder
    Answer: c   LO: 23, 25; factual   pages: 333, 336-337, 345

93. All of the following statements about gender differences in childhood disorders have been supported by evidence *except*:
    a. boys are more likely than girls to suffer from most major childhood diseases, which can predispose a child to several of the childhood disorders
    b. adults are more tolerant of deviance in boys than in girls
    c. girls express their distress and deviance in more socially acceptable ways than boys
    d. that rates of depression and anxiety increase for girls in adolescence, whereas boys do not show this increase and may even have decreased rates of most disorders.
    Answer: b   LO: 26; factual, conceptual   page: 348

94. Which of the following childhood disorders is found more often in girls than in boys?
    a. attention deficit/hyperactivity disorder
    b. separation anxiety disorder
    c. autism
    d. mental retardation
    Answer: b   LO: 26; factual   pages: 333, 348

95. As noted in the text, depression can affect parenting by reducing each of the following *except* the parent's:
    a. self-esteem.
    b. ability to love his or her child.
    c. energy levels for dealing with the child's needs.
    d. ability to respond to the child.
    Answer: b   LO: 1; factual, conceptual   page: 351

Chapter 9

Essay Questions

96. Imagine that you are an obstetrician. In your "spare" time, you volunteer as a speaker for high school students to educate them about pregnancy. Consider what you have learned about disorders that are attributed, at least in part, to neurological problems that may have originated during the mother's pregnancy or at birth, either through intentional behavior (e.g., consuming alcohol) or accident (e.g., contracting rubella). What are these disorders? Discuss the three that you believe would be most important for your high school audience to know about, describing the symptoms, causes, consequences, and prognosis (what would affect that prognosis?). How would you ensure that these students were taking proper precautions?

    The student needs to address the effects on the fetus of environmental toxins to which the pregnant mother may be exposed, as well as illnesses (such as rubella), or intentional actions, such as consuming alcohol or other drugs; genetic heritage is also relevant to this discussion. Each of the teratogens, as well as the genetic link, should be followed toward its ultimate effect on the child in terms of the particular disorder, whether ADHD, conduct disorder, ODD, fetal alcohol syndrome, Down syndrome, etc. The student will need to present the typical profile of a child with each of the disorders, including physical, behavioral, cognitive, and social functioning. The prognosis should look at whether a problem is organic or cultural-familial and should address some issues of how to treat it accordingly. Finally, the student should explain a way to monitor the practices of the "audience."

97. Fetal alcohol syndrome is one of the most preventable of all childhood disorders. Explain what this disorder is, the characteristics of a child who has the disorder, the prognosis for such a child, and what causes the disorder. As stated, this disorder is preventable! How would you go about eradicating it?

    The student should give an explanation of the disorder that includes the effects on the unborn fetus of the pregnant mother consuming alcohol (since we do not know how much is too much, a pregnant woman should not drink any alcohol), and all of the neurological, cognitive, behavioral, emotional, and social consequences in terms of development and daily living. Prognosis for this disorder is poor. The student should come up with some reasonable education plan (or other creative idea within the boundaries of ethics and morality) to prevent FAS.

Childhood Disorders

98. Imagine that you are working in a home for the mentally retarded. Remember that the text defines mental retardation as "subaverage intellectual functioning, indexed by an IQ score of below 70 and deficits in adaptive behavioral functioning." With this in mind, list and describe the four levels of mental retardation and how they limit (or don't limit) persons in those categories, so you would know what you might or might not be able to expect from the people you work with. What biological factors are implicated in mental retardation? What are the precise effects of each of those factors on the individual? What treatments are effective, in terms of psychotherapy, drugs, and education, in minimizing the negative consequences of the retardation? Explain which forms of treatment you would use for the mentally retarded people with whom you are working and why you would use those particular treatments.

   The student needs to explain the four levels of mental retardation from mild to profound and the limitations imposed by each, as well as the capabilities of individuals at each level. Biological factors of PKU, Tay-Sachs, chromosomal disorders, rubella, herpes, syphilis, drugs, etc. should all be addressed in terms of what they are and their ultimate effect in terms of leading to retardation and the specific forms of retardation involved. The student should note the drugs that have some effect on reducing symptoms but should focus on the behavioral interventions that have proven most successful; the issue of whether to mainstream children or keeping them in separate classrooms should be examined. Then the student should indicate which treatment(s) the student would prefer and provide a rationale for their use.

99. Behavior therapy appears to be the most effective treatment for the disorders discussed in this chapter. Describe the behavior techniques a psychologist would use to treat a child with each of the following: (1) attention deficit/hyperactivity disorder; (2) separation anxiety disorder; (3) enuresis; and (4) autism. What evidence is there that these interventions are effective (describing at least one of the studies discussed in the text)? The text noted that some theorists believe adding a cognitive component to these therapies is helpful? Describe what that cognitive component is, how it works, and for each of these disorders whether you agree that it would be helpful.

   The specific techniques used with each of these disorders should be described (e.g., setting a contract with an ADHD child and providing chips to be exchanged for specified rewards when she or he behaves well, and that are taken away when she or he does not behave well). All of these should mention the importance of training the parents to carry through on the training at home. Ivar Lovaas' work at UCLA could be mentioned as an excellent example of how persistence on the part of the psychologists and parents was effective in helping almost half of the autistic children in the study achieve a state of normalcy by age 7. In terms of a cognitive component, the student should discuss the effects of teaching "self-talk."

Chapter 9

100. At the end of the chapter, the author talks about what to do if *your parent* has a psychological disorder and the effects you anticipate that might have on you. Discuss the risk factors inherent in having a parent with a psychological disorder, both in terms of what that means genetically and environmentally (growing up in a home with a psychologically impaired parent). What factors would work to protect a child against any ill effects of such a set of circumstances? As an adult, what could you do to seek assistance, either for yourself or for a child you know who is in such a situation?

    Here the student needs to address the small risk factor of genetic transmission and the reasons the risk is relatively minimal. Also, the environmental influences of growing up in a family where the parent(s) has (have) impaired functioning but it is important here to consider the influence of familial support from other relatives (including the other parent), an adult mentor, the child's own resilience factors, and the love that even a psychologically impaired parent can offer. The text suggests support groups, especially for alcohol problems. Most local phone books have a listing of 800 numbers for support and information, and the student should get creative in talking about ways to find help.

Chapter 10   Eating Disorders

1. According to Hawkins, Turell, and Jackson (1983), over 70% of American females have dieted by age:
   a. 10.
   b. 15.
   c. 18.
   d. 20.
   Answer: a   LO: 1; factual   page: 354

2. Which of the following is *not* one of the methods of weight loss mentioned in the text?
   a. yo-yo dieting
   b. wiring the jaw shut
   c. liposuction
   d. eating a healthy diet
   Answer: d   LO: 1; factual   page: 355

3. According to the text, the driving force behind most people's attempts to lose weight is the desire to:
   a. avoid high blood pressure and stroke.
   b. avoid heart disease and diabetes.
   c. live longer.
   d. be more attractive and increase self-esteem.
   Answer: d   LO: 1; factual   page: 355

4. Which of the following is *true* concerning pressures to be thin?
   a. Pressures to be thin come primarily from the media and toy manufacturers.
   b. Although some women give in to pressure to conform to societal expectations, most do not moderate their eating habits to any large extent when in public.
   c. In recent years, more men have succumbed to the pressure to have a lean, toned body.
   d. The reality is that weight is only tangentially linked to a person's self-esteem.
   Answer: c   LO: 1; factual, conceptual   page: 355

5. Which of the following is *not* discussed in the text as an eating disorder?
   a. anorexia nervosa
   b. obesity
   c. bulimia nervosa
   d. binge-eating disorder
   Answer: b   LO: 1; factual   page: 356

Chapter 10

6. When concerns about eating and weight become so overwhelming and behaviors oriented toward eating or avoiding eating get totally out of control, a person is said to have:
   a. an eating disorder.
   b. anorexia nervosa.
   c. bulimia nervosa.
   d. obesity.
   Answer: a   LO: 1; conceptual   page: 356

7. The eating disorder that is characterized by a pursuit for thinness that leads people to starve themselves is called:
   a. binge-eating disorder.
   b. excessive dieting.
   c. bulimia nervosa.
   d. anorexia nervosa.
   Answer: d   LO: 2; conceptual   page: 356-357

8. Sarah is 18. Because of her record-breaking speed and excellent academic performance, she received a track scholarship at a prestigious women's college, and so she is about to leave home for the first time. The thought of leaving her friends and the small town where she grew up and having to meet new people is terrifying for her. Her parents attribute her drop in weight from 120 to 100 lbs, her apparent lack of appetite, and the fact that her menstrual periods have stopped to her anxiety over the new challenges she is facing. Her mother, who tends toward fits of depression, would prefer that Sarah remain at home. From this scenario, we might determine that Sarah has:
   a. anxiety disorder.
   b. anorexia nervosa.
   c. major depression.
   d. normal "jitters" about going off to college.
   Answer: b   LO: 2; applied   pages: 356-358

9. The eating disorder that is characterized by a cycle of binge-eating followed by extreme behaviors to prevent weight gain, such as self-induced vomiting is called:
   a. binge-eating disorder.
   b. obesity.
   c. bulimia nervosa.
   d. anorexia nervosa.
   Answer: c   LO: 2; conceptual   page: 356

Eating Disorders

10. The eating disorder characterized by uncontrollable periods of stuffing oneself with food beyond the point of physical need is called:
    a. binge-eating disorder.
    b. obesity.
    c. bulimia nervosa.
    d. anorexia nervosa.
    Answer: a   LO: 2; conceptual   page: 356

11. Kimberly refuses to maintain the minimal body weight she needs that is normal for her age and height, and that would keep her health. Which disorder does she have?
    a. binge-eating disorder
    b. excessive dieting
    c. bulimia nervosa
    d. anorexia nervosa
    Answer: d   LO: 2; applied   page: 356

12. Which of the following is *not* one of the DSM-IV criteria for anorexia nervosa?
    a. being at least 20% below the ideal weight for his or her age and height
    b. amenorrhea in females who have begun menstruating
    c. having intense fears of becoming fat
    d. having a distorted image of their body
    Answer: a   LO: 2; factual   page: 356

13. The most obvious symptom of anorexia nervosa involves:
    a. weight loss.
    b. depression.
    c. anxiety.
    d. thought disorder.
    Answer: a   LO: 2; factual, conceptual   page: 356

14. The two types of anorexia recognized by DSM-IV are:
    a. simple anorexia and anorexia nervosa.
    b. anorexia and bulimia.
    c. restricting type and binge/purge type.
    d. self-imposed and environmentally induced.
    Answer: c   LO: 2; factual   page: 356

Chapter 10

15. Which statement is *false* about the binge/purge type of anorexia?
    a. The person engages in binge eating.
    b. The person meets the criteria DSM-IV for anorexia.
    c. The person engages in purging activities.
    d. The person consumes large amounts of food when binging.
    Answer: d   LO: 2; factual   page: 357

16. Which of the following is *true* concerning the differences between the restricting type of anorexia and the binge/purge type?
    a. People with the binge/purge type of anorexia are less trusting of others.
    b. People with the binge/purge type of anorexia are less willing to acknowledge that they have a problem.
    c. People with the binge/purge type of anorexia have fewer problems with emotional lability.
    d. There is a more chronic course to the binge/purge type of anorexia than to the restricting type.
    Answer: d   LO: 2; factual   pages: 356-357

17. Which condition is more commonly seen in the restricting type of anorexia, as opposed to the binge/purge type?
    a. problems with unstable moods
    b. deep mistrust of others
    c. alcohol and drug abuse
    d. self-mutilation
    Answer: b   LO: 2; factual   page: 358

18. Who coined the term *anorexia nervosa* and first noted its prevalence among females and its timing of onset?
    a. Sir William Gull
    b. Charles Laseque
    c. Hilda Bruch
    d. Salvador Minuchin
    Answer: a   LO: 2, 3, 4; factual   page: 359

19. Which of the following is *not* considered a serious physical consequences of anorexia?
    a. death
    b. cardiovascular complications
    c. colon abnormalities
    d. kidney damage
    Answer: c   LO: 3; factual   pages: 358-359

Eating Disorders

20. Which of the following is *true* concerning the prevalence of anorexia nervosa?
    a. It affects approximately 2% of the population.
    b. Somewhere between 90 to 95% of people diagnosed with anorexia nervosa are female.
    c. Anorexia nervosa usually begins immediately before the onset of puberty.
    d. The death rate among anorexics is about 10%.
    Answer: b   LO: 3; factual   page: 358

21. Accounts of anorexia are seen as early as:
    a. 1225 in England.
    b. 1684 in England.
    c. 1873 in England.
    d. 1940 in the United States.
    Answer: a   LO: 3, 4; factual   page: 360

22. Which of the following is *not* included in the DSM-IV definition of a binge?
    a. It includes a feeling of a lack of control over one's eating.
    b. It occurs in a discrete period of time.
    c. It must include a minimum of 1500 calories.
    d. It includes eating an amount of food that is definitely larger than most people would eat under similar circumstances.
    Answer: c   LO: 5; factual   page: 360

23. Which of the following is *not* a method used by someone with the purging type of bulimia?
    a. abuse of laxatives
    b. excessive exercise
    c. self-induced vomiting
    d. abuse of diuretics
    Answer: b   LO: 5; factual, conceptual   page: 360

24. Which of the following is most likely to be able to hide her bulimia?
    a. The bulimic who is obsessively clean and leaves no mess after vomiting.
    b. The bulimic who purges by use of laxatives.
    c. The bulimic who uses excessive exercise to control her weight.
    d. The bulimic who carefully brushes her teeth and uses mouthwash after vomiting.
    Answer: c   LO: 5; conceptual   page: 360

Chapter 10

25. The overriding perception of the bulimic with respect to binging is:
    a. the lack of control.
    b. the type of food consumed.
    c. the need to hide the fact she or he is binging.
    d. the need to purge.
    Answer: a LO: 5; conceptual page: 360

26. Which is a symptom of the binge/purge type of anorexia, *but not* a symptom of bulimia?
    a. amenorrhea
    b. lack of control over eating
    c. food binges
    d. excessive concern about losing weight
    Answer: a LO: 7; factual, conceptual page: 361

27. Audrey has an eating disorder that does *not* involve binge eating. It would be:
    a. purging type of bulimia.
    b. restricting type of anorexia.
    c. non-purging type of bulimia.
    d. binge/purge type of anorexia.
    Answer: b LO: 7; applied page: 356, 361

28. Which of the following statements about anorexia and bulimia is *false*?
    a. Both anorexia and bulimia are more common on college campuses, with as many as 25% of women meeting the diagnostic criteria for one of the eating disorders.
    b. People with bulimia do not have a distorted body image, as do people with anorexia.
    c. People are more likely to die from anorexia than from bulimia.
    d. Amenorrhea is a symptom of anorexia, but not bulimia.
    Answer: a LO: 7; factual, conceptual page: 362

29. The most serious medical complication stated in the text that arises from bulimia is that
    a. an imbalance in the body's electrolytes that can lead to heart failure.
    b. the constant use of laxatives and diuretics can lead to colon cancer.
    c. the gastric acids from induced vomiting rot the teeth and lead to malnutrition.
    d. dehydration resulting from use of diuretics leads to renal failure.
    Answer: a LO: 6; factual page: 362

30. Binge/eating disorder differs from bulimia in that the person with binge/eating disorder:
    a. limits the times when she or he will binge.
    b. is better able to control his or her food intake.
    c. does not regularly engage in purging or excessive exercise.
    d. feels less anxiety about binging.
    Answer: c LO: 8; factual, conceptual page: 363

Eating Disorders

31. People with which of the following eating disorders are *most likely* to be significantly overweight?
    a. anorexia nervosa, restricting type
    b. bulimia nervosa, purging type
    c. binge/eating disorder
    d. bulimia nervosa, nonpurging type
    Answer: c   LO: 8; factual, conceptual   page: 363

32. Which of the following is *true* about binge/eating disorder?
    a. Although only 2% of the general public suffers from this disorder, at least half of the people currently in weight loss programs may have binge/eating disorder.
    b. Binge/eating disorder is not one of the officially recognized forms of eating disorder in the DSM-IV.
    c. Unlike anorexia and bulimia, men are more likely than women to have binge/eating disorders.
    d. People with binge/eating disorders have high rates of anxiety and alcohol abuse, and lower rates of depression than anorectics, bulimics, or the general public.
    Answer: b   LO: 8; factual   pages: 363-364

33. Which of the following statements about dieting is *false*?
    a. Dieting increases irritability and emotional reactivity.
    b. Dieting increases people's ability to read their body's cues about hunger and satiety.
    c. Dieting slows down the metabolic rate, reducing the body's need for food.
    d. The majority of people can lose weight through weight-loss programs, such as liquid diets as well as drug and behavior therapies.
    Answer: b   LO: 9; factual   page: 364

34. In a study by Herman and Mack (1975), participants were asked to "rate" three flavors of ice cream after consuming two milkshakes, one milkshake, or no milkshakes. The researchers noted that:
    a. the number of milkshakes people consumed had no effect on how much ice cream they consumed.
    b. chronic dieters in the study who had no milkshake at all ate the most amount of ice cream.
    c. chronic dieters in the study who had one milkshake ate the most amount of ice cream.
    d. chronic dieters in the study who had two milkshakes ate the most amount of ice cream.
    Answer: d   LO: 9; factual   page: 364

Chapter 10

35. Which of the following is *true* concerning the binge/purge cycle in bulimia?
   a. Bulimics who use this technique for weight reduction begin the cycle about 6 months after they begin binge eating.
   b. Purging increases the bulimics distress and guilt over binging.
   c. After the binge/purge cycle has been established, purging is related more to the bulimic's sense of guilt than to avoid weight gain.
   d. The binge/purge pattern becomes a way of life that interferes with the bulimic's social life and daily functioning.
   Answer: d   LO: 10; factual, conceptual   page: 365

36. In regard to the progression from excessive dieting to developing anorexia, which of the following is *false*?
   a. They believe the only way to control their eating is not to eat at all.
   b. They become obsessed with following strict rules about eating and exercise.
   c. They have a sense of feeling overtaken and controlled by their rules for eating.
   d. Eventually, the anorectic's self-esteem becomes dependent on his or her ability to control his or her food intake.
   Answer: c   LO: 9; factual, conceptual   page: 365

37. Which of the following groups was discussed in the text as being at increased risk for unhealthy eating habits and full-blown eating disorders?
   a. movie actors/actresses
   b. stage actors/actresses
   c. models
   d. athletes
   Answer: d   LO: 10; factual   page: 365

38. Which of the following was identified by female athletes as being a "trigger" for their eating disorders?
   a. early onset of puberty
   b. late onset of puberty
   c. peer pressure
   d. pressure from parents or coaches
   Answer: a   LO: 10; factual   pages: 365-366

39. The study by Sundgot-Borgen (1993) addressing eating disorders in female athletes found which sorts to have the highest rates of such disorders?
   a. cycling, running, and swimming
   b. figure skating and gymnastics
   c. tennis and swimming
   d. volleyball and soccer
   Answer: b   LO: 10; factual   page: 366

-228-

Eating Disorders

40. Which of the following statements about gender differences in eating disorders is *false*?
    a. Homosexual men are more likely than heterosexual men to have eating disorders.
    b. Young women attending college are more likely than working women of the same age to develop an eating disorder.
    c. Both men and women with eating disorders have higher rates of substance abuse.
    d. Women are more likely than men to have a history of being overweight and binge-eating before their anorexia or bulimia developed.
    Answer: d   LO: 11; factual   pages: 368-369

41. Which of these explanations was given in the text for women developing anorexia or bulimia?
    a. Nearly 75% of women under the age of 35 report frequent dissatisfaction with their appearance, particularly in terms of believing they are overweight.
    b. Women who exercise are more likely to do so for improving their health and their appearance than they are as a method of weight control.
    c. Because of the pressures of our Western culture, adolescent girls and young women develop eating disorders as a way to "drop out" and be taken care of.
    d. Being excessively thin is a way to escape the need to be attractive and thus allows the girl or woman to avoid developing intimate relationships.
    Answer: c   LO: 11; factual, conceptual   pages: 368-369

42. Historical psychologists have linked eating disorders with:
    a. standards of beauty for women.
    b. how affluent or poor a society is.
    c. media influence dating back to times of wandering minstrels.
    d. level of education.
    Answer: a   LO: 12; factual, conceptual   page: 369

43. Which of the following statements about cultural factors in eating disorders is *false*?
    a. Eating disorders are uncommon in many less developed countries.
    b. Eating disorders are more common among the upper and middle classes than among people in lower socioeconomic classes.
    c. The rates of eating disorders have increased among Caucasians in recent years but have remained consistently low among ethnic minority groups.
    d. When the most influential members of a society view a heavy weight as beautiful, eating disorders are uncommon, but obesity is common.
    Answer: c   LO: 12; factual   pages: 369-370

Chapter 10

44. Which of the following symptoms of anorexia is *not* typically found in anorexic patients in Eastern cultures?
    a. amenorrhea
    b. fear of becoming fat
    c. excessive exercise (in the binge-purge type)
    d. deep mistrust of others
    Answer: b   LO: 12; factual   page: 370

45. Which of the following was *not* one of the factors mentioned in the case study of the young woman with bulimia nervosa as an "emotional underpinning" of her eating disorder?
    a. hunger
    b. an emptiness of self
    c. a desire for food
    d. a desire for approval
    Answer: c   LO: 13; factual, conceptual   page: 370

46. Hilda Bruch (1973, 1978, 1982), described the families of girls with eating disorders as being:
    a. parent focused.
    b. neglecting.
    c. enmeshed.
    d. overly focused on negative feelings.
    Answer: a   LO: 13; factual, conceptual   page: 371

47. Which of the following is *not* an aspect of Hilda Bruch's theory of eating disorders?
    a. Girls develop eating disorders because they have parents who expect them to be both a "modern woman" but also to conform to traditional female roles; these girls strive to be perfect in all ways, but eventually want to "drop out of the race" and be taken care of, which is facilitated by having an eating disorder.
    b. Girls who develop eating disorders have parents who are overinvested in their daughters' compliance and achievements, who are overcontrolling, and who will not allow the expression of negative emotions.
    c. Because of the parenting they receive, girls with eating disorders learn to monitor closely the needs and desires of others and to comply with others' demands.
    d. Girls develop eating disorders because their mothers may need them to remain dependent, because the mother's identity is tied too closely to her daughter.
    Answer: a   LO: 13; factual, conceptual   page: 371

Eating Disorders

48. Salvador Minuchin (Minuchin, Rosman, & Baker, 1978) described families of anorexics as:
    a. extremely closed off from each other and from the outside world, with rigid boundaries that prohibit communication.
    b. extremely interdependent and intense, with weak, easily crossed boundaries between the identities of individual family members.
    c. demanding perfection from a compliant daughter who wants to please her parents but is incapable of doing so.
    d. overcontrolling and demanding, who will not allow the expression of feelings, particularly negative feelings.
    Answer: b   LO: 13; factual, conceptual   page: 371

49. Bulimia frequently co-occurs with which of the following?
    a. obsessive-compulsive disorder
    b. depression
    c. mania
    d. schizophrenia
    Answer: b   LO: 6; factual   pages: 371, 374

50. Which of the following is *not* a characteristic of anorexic girls described in the text?
    a. They have fundamental deficits in their sense of self and identity.
    b. They feel they are always acting in response to others.
    c. They are supersensitive to their feelings, for which they feel guilty.
    d. They do not accurately identify bodily sensations.
    Answer: c   LO: 13; factual, conceptual   page: 372

51. Which of the following is *not* a reason stated in the text that adolescent girls are particularly at risk for eating disorders?
    a. They fear separation from their families.
    b. They fear intimate relationships with peers.
    c. They feel rage against their parents for overcontrolling them.
    d. They lack control over their lives and their bodies.
    Answer: d   LO: 13; factual, conceptual   pages: 372-373

52. The critical element stated in the text for why girls develop eating disorders is:
    a. their families have high levels of conflict.
    b. expression of negative emotions is discouraged.
    c. control and perfectionism are paramount in their lives.
    d. they are unaware of their own bodily sensations.
    Answer: d   LO: 14; factual, conceptual   page: 372

Chapter 10

53. One of the major research limitations in determining the types of parenting that may lead to eating disorders in children is:
    a. there is a wide disparity in terms of the types of parenting styles that children and adolescents with eating disorders have, so it is difficult to categorize them.
    b. since all the studies are retrospective, not prospective, it is difficult to look at causal relationships.
    c. there are many conflicting findings, particularly in terms of control issues, so that it is difficult to determine exactly which style leads to which disorder and if it does so consistently.
    d. there is more evidence pointing to a biological basis for the eating disorders than a psychosocial basis.
    Answer: b   LO: 13; factual, conceptual   page: 373

54. All of the following are found in people with eating disorders and their families but are also found in people with depression and anxiety, *except*:
    a. discouragement of the expression of negative emotions in the family.
    b. a tendency to judge oneself and others according to harsh evaluations and dichotomous thinking.
    c. a history of sexual abuse.
    d. a lack of awareness of one's own bodily sensations.
    Answer: d   LO: 15; factual, conceptual   page: 372

55. Which is the most likely reason that boys are less likely than girls to develop eating disorders?
    a. More value is placed on boys than on girls gaining independence and separating from their families.
    b. Girls are physiologically more vulnerable to eating disorders.
    c. There is more pressure for females to look attractive than males; males have more pressure to achieve.
    d. Girls are more likely to somatize and thus develop an eating disorder; boys are more likely to become aggressive and/or turn to drugs.
    Answer: a   LO: 14; factual, conceptual   page: 373

56. With respect to the connection between eating disorders and sexual abuse:
    a. researchers have found that people with eating disorders tend to have higher rates of sexual abuse than people with anxiety, but not those with depression.
    b. survivors of sexual abuse feel so insecure about their body image that they become anorexic in an attempt to appear more attractive.
    c. researchers have found that people with eating disorders tend to have higher rates of sexual abuse than people with no psychological disorders.
    d. researchers have found that people with eating disorders have higher rates of sexual abuse than people with depression.
    Answer: c   LO: 15; factual, conceptual   page: 374

Eating Disorders

57. Twin studies exploring biological factors of eating disorders have found:
    a. there is no statistically significant genetic relatedness between the two.
    b. a higher concordance rate for female bulimics than for female anorectics.
    c. the significant relationship between eating disorders and depression leads some researchers to believe eating disorders are variants of mood disorders.
    d. there are ten times as many first degree relatives of anorexic patients with eating disorders than there are in nonpsychiatric control groups.
    Answer: c   LO: 16; factual   page: 374

58. Researchers have found a strong link between eating disorders and which of the following?
    a. schizophrenia
    b. affective disorders
    c. personality disorders
    d. dissociative disorders
    Answer: b   LO: 17; factual   page: 374

59. A biological abnormality found in people with anorexia is:
    a. increased functioning in the caudate nucleus.
    b. low levels of norepinephrine.
    c. decreased metabolism in the frontal cerebrum.
    d. lowered functioning of the hypothalamus.
    Answer: d   LO: 16; factual   page: 375

60. A criticism of viewing eating disorders as one way to manifest mood disorders is that:
    a. they are not strongly enough related to allow for such a connection.
    b. depression has unique characteristics that must be addressed in therapy.
    c. by doing so we overlook the specific factors that lead toward one or the other.
    d. the depression gets treated while the eating disorder is often overlooked.
    Answer: c   LO: 17; factual   page: 375

61. With respect to the relationship between biological abnormalities and eating disorders:
    a. researchers have been able to determine through controlled laboratory studies that many biological abnormalities lead to eating disorders.
    b. researchers have been able to demonstrate through controlled laboratory studies that the eating disorders cause the biological abnormalities.
    c. controlled experiments addressing this relationship on humans are unethical, but research on mice seems to indicate that biological abnormalities lead to anorexia.
    d. as with correlational data generally, it is impossible to determine if the biological abnormalities are the cause or the consequence of the eating disorders.
    Answer: d   LO: 18; conceptual   page: 375

Chapter 10

62. Lakeisha weighs 85 lbs due to her anorexia. Which of the following issues is likely to present a major difficulty with respect to conducting therapy with her?
    a. control
    b. body image
    c. transference
    d. ethics
    Answer: a   LO: 19; applied   page: 376

63. Lance has had anorexia for the past two years. Which of the following ideas is most accurate with respect to treating him for this disorder?
    a. Lance would be expected to cooperate because he is extremely compliant.
    b. Lance would be expected to cooperate because his life is at stake.
    c. Lance would not be expected to cooperate because of the rage he feels.
    d. Lance would not be expected to cooperate because he must maintain control.
    Answer: d   LO: 19; applied   page: 376

64. The most important thing a therapist must do in therapy is:
    a. get the client to give up control.
    b. win and maintain the client's trust and participation.
    c. convince the family to develop more clear-cut boundaries.
    d. win and maintain the family's trust and participation.
    Answer: b   LO: 19; factual, conceptual   page: 376

65. The first job of the therapist in treating an anorexic is often:
    a. doing whatever is necessary to save her life.
    b. gain her trust and confidence.
    c. gain the family's trust and confidence.
    d. convincing her that she is killing herself.
    Answer: a   LO: 19; factual, conceptual   page: 376

66. Dr. Rhodes is about to begin treatment with Stephanie, who has been hospitalized due to medical complications resulting from anorexia. Dr. Rhodes will most likely begin the work of engaging Stephanie in facing and solving her psychological issues:
    a. during her hospitalization.
    b. after she has regained enough weight to focus on the therapy.
    c. after she has been released from the hospital.
    d. after the therapist has had several sessions with the family to be sure they will cooperate.
    Answer: a   LO: 19; applied   page: 376

Eating Disorders

67. The two types of therapy that are used most often to treat anorexia are:
    a. psychodynamic therapy and use of selective serotonin reuptake inhibitors (SSRIs).
    b. family therapy and use of selective serotonin reuptake inhibitors (SSRIs).
    c. family therapy and behavior therapy.
    d. behavior therapy and cognitive therapy.
    Answer: c		LO: 19; factual, conceptual		page: 376

68. Behavior therapy for treating anorexia typically uses:
    a. aversive conditioning to stop the patient from engaging in harmful behaviors.
    b. systematic desensitization for the anxiety produced by gaining weight.
    c. flooding by causing the patient to binge and showing her that there are no negative consequences.
    d. reinforcement for gaining weight and relaxation to relieve anxiety caused by eating.
    Answer: d		LO: 19; factual, conceptual		page: 376

69. Which of the following is an effective treatment for anorexia *and* has the lowest relapse rate of the following treatments?
    a. MAO inhibitors
    b. behavior therapy
    c. tricyclic antidepressants
    d. family therapy
    Answer: d		LO: 19; factual, conceptual		page: 377

70. A drawback of behavior therapy for treating anorexia is that:
    a. it is difficult to teach the family appropriate techniques for helping the patient.
    b. there is a high relapse rate because the emotional issues accompanying the anorexia are not confronted.
    c. it requires constant reinforcement to be effective in the long term.
    d. it works best when combined with drugs, but drugs are not something to give a patient whose health is already compromised through starvation.
    Answer: b		LO: 19; factual, conceptual		page: 377

71. Which of the following is *false* about families of anorexics?
    a. They have been supporting the daughter's avoidance of food.
    b. Their actions contribute to the daughter's sense of being controlled.
    c. Their expectations of their daughters are unreasonable.
    d. Most families need to lower their level of anxiety about their daughter's disorder.
    Answer: d		LO: 19; factual, conceptual		page: 377

Chapter 10

72. Which of the following patients has the best prognosis for achieving and maintaining normal eating patterns?
    a. Selena, a 14-year-old girl who has been anorectic for the past 4 months.
    b. Andrea, a 30-year-old graduate student who has been anorectic for 12 years.
    c. Cheryl, an 18-year-old college freshman whose family will not stop their infighting.
    d. Peggy, a 20-year-old gymnast, who is concerned about competition from younger gymnasts.
    Answer: a   LO: 19; applied   page: 377

73. In family therapy, Salvador Minuchin would be most likely to focus on:
    a. the necessity to get the anorexic to eat.
    b. family patterns that lead to the daughter's eating disorder.
    c. ways of reinforcing the anorexic and her parents for appropriate eating behaviors.
    d. teaching the parents to take control of the therapy sessions.
    Answer: b   LO: 19; factual, conceptual   page: 377

74. Pearl is receiving individual therapy from Dr. Bailey for anorexia. One of the major focuses of this therapy is likely to be that Dr Bailey will:
    a. define Pearl's feelings for her.
    b. help Pearl understand that her feelings have been inaccurate.
    c. teach Pearl to read her feelings accurately.
    d. teach her to trust her parents.
    Answer: c   LO: 19; applied   page: 377

75. Which of the following is *not* a goal of therapy with clients who suffer from anorexia?
    a. confronting their distorted cognitions about their body
    b. changing their distorted cognitions about their body
    c. teaching them to read their feelings accurately
    d. helping them to trust and rely on their parents
    Answer: d   LO: 19; factual, conceptual   page: 377

76. Which of the following is an example of the distorted thinking pattern in eating disorders referred to as overgeneralization?
    a. "I just can't control myself. Last night when I had dinner in a restaurant, I ate everything in sight, event though I told myself ahead of time I would be careful."
    b. "When I used to eat carbohydrates, I was fat. Therefore, I must avoid carbohydrates so I won't become obese."
    c. "Gaining 5 pounds would push me over the brink!"
    d. "If I'm not in complete control, I lose all control. If I can't master this area of my life, I'll lose everything."
    Answer: b   LO: 19; applied   page: 377

Eating Disorders

77. Which of the following is an example of the distorted thinking pattern in eating disorders referred to as dichotomous reasoning?
    a. "The only way I can be in control is through eating."
    b. "If others comment on my weight gain, I won't be able to stand it."
    c. "If I don't establish a daily routine, everything will be chaotic and I won't accomplish anything."
    d. "If I eat a sweet, it will immediately be pasted onto my hips."
    Answer: c   LO: 19; applied   page: 377

78. Which of the following is an example of the distorted thinking pattern in eating disorders referred to as magnification?
    a. "I am special if I'm thin."
    b. "I've gained 5 pounds, so I can't wear my shorts anymore."
    c. "If I gain one pound, I'll go on and gain a hundred pounds."
    d. "I'm embarrassed when other people see me eat."
    Answer: b   LO: 19; applied   page: 377

79. Which of the following is *false* concerning treatment of anorexia?
    a. Most therapists combine different modes of therapy to meet client's individual needs.
    b. Once a client has had an extended period of restored weight and healthy eating patterns, there is no longer a high risk of relapse.
    c. Psychotherapy helps many anorexics, but is a long process that takes many years.
    d. Despite having achieved normal weight and healthy eating patterns, anorectics often continue to have self-esteem deficits, family problems, and periods of depression.
    Answer: b   LO: 19; factual, conceptual   page: 377

80. Which of the following statements about psychotherapy for bulimia is *false*?
    a. Studies comparing cognitive-behavioral therapy (CBT) to drug therapies found CBT is at least as effective as drug therapy in the short term but is more likely than drug therapy to prevent relapse in the long term.
    b. Studies show that CBT is more effective than interpersonal therapy, supportive-expressive therapy, and behavior therapy at eliminating disturbed attitudes toward shape and weight, and extreme attempts to diet.
    c. Studies comparing CBT to other psychotherapies found that clients maintain the gains they make during therapy longer if they are treated with CBT, as opposed to other therapies.
    d. CBT and behavior therapy are more effective than interpersonal therapy and supportive-expressive therapy at eliminating self-induced vomiting.
    Answer: c   LO: 20; factual, conceptual   page: 379

Chapter 10

81. Studies on cognitive-behavior therapy (CBT) indicate that the central features of bulimia are:
    a. the bulimic's extreme concerns about shape and weight.
    b. the bulimic's power struggle with her parents and her need for control.
    c. an underlying depression coupled with a genetic predisposition to the disorder.
    d. the bulimic's enjoyment of food and her family's dysfunctional communication patterns.
    Answer: a   LO: 20; factual, conceptual   page: 379

82. Rhoda tells her cognitive-behaviorist therapist, "Food was the first thing I loved that loved me back." She feels insecure in social situations and feels like a total failure with her life, even though she's a vice-president of the advertising firm where she works. When she eats with clients, she can't wait for them to leave the table to go to the ladies' room so she can finish what's on their plates, and when they come back, she excuses herself and goes to the ladies' room to vomit, so she won't gain weight from eating three leftover desserts. The therapist will most likely:
    a. teach Rhoda to monitor her thoughts as she eats and then help her confront those thoughts.
    b. agree with her that food has been a comforting force in her life, but now it's time to reassess how comforting it is for her.
    c. teach Rhoda how to relax when she is with clients so it will not be necessary for her to binge on their leftovers.
    d. send Rhoda to a dentist for "shock" therapy when she learns how expensive it will be to repair (or replace) her corroded teeth.
    Answer: a   LO: 20; applied   page: 379

83. Which of the following is *true* about cognitive-behavioral therapy?
    a. Clients show some decrease in depression and anxiety, but there is a high relapse rate with respect to binging and purging.
    b. It is not as effective as behavior therapy in eliminating extreme dieting.
    c. After 10 to 20 sessions over a period of 3 to 6 months, about half of the clients completely stop the binge-purge cycle.
    d. As the client learns to monitor her eating habits, she spontaneously begins to resolve some of the personal issues that led to the disorder.
    Answer: c   LO: 20; factual, conceptual   page: 379

84. Annette is seeing Dr. Reich for help with her eating disorder. During the sessions, Annette discusses her problems in relationships with others and works on solving those problems. The type of therapy Dr. Reich is using with Annette is:
   a. behavior therapy.
   b. interpersonal therapy.
   c. supportive-expressive therapy.
   d. cognitive therapy.
   Answer: b   LO: 20; applied   page: 379

85. William has been seeing Dr. Fromm for help with his eating disorder. In the therapy sessions, Dr. Fromm uses a highly nondirective manner to help William talk about problems related to the eating disorder, including those related to his interpersonal relationships. The type of therapy Dr. Fromm is using with William is:
   a. behavior therapy.
   b. interpersonal therapy.
   c. supportive-expressive therapy.
   d. cognitive therapy.
   Answer: c   LO: 20; applied   page: 379

86. Which of the following is *true* about the various modes of psychotherapy used for treating bulimia?
   a. In the long-term, CBT is the most effective treatment modality, with the lowest rate of relapse.
   b. Interpersonal and supportive-expressive are not as effective as CBT in the short term, but are more effective in the long term because they get to the root of the client's problems.
   c. Cognitive therapy has the lowest relapse rate because it helps the client challenge her beliefs about how wonderful food is.
   d. CBT, behavior therapy, cognitive therapy, interpersonal therapy, and supportive expressive therapy all appear to be equally effective for treating bulimia in the long term.
   Answer: d   LO: 20; factual, conceptual   page: 379

87. All of the following have been shown to be effective drug therapies for bulimia *except*:
   a. lithium.
   b. tricyclic antidepressants.
   c. MAO inhibitors.
   d. SSRIs.
   Answer: a   LO: 21; factual   page: 379

Chapter 10

88. Which of the following bulimic behaviors has *not* been successfully treated by use of tricyclic antidepressants?
    a. reduction of binge eating
    b. reduction of vomiting
    c. reduction of severe dieting
    d. increase in sense of control
    Answer: c   LO: 21; factual   page: 379

89. Which of the following is *true* concerning the use of MAO inhibitors for treating bulimia?
    a. They are effectively used for treating the disorder and are often prescribed for it.
    b. They are not effective for treating bulimia.
    c. Although they are effective, they are not typically prescribed because their side effects require severe dietary restrictions.
    d. They are just as effective as placebos for treating bulimia.
    Answer: c   LO: 21; factual   page: 379

90. Which of the following drug therapies has shown some effectiveness in treating anorexia?
    a. MAO inhibitors
    b. tricyclic antidepressants
    c. SSRIs
    d. They have all been shown to be effective.
    Answer: c   LO: 21; factual   page: 379

91. An ironic paradox of the eating disorder in industrialized countries is that:
    a. as the "ideal" body shape is getting thinner, the average person is getting fatter.
    b. as the "ideal" body shape gets somewhat heavier, the average person gets even heavier still.
    c. as the "ideal" body shape gets thinner, the average person damages his or her health by trying to achieve that "ideal."
    d. people have become so oversaturated with "thin is in," that it no longer has much effect on the average person's eating behaviors.
    Answer: a   LO: 22; conceptual   page: 380

Eating Disorders

92. Which of the following is *false* about the relationship between eating disorders and mood disorders?
    a. The families of people with eating disorders have higher rates of depression compared with the families of people without eating disorders.
    b. Seventy-five percent of people with an eating disorder can also be diagnosed with a mood disorder.
    c. People with eating disorders and people with mood disorders have abnormal functioning in the hypothalamus.
    d. Cognitive-behavioral therapy is an effective treatment for both anorexia and depression.
    Answer: d   LO: 22; factual, conceptual   page: 380

93. Which of the following is *the most critical factor* in developing an eating disorder?
    a. biological predisposition
    b. environmental pressures
    c. personality factors
    d. It is probably necessary for all of them to interact with each other for a person to develop an eating disorder.
    Answer: d   LO: 22; factual, conceptual   page: 380

94. In response to the question asked in the text of, "What is so bad about being obese?" one might reasonably conclude that:
    a. it may not be obesity itself, but something such as lack of exercise that is the health problem.
    b. obesity is more of a health problem for women than it is for men.
    c. obesity is a major health problem for men and women.
    d. obesity is not a problem.
    Answer. a   LO: 1; factual   page: 382

95. The text suggests that overweight people should:
    a. diet regularly, but not to extremes.
    b. exercise regularly.
    c. decrease their intake of complex carbohydrates.
    d. aim for a weight just below where they want to be as an incentive to get where they want their weight to be.
    Answer: b   LO: 22; factual, conceptual   page: 382

Chapter 10

Essay Questions

96. Imagine that you have been asked to talk to your younger sister's ninth grade class about eating disorders because her teacher has become alarmed with how many of the girls are on self-induced weight-reduction diets. You want all of the students (girls *and* boys) to understand the different types of eating disorders and the dangers that are involved with them. To do this, you will need to compare and contrast anorexia nervosa (both restricting and binge-purge types) with bulimia nervosa (both purging and nonpurging) in terms of diagnostic criteria, health risks posed, origins of the disorders, and prognosis and treatments for each. What would you suggest to these young people about their eating habits?

    The student should delineate the diagnostic criteria that characterize each disorder, noting where they are similar and how they diverge. Health risks specific to each disorder and the potential that each of them can be fatal should be covered. Biological, familial, and societal factors involved in developing each disorder should be discussed, as well as the specific types of treatment, focusing on the importance of family systems and getting the anorexic patient to eat. Differences in treatment effectiveness between anorexia and bulimia should also be discussed. The prognosis for all four types should be addressed. The student should then suggest proper eating habits for teenagers.

97. Recently, you have become involved in the International Students' Club on campus, and you have noticed that students from around the world have different attitudes about food, dieting, and body image. This reminds you of the biopsychosocial factors you learned about in your Abnormal Psychology class. You decide to explore the biopsychosocial factors that contribute to eating disorders so you can share these ideas in your class. Discuss each of the factors individually and how they interact with each other to create the problem. What do you think would be the most effective way to eliminate these disorders?

    A proper answer will discuss biological components of the disorders and their relationship to other clinical syndromes, such as depression, and address the psychological underpinnings, notably in terms of family issues for each. Extremely important here are the cultural factors that contribute to development of eating disorders (e.g., societal apotheosis of a thin figure for women), and critically evaluate those for which evidence is mixed (e.g., being a Caucasian). The evidence should be presented (e.g., people rate women who are thinner as more feminine; people in Eastern cultures do not exhibit the distorted body image as do people in Western cultures; or, some studies have found lower rates of eating disorders among African-Americans and Hispanics, others have not, and lower rates are not found among African-Americans and Hispanics of higher socioeconomic status). Students should also discuss the synergistic effects of the biological, psychological, and social factors, and present a thoughtful plan to use this information to eliminate eating disorders.

Eating Disorders

98. You have noticed that the text discusses binge-eating disorder, although it is not included as a specific diagnosable disorder in DSM-IV. This arouses your curiosity about how disorders do or do not get included in this important manual for mental health workers. To help you understand this process, explain what binge-eating disorder is and why it has been omitted (or, more accurately, included in the appendix rather than on Axis I) and why you believe it should or should not be considered an actual disorder.

    Binge-eating disorder does not have the same focus on being thin that are seen in anorexia and bulimia and, in fact, many people with the disorder are overweight. It has been excluded because there is not enough research to sanction the diagnosis. The student should present a convincing argument on why it should or should not be included as a diagnostic category in DSM, including its prevalence.

99. Examine the argument that eating disorders are a product of culture and family dynamics. Which cultural factors contribute to the development of eating disorders, and what is the evidence for their role? What sort of family dynamics interact with these cultural factors to promote the development of eating disorders?

    Cultural factors that contribute to the development of eating disorders (e.g., societal apotheosis of a thin figure for women) should be addressed and critically evaluated in terms of those that find support and those for which evidence is mixed (e.g., being a Caucasian). The evidence should be presented (e.g., people rate women who are thinner as more feminine; people in Eastern cultures do not exhibit the distorted body image as do people in Western cultures; or some studies have found lower rates of eating disorders among African-Americans and Hispanics, others have not, and lower rates are not found among African-Americans and Hispanics of higher socioeconomic status). The various family patterns that foster each of the disorders (e.g., lack of boundaries, mothers' need to keep daughters dependent, etc.) should be discussed. The interaction between cultural and familial values should then be addressed--how cultures set up certain standards that may be played out, distorted, or even exaggerated in some dysfunctional families. The different family dynamics for each of the disorders needs to be explored.

Chapter 10

100. You have been asked to work with Karin Karpin in the hospital. She is 5'5" tall and weighs 92 lbs. When you first meet her, she is rude to you, accuses you of creating a problem so you can make a ton of money, assures you that there is nothing wrong with her because she is almost at the weight she wants to be, she is in perfect control of her eating habits, and she is going to leave the hospital as soon as she is out of restraints. As you talk to her, you hear her parents arguing out in the hall. Her father is concerned that she is about to die, and her mother denies that any problem exists; as they argue, Karin faints. What would be the first steps you take in treating her, and how would you go about working with Karin to ensure that she lives a long and healthy life?

The first step here is to stabilize Karin's medical condition caused by the anorexia and to get nutrition into her body. The student should then go through the family systems approaches to working within the family to rebalance the family dynamics, set boundaries, realign issues of control, etc. Behavioral techniques, particularly those using reinforcement to get Karin to eat, should be addressed. Long-term follow-up will be necessary here.

Chapter 11   Sexual Disorders

1. As stated in the text, the one underlying commonality of the sexual disorders is that they:
   a. are all considered to be sexually deviant.
   b. all involve behaviors or beliefs that are a source of distress.
   c. affect men and women in parallel, if not the same, ways.
   d. are all much more common than society is comfortable admitting.
   Answer: b   LO: 1; factual, conceptual   page: 386

2. Which of the following *is not* one of the distinct categories of sexual disorders?
   a. sexual dysfunction
   b. paraphilias
   c. self-abuse
   d. gender identity disorder.
   Answer: c   LO: 1; factual   page: 386

3. Transsexualism is another name for:
   a. homosexuality.
   b. bisexuality.
   c. paraphilia.
   d. gender identity disorder.
   Answer: d   LO: 1; factual   page: 386

4. Sexual activities that focus on nonhuman objects, children or nonconsenting adults, or on suffering or humiliation are termed:
   a. sadomasochistic.
   b. paraphilias.
   c. sexually deviant.
   d. abnormal sexuality.
   Answer: b   LO: 1; factual   page: 386

5. The most common of the sexual disorders is:
   a. sexual dysfunction.
   b. paraphilia.
   c. gender identity disorder.
   d. transsexualism.
   Answer: a   LO: 1; factual   page: 386

Chapter 11

6. The least common sexual disorder is:
   a. sexual dysfunction.
   b. paraphilia.
   c. vaginismus.
   d. transsexualism.
   Answer: d   LO: 1; factual   page: 386

7. The sexual dysfunctions are:
   a. a set of disorders in which people have trouble engaging in and enjoying sexual interchanges with other people.
   b. deviant behaviors that are typically kept hidden for fear that the person with the disorder may be arrested.
   c. physical disorders that affect a person's ability to engage in sexual intercourse with another person.
   d. psychological disorders that inhibit a person's ability to engage in sexual intercourse with another person.
   Answer: a   LO: 1; factual, conceptual   page: 386

8. The physiological change occurring with penile erection and vaginal lubrication is known as _____ and first occurs during the _____ phase of the sexual response cycle.
   a. myotonia; desire
   b. vasocongestion; plateau
   c. engorgement; desire
   d. vasocongestion; excitement
   Answer: d   LO: 1; factual   page: 387

9. Which of the following *is not* one of the phases of the sexual response cycle?
   a. foreplay
   b. arousal
   c. orgasm
   d. plateau
   Answer: a   LO: 1; factual   page: 387

10. Sandy and Chris are engaging in sexual intercourse. The phases of the sexual response cycle they would normally be expected to experience are:
    a. foreplay, excitement, and orgasm.
    b. desire, excitement, plateau, orgasm, and resolution.
    c. stimulation, arousal, orgasm, and resolution.
    d. stimulation, plateau, orgasm, and completion.
    Answer: b   LO: 1; applied   page: 387

Sexual Disorders

11. Which phase of the sexual response cycle is typically only experienced by men?
    a. excitement
    b. orgasm
    c. resolution
    d. refractory
    Answer: d   LO: 1; factual   page: 387

12. Vasocongestion refers to:
    a. muscular tension that allows the penis to become hard.
    b. muscular tension that excites the parties to engage in coitus.
    c. filling of blood vessels and tissues with blood.
    d. augmentation of bodily fluids including blood, saliva, and semen.
    Answer: c   LO: 1; factual   page: 387

13. During vasocongestion:
    a. males experience erection of the penis, and females experience enlargement of the clitoris, swelling of the labia, and moistening of the vagina.
    b. males and females experience similar responses of muscle tension, which culminate in muscular contractions.
    c. the male experiences erection of the penis; females experience psychological excitement but no physiological changes.
    d. the female experiences enlargement of clitoris, swelling of labia, and moistening of vagina; males experience psychological excitement but no physiological changes.
    Answer: a   LO: 1; factual   page: 387

14. The phase of the sexual response cycle in which excitement is at a high but stable level is the _____ phase.
    a. desire
    b. arousal
    c. plateau
    d. resolution
    Answer: c   LO: 1; factual   page: 387

15. Which of the following is *false* concerning sexual patterns?
    a. Problems in sexual functioning are extremely common.
    b. Women exhibit considerably more variability in terms of sexual response patterns than do men.
    c. Individuals vary greatly in terms of personal sexual response patterns.
    d. Women and men, overall, exhibit pretty much the same sexual response patterns.
    Answer: d   LO: 1; factual   page: 387

Chapter 11

16. With respect to the stages of the sexual response cycle:
    a. males experience all of these stages, whether through coitus, masturbation, or some other activity, but females only experience them through coitus.
    b. females experience all of these stages, whether through coitus, masturbation, or some other activity, but males only experience them through coitus.
    c. males and females experience the same stages, whether through coitus, masturbation, or some other activity.
    d. males experience all of the stages during any form of sexual activity, but females only experience *all* of the stages through masturbation.
    Answer: c   LO: 1; factual, conceptual   page: 387

17. Dale and Nan are in therapy because of their sexual problem. If they are like most couples who are involved in sex therapy, their problem would be:
    a. lack of sexual desire.
    b. inability to experience orgasm.
    c. pain or discomfort during sex.
    d. discomfort with their sexual orientation.
    Answer: a   LO: 2; applied   page: 388-389

18. Which of the following is *not* a way in which sexual desire is manifested?
    a. sexual thoughts and fantasies
    b. an individual's interest in initiating or participating in sexual activities
    c. awareness of sexual cues from others
    d. concern about the moral ramifications of engaging in sex
    Answer: d   LO: 2; conceptual   page: 388

19. Having little desire for sex is termed:
    a. hypersexuality.
    b. hyperactive sexual desire.
    c. hypoactive sexual desire.
    d. anhedonia.
    Answer: c   LO: 2; factual, conceptual   page: 389

20. A diagnosis of hypoactive sexual desire would be given when an individual:
    a. does not desire sexual relations because she is too tired from overwork.
    b. has been diagnosed with an inability to achieve orgasm.
    c. is obsessed with thoughts of sex most of his waking (and some of his sleeping) hours.
    d. who used to enjoy sex has lost interest in it, despite the presence of a willing and desirable partner.
    Answer: d   LO: 2; factual, conceptual   page: 389-390

Sexual Disorders

21. Joe has noticed, over the past few years, that he no longer has any desire for sex. His wife, Patsy, has tried everything she can think of, including sexy lingerie, whipped cream, erotic movies, and even hiring a strip tease dancer to perform at his fiftieth birthday party. He's an attentive and loving husband, comes straight home from work, and spends all of his non-working hours with Patsy, their children, and their grandchildren, so she knows he's not going elsewhere for sexual gratification. Joe would be diagnosed with:
    a. generalized hypoactive sexual desire.
    b. situational hypoactive sexual desire.
    c. sexual aversion disorder.
    d. male erectile disorder.
    Answer: a   LO: 2; applied   pages: 389-390

22. Ginger and Frank have just celebrated their twenty-fifth anniversary. They were high school sweethearts. He was captain of the football team, and she was captain of the cheerleader squad. They were voted the "Most Perfect Couple." Gradually, over the years, Ginger has lost her girlish figure, and Frank has put on a "beer belly," and although they remain devoted to each other, neither finds the other sexually attractive. Frank justifies his affairs with other women as a way to keep him happy and thus a better husband; Ginger had a brief affair a few years ago, but felt so guilty that all she does now is fantasize about being carried off by Mel Gibson and Brad Pitt. Ginger and Frank are experiencing:
    a. generalized hypoactive sexual desire.
    b. situational hypoactive sexual desire.
    c. sexual aversion disorder.
    d. male erectile disorder.
    Answer: b   LO: 2; applied   pages: 389-390

23. For many years, Catherine had repressed the memory of being sexually abused by her older brother. She has one daughter, Jennifer, but feels sex is disgusting and animalistic, and barely had any sexual relations with her husband since Jennifer was born. It was not until Jennifer entered puberty that Catherine began to remember the abuse. Catherine is likely experiencing:
    a. generalized hypoactive sexual desire.
    b. situational hypoactive sexual desire.
    c. sexual aversion disorder.
    d. male erectile disorder.
    Answer: c   LO: 2; applied   page: 390

Chapter 11

24. The term for not experiencing the normal physiological changes incident to the excitement phase of the sexual response cycle is:
    a. hypoactive sexual desire.
    b. sexual arousal disorder.
    c. myotonia.
    d. dyspareunia.
    Answer: b   LO: 3; factual   page: 390

25. Female sexual arousal disorder involves:
    a. feelings of disgust associated with sexual intercourse.
    b. a recurrent inability to attain or maintain the swelling-lubrication response of sexual excitement.
    c. a recurrent inability to feel emotionally excited by her partner during foreplay.
    d. a recurrent inability to feel physically aroused, as experienced through tingling sensations and muscle tension.
    Answer: b   LO: 3; factual   page: 391

26. The recurrent inability of a man to attain or maintain an erection until the completion of sexual activity is referred to as:
    a. hypoactivity.
    b. penile disorder.
    c. male erectile disorder.
    d. delayed ejaculation.
    Answer: c   LO: 3; factual   page: 391

27. Which of the following is *not true* concerning male erectile dysfunction?
    a. It is a common problem with as many as 30,000,000 men in the United States having erectile problems at some time in their lives.
    b. Primary male erectile dysfunction disorder is diagnosed for men who have never been able to sustain an erection for the desired amount of time.
    c. Secondary male erectile dysfunction disorder is diagnosed for men who in the past were been able to sustain an erection but no longer can.
    d. Over 10% of men in the United States have problems sufficient to warrant a diagnosis of male erectile disorder.
    Answer: d   LO: 3; factual   page: 391

Sexual Disorders

28. Which of the following is *true* concerning sexual dysfunctions?
    a. It is significantly more common for men than for women to have anorgasmia.
    b. The most common form of orgasmic disorder for men is male orgasmic disorder.
    c. Women who are not able to achieve orgasm from sexual activity with their partner are generally not able to achieve orgasm with other types of stimulation.
    d. Many women treated for anorgasmia are able to achieve orgasm when they receive adequate stimulation.
    Answer: d   LO: 4; factual, conceptual   page: 392

29. The most common form of orgasmic disorder in males is:
    a. premature ejaculation.
    b. male orgasmic disorder.
    c. delayed gratification.
    d. anorgasmia.
    Answer: a   LO: 4; factual   page: 392

30. A man who persistently ejaculates with minimal sexual stimulation before they wish to ejaculate has:
    a. premature ejaculation.
    b. male orgasmic disorder.
    c. delayed gratification disorder.
    d. anorgasmia.
    Answer: a   LO: 4; factual, conceptual   page: 392

31. A recurrent delay in, or absence of, orgasm following the excitement phase of the sexual response cycle is referred to as:
    a. dyspareunia.
    b. premature ejaculation.
    c. male orgasmic disorder.
    d. sexual delay disorder.
    Answer: c   LO: 4; factual, conceptual   page: 393

32. Which of the following is *true* concerning male orgasmic disorder?
    a. This disorder refers to a complete inability to achieve orgasm.
    b. Men with this disorder can usually ejaculate with manual or oral stimulation.
    c. This is a device used by men to pressure their sex partners into performing oral sex.
    d. This is a rare disorder, with only about 1% of men experiencing it their lifetime.
    Answer: b   LO: 4; factual, conceptual   page: 393

Chapter 11

33. Pain during sexual intercourse is known as:
   a. myotonia.
   b. dyspareunia.
   c. vaginismus.
   d. anorgasmia.
   Answer: b   LO: 5; factual   page: 393

34. Which of the following is *true* concerning dyspareunia?
   a. It is more common in women than it is in men.
   b. The term relates to uterine pain for women and penile pain for men.
   c. The primary cause of the pain for women is deep penile thrusting.
   d. The primary cause of the pain for men relates to erectile dysfunction.
   Answer: a   LO: 5; factual, conceptual   page: 393

35. Which of the following is *true* concerning vaginismus?
   a. It is extremely common in women, and relatively rare in men.
   b. In some individuals, even the anticipation of coitus can result in vaginismus.
   c. It involves contraction of vaginal muscles for women, penile muscles for men.
   d. It occurs in sexual situations but does not in medical examinations.
   Answer: b   LO: 5; factual   page: 393

36. Which of the following statements about the causes of sexual dysfunction is *true*?
   a. In men, low levels of prolactin and estrogen can cause sexual dysfunction.
   b. In women, changes in reproductive hormone levels cause consistent fluctuations in levels of sexual desire.
   c. Biologically caused sexual dysfunctions typically appear suddenly and are global and consistent.
   d. None of the above is true.
   Answer: d   LO: 6; factual   page: 394

37. The text suggests that the most common cause of a sexual dysfunction may be:
   a. biological.
   b. psychological.
   c. societal.
   d. another sexual dysfunction.
   Answer: d   LO: 6; factual, conceptual   page: 394

Sexual Disorders

38. Which of the following is among the most common biological causes of sexual dysfunction?
    a. heart attack
    b. diabetes
    c. high levels of testosterone
    d. low levels of estrogen
    Answer: b   LO: 6; factual   page: 394

39. Which of the following is *not* typically a biological cause of sexual dysfunction in women?
    a. inconsistent hormone levels
    b. radiation therapy
    c. vaginal infections
    d. antihistamines
    Answer: a   LO: 6; factual   pages: 394-395

40. Which of the following is *true* about sexual activity in old age?
    a. There is a major decline in sexual activity, and by the age of 80, it is a rare occurrence.
    b. So long as they remain in good health, men will evidence little if any reduction in sexual activity even in their late years.
    c. Although many elderly people remain sexually active, there is typically a decrease in desire, arousal, and sexual activity as people get older.
    d. Men often experience little, if any, decline in their sexual activities over time (provided they have a stimulating partner), but women experience a major decline (even with a stimulating partner).
    Answer: c   LO: 6; factual, conceptual   page: 395

41. Which of the following is *not* a way suggested in the text for determining whether a man is having nocturnal erections?
    a. Have his wife or significant other observe his penile activity during the night.
    b. Observe whether he awakens in the morning with an erection.
    c. Use a device that wraps around the man's penis to detect penile pressure.
    d. Attach a ring of postage stamps to the base of the penis before he goes to sleep.
    Answer: a   LO: 6; factual   page: 395

42. A major reason stated in the text for women to experience anorgasmia is:
    a. moral concerns about sex.
    b. lack of communication with her partner.
    c. lack of knowledge about sex.
    d. fear.
    Answer: b   LO: 7; factual   page: 396

Chapter 11

43. Which of the following is *not* an interpersonal problem discussed in the text that can cause sexual dysfunction?
    a. communication between the partners
    b. anger and distrust by one or both partners directed toward the other partner
    c. an imbalance of power in the relationship
    d. concerns over the immorality of the sex act
    Answer: d   LO: 7; factual, conceptual   pages: 396-397

44. Which of the following is *false* concerning women and men who seek treatment for hypoactive sexual desire disorder?
    a. Men and women are equally as likely to report problems in their marital relationships.
    b. Women are more likely than men to report stressful events in their lives and higher psychological distress.
    c. Men seeking treatment are more likely than women to have other types of sexual dysfunction in addition to low desire.
    d. For men, issues of sexual functioning appear to have precipitated their entry into treatment, whereas for women hypoactive sexual desire is linked to many other psychosocial problems.
    Answer: a   LO: 7; factual, conceptual   page: 397

45. Which of the following is *not* a factor discussed in the text that might bring on sexual dysfunction?
    a. relationship factors
    b. environmental toxins
    c. attitudes and cognitions
    d. trauma
    Answer: b   LO: 7; factual   pages: 396-397

46. Which of the following men might be expected to be the most likely to experience hypoactive sexual desire with his partner because he is unable to cope with the fact that she was raped?
    a. Joe, who says, "My wife, Joanne, and I have been best friends since first grade."
    b. Manny, who says, "Rape is not a crime about sex; it's about power, control and anger."
    c. Sidney, who says, "There really is no such thing as rape. Most of the time a woman enjoys it but doesn't feel comfortable saying so."
    d. Arden, who says, "I am so angry and so hurt that this was done to my wife. Part of me wants to cry, part of me wants to go out and kill that guy."
    Answer: c   LO: 7; applied   page: 397

Sexual Disorders

47. An attitude that interferes with sexual functioning that appears to be rampant among middle-aged and younger adults is:
    a. negative gender stereotypes.
    b. performance anxiety.
    c. fear of sex itself.
    d. that it is not emotionally safe to give up control through orgasm.
    Answer: b LO: 7; conceptual page: 398

48. "Spectatoring" involves:
    a. couples engaging in sexual intercourse while others are watching.
    b. voyeurs watching people engage in sex without the people knowing this.
    c. exhibitionists revealing themselves to large groups of people at the same time.
    d. individuals closely monitoring their own behaviors and feelings while engaging in sexual relations with another person.
    Answer: d LO: 7; factual page: 398

49. Which of the following statements is *true*?
    a. Performance anxiety cannot only hinder sexual enjoyment and retard orgasm, it can also lead to premature ejaculation is some men.
    b. Having severely negative attitudes toward sex can hinder one's level of sexual desire, but it cannot lead to such biological conditions as dyspareunia.
    c. Women undergoing menopause frequently experience an increase in their levels of sexual desire.
    d. Men who have more frequent and more varied sex are less likely to gain ejaculatory control than other men.
    Answer: a LO: 7; factual, conceptual page: 398

50. There is a biblical admonition against "wasting [a man's] seed," which has been interpreted as a prohibition against masturbation. As noted in the text, this attitude is also expressed by:
    a. the ancient Greek physician, Hippocrates.
    b. traditional medical systems from China and India.
    c. the hieroglyphic writings of the ancient Egyptians.
    d. the eighteenth century German and French physicians.
    Answer: b LO: 8; factual page: 399

Chapter 11

51. A syndrome known as _____, thought to result from semen loss, has been reported by several Asian cultures. This involves acute anxiety, a feeling of panic and impending death, and a delusion that the penis is shrinking into the body and disappearing.
    a. Koro
    b. Amok
    c. *ataque de nervios*
    d. Sasaki
    Answer: a   LO: 8; factual   page: 399

52. Which of the following is *not* a reason given in the text as to why men and women of lower socioeconomic status would experience more sexual dysfunction and less sexual pleasure?
    a. greater psychological stress
    b. worse physical health
    c. less education about their bodies
    d. closer family systems
    Answer: d   LO: 8; factual   page: 399

53. Which of the following is an accurate match between a sexual dysfunction and the proper biological treatment for it?
    a. premature ejaculation: apomorphine
    b. male erectile disorder: clomipramine
    c. premature ejaculation: yohimbine
    d. male erectile disorder: apomorphine
    Answer: d   LO: 9; factual   page: 400

54. Which of the following is *true* concerning use of drugs and sexual functioning?
    a. A person who takes insulin for diabetes will generally need to adjust to having a less-than-satisfactory sex life, since diabetes negatively affects sexual functioning.
    b. Discontinuing the use of recreational drugs can often cure a sexual dysfunction.
    c. Antidepressant drugs, such as clomipramine and sertraline, often produce premature ejaculation in men.
    d. Ironically, while chewing the bark of the yohimbehe tree has been noted to increase sexual functioning in Africa, its derivative drug, yohimbine, has the opposite effect on men in industrialized nations.
    Answer: b   LO: 9; factual   page: 400

Sexual Disorders

55. Sex therapy can be particularly useful when:
    a. either the man or the woman (or both) have a physiological problem that contributes to their sexual dysfunction.
    b. a man cannot cure an erectile disorder by using drugs.
    c. the sexual dysfunction is due, at least in part, to inadequate sexual practices of one or both partners.
    d. there is a great deal of emotional conflict between the sex partners.
    Answer: c   LO: 10; factual, conceptual   page: 400

56. The type of sex therapy in which one partner is active and carries out a set of exercises to stimulate the other partner, while the other partner is the passive recipient who receives pleasure that the exercises bring is called:
    a. the stop-start technique.
    b. sensate focus therapy.
    c. the squeeze technique.
    d. pleasure stimulation therapy.
    Answer: b   LO: 10; factual, conceptual   page: 400

57. Which of the following is *not* part of the initial phases of sensate focus therapy?
    a. the couple spends time gently touching each other, but not around the genitals.
    b. the couple stimulates each others' breasts and genitals until they are fully aroused, and then they gently engage in intercourse.
    c. the partner with the problem is instructed to focus on the pleasure that partner is experiencing.
    d. the partner with the problem is instructed to communicate with his or her partner about what feels good.
    Answer: b   LO: 10; factual, conceptual   pages: 400-401

58. Which of the following is *not* a goal of teaching a client to masturbate?
    a. for the person to explore his or her own body
    b. for the person to discover what is arousing
    c. for the person to become less inhibited about his or her sexuality
    d. for the person to enjoy sex without needing to discuss it with his or her partner
    Answer: d   LO: 10; factual, conceptual   page: 401

Chapter 11

59. The stop-start technique is used primarily to help:
    a. a paraphiliac stop engaging in that paraphiliac behavior and start engaging in normal sexual behavior
    b. men who have premature ejaculations control their ejaculations
    c. women with vaginismus gain some control over their vaginal contractions
    d. women with dyspareunia learn they can stop sexual interactions when they feel pain and start them again when the pain passes
    Answer: b   LO: 10; factual   page: 401

60. The goals of the stop-start technique are:
    a. for the man to gain control over his ejaculations and to enjoy the sensation of being in the woman's vagina.
    b. for the woman to gain control over her vaginismus and for the man to gain control over his ejaculations.
    c. for the woman to gain control over her dyspareunia and to enjoy the sensation of having the man's penis in her vagina.
    d. for both the man and the woman to control their respective orgasms so they can climax together.
    Answer: a   LO: 10; factual, conceptual   pages: 401-402

61. The technique used most often for vaginismus is:
    a. the squeeze technique.
    b. the stop-start technique.
    c. deconditioning of vaginal contractions.
    d. sensate focus therapy.
    Answer: c   LO: 10; factual   page: 402

62. Deconditioning a woman's automatic tightening of her vaginal muscles is an especially effective treatment for:
    a. dyspareunia.
    b. myotonia.
    c. vaginismus.
    d. anorgasmia.
    Answer: c   LO: 10; factual   page: 402

Sexual Disorders

63. Which statement is *false* about individual psychotherapy as it relates to sexual dysfunction?
    a. Individual psychotherapy is the preferred modality since it allows the person with the dysfunction to work on it in a supportive context without embarrassment.
    b. Cognitive-behavioral interventions address attitudes and scripts that interfere with a person's sexual functioning.
    c. Psychodynamic therapies explore childhood experiences that contributed to a person's negative attitudes toward sex.
    d. Behavioral techniques of sex therapy teach the client new sexual skills and provide material for discussion in therapy sessions.
    Answer: a   LO: 10; factual, conceptual   page: 403

64. Couples therapy is especially useful:
    a. to teach couples who don't know how to stimulate each other effective stimulation techniques.
    b. to help couples enjoy incongruities between partners' expectations for sexual encounters.
    c. to help couples solve problems in their relationship that interfere with sexual enjoyment.
    d. to help the partners reduce genital dryness.
    Answer: c   LO: 10; factual, conceptual   page: 405

65. Which of the following statements is *true* with respect to homosexual relationships as stated in the text?
    a. Lesbians are less likely than heterosexual women to complain of dyspareunia or vaginismus, but may be more likely to have an aversion to oral sex.
    b. As a result of the AIDS epidemic, gay men have to deal with the cognitive dissonance of high sexual arousal but fear of getting the AIDS virus.
    c. There are no extraordinary issues surrounding the homosexual orientation that would make dealing with a lesbian or gay client different from working with a straight client.
    d. Because of their sexual orientation, it is necessary for a couples therapist to formulate different techniques for dealing with homosexual couples.
    Answer: a   LO: 11; factual, conceptual   page: 405

Chapter 11

66. Sex is a vital component of life and is necessary for any species to continue. Consequently, in some states, such as California, all licensed therapists (MFCCs, clinical psychologists, psychiatrists, MSWs) are required to take courses in human sexuality and to acquire a comfort zone for dealing with the intimate details of a person's (or couple's) life. Understanding this, consider the appropriate response to a couple who advise you that they believe sex is evil.
    a. Their belief will have to be challenged using cognitive-behavioral therapy.
    b. The therapist needs to work within the couple's belief system, determine their current repertoire of sexual activity, and build on that according to their comfort.
    c. The therapist needs to accept the couple's belief system and assure them that it may be best for them to refrain from any form sex.
    d. The therapist needs to accept the couple's belief system and advise them to be content holding each other and refrain from more complex sexual behaviors.
    Answer: b   LO: 11; factual, conceptual   page: 405

67. Which of the following is *not* true about variations in preferences for sexually arousing stimuli?
    a. Most of the time they merely add "spice to life."
    b. What is considered acceptable sexual activity depends on the particular culture.
    c. Judgments about what are normal and abnormal sexual behaviors are subjective.
    d. Most people diagnosed with a paraphilia use their atypical sexual act as a secondary form of sexual arousal.
    Answer: d   LO: 12; factual, conceptual   page: 406

68. Which of the following is *not* a paraphilia?
    a. sadism
    b. voyeurism
    c. transsexualism
    d. pedophilia
    Answer: c   LO: 12; factual   page: 407

69. As stated in the text, the most benign of the paraphilias is:
    a. exhibitionism.
    b. voyeurism.
    c. fetishism.
    d. pedophilia.
    Answer: c   LO: 13; factual   page: 407

Sexual Disorders

70. The focus of sexual activity for a person with a fetish is:
    a. a young boy.
    b. a young girl.
    c. a nonhuman object.
    d. a fantasy.
    Answer: c   LO: 13; factual, conceptual   page: 407

71. As stated in the text, the most severe paraphilia is:
    a. sadomasochism.
    b. pedophilia.
    c. voyeurism.
    d. fetishism.
    Answer: b   LO: 13; factual, conceptual   page: 407

72. An elaborate form of fetishism is:
    a. transsexualism.
    b. homosexuality.
    c. tokenism.
    d. transvestism.
    Answer: d   LO: 13; factual   page: 408

73. One of the most common secondary diagnoses of persons with other types of paraphilias is:
    a. fetishism.
    b. transvestism.
    c. sadomasochism.
    d. pedophilia.
    Answer: a   LO: 13; factual   page: 408

74. _____ refers to gaining sexual gratification by inflicting pain on one's sexual partner; _____ involves gaining sexual gratification by suffering pain or humiliation during sex.
    a. Sadism; masochism
    b. Bondage; domination
    c. Masochism; sadism
    d. Abuse; acceptance
    Answer: a   LO: 13; factual, conceptual   page: 408

Chapter 11

75. Which of the following is *true* about sadomasochistic sex?
    a. Women are more likely to be the sadist, while men are more likely to be the masochist.
    b. The partner who is the victim in these encounters is generally a masochist and thus a willing victim.
    c. The sexual rituals of sadists and masochists typically involve practices of bondage and domination.
    d. Particularly in the case of voluntary participation by both partners, there is little, if any chance, of serious danger to either.
    Answer: c   LO: 13; factual, conceptual   page: 409

76. In _____ the person secretly watches another person undressing, bathing, or engaged in sex as a preferred or exclusive form of sexual arousal, while in _____ the person is sexually aroused by exposing his or her genitals to involuntary observers.
    a. sadism; masochism
    b. voyeurism; exhibitionism
    c. exhibitionism; voyeurism
    d. voyeurism; frotteurism
    Answer: b   LO: 13; factual, conceptual   page: 409

77. Which of the following is *false* about the "typical" exhibitionist?
    a. He will confront a woman in a public place, expose his genitals, and masturbate.
    b. They are more likely than most sex offenders to get caught.
    c. They are "calling out for help" since they invite arrest by returning to the crime scene.
    d. They are likely to continue their behavior after having been caught.
    Answer: c   LO: 13; factual, conceptual   pages: 409-410

78. Andrew achieves his primary source of sexual gratification from rubbing and fondling the body parts of nonconsenting adults. He would be diagnosed with:
    a. exhibitionism.
    b. voyeurism.
    c. frotteurism.
    d. pedophilia.
    Answer: c   LO: 13; applied   page: 410

79. Robert is 36 years old. He is sexually attracted to children and prefers to engage in sex activity with them rather than with other adults. He would receive the DSM-IV diagnosis of:
    a. child molester.
    b. pediatrician.
    c. pedophile.
    d. pervert.
    Answer: c   LO: 14; applied   page: 410

Sexual Disorders

80. Which of the following statements is *false*?
    a. Pedophiles have typically been abused as children.
    b. Pedophiles are typically homosexual.
    c. Pedophiles typically have poor interpersonal skills.
    d. Pedophiles must be, by definition, at least 5 years older than their victim(s).
    Answer: b LO: 14; factual, conceptual page: 410

81. Which of the following is *true* concerning the legal and psychiatric conceptions of child molestation?
    a. Both concur that the sexual encounters are committed by persons over the age of 18 with a person under the age of 18.
    b. A diagnosis of pedophilia requires the perpetrator to be over 16 and at least 5 years older than the victim, who is under 13.
    c. Laws in the United States define child molestation or statutory rape to include adults over 21 having nonconsensual sex with a person under the age of 18.
    d. Laws in the United States define child molestation or statutory rape to include adults over 21 having sex with any person under the age of 16.
    Answer: b LO: 14; factual, conceptual page: 410

82. Which of the following is *false* concerning the behavior of pedophiles?
    a. They often threaten the child with harm or threaten to hurt someone the child loves if the child tells about the liaison.
    b. They often try to convince the child that they are showing the child love.
    c. The contact most often consists of the pedophile exposing and touching the child's genitals, sometimes involves oral sex, but rarely actually involves penile insertion.
    d. Many pedophiles develop elaborate plans for gaining access to the child.
    Answer: c LO: 14; factual, conceptual page: 410

83. Which of the following is *false* concerning the statistical information on pedophilia?
    a. It is estimated that approximately 400,000 children are sexually abused each year in the United States.
    b. Approximately 60% of the children who are sexually abused are under 12 years of age.
    c. It is estimated that only 5% of child sexual abuse cases are reported.
    d. Most abusers are heterosexual men who abuse female family members or other children they already know.
    Answer: c LO: 14; factual page: 410

Chapter 11

84. Which of the following is *not* one of the factors that increases a child's risk for long-term psychological distress following abuse by a pedophile?
    a. having been penetrated by the pedophile
    b. having been abused by a complete stranger rather than a family member
    c. having a mother who doesn't believe the child has been abused
    d. having frequent abuse over a long period of time
    Answer: b   LO: 14; factual, conceptual   page: 411

85. Which of the following is *false* about the view of mental health professionals concerning pedophiles?
    a. They are split on whether pedophiles should be considered as suffering from a treatable psychological disorder or a criminal offense for which they should be incarcerated.
    b. They agree that despite the label given to the behavior, pedophiles should be prevented from performing the behavior.
    c. Some believe there is an excellent prognosis for the disorder through cognitive-behavioral and behavior therapies and the disorder can be cured.
    d. Some clinicians are unable to empathize with pedophiles and thus cannot treat them.
    Answer: c   LO: 14; factual, conceptual   page: 411

86. According to behavioral theories, how does a paraphilia develop?
    a. Paraphilia develops when the person has been rewarded by others for engaging in paraphiliac behaviors and punished for engaging in "normal" sexual behaviors.
    b. Children who have been abused develop paraphiliac behaviors as a reaction to their abuse.
    c. The paraphiliac object and the person's usual sexual partner must be paired for the person to develop sexual arousal to the paraphiliac object.
    d. The chance pairing of the paraphiliac object and sexual arousal leads the person to develop a classically conditioned sexual response to the paraphiliac object.
    Answer: d   LO: 15; factual, conceptual   pages: 411-412

87. Which of the following is *false* about treatment for paraphilias?
    a. Most paraphilics seek treatment for their behaviors because they feel great shame and guilt.
    b. If a paraphiliac has not sought treatment for his problem, it is often forced upon him after he has been arrested for breaking the law.
    c. Incarceration for these behaviors does little to change them.
    d. The recidivism rate among convicted sex offenders is very high.
    Answer: a   LO: 14; factual, conceptual   page: 412

88. Aversion therapy for paraphilia involves:
   a. convincing the paraphiliac through cognitive techniques that society finds his or her behavior so aversive that he or she cannot be accepted by society until the behavior ends.
   b. all of the family members and friends of the paraphiliac rejecting him or her until he or she gives up the paraphiliac behavior.
   c. extinguishing the paraphiliac's response to the paraphiliac object by pairing the object with an unpleasant stimulus.
   d. flooding the paraphiliac with his or her object of desire until he or she habituates to and no longer is sexually aroused by it.
   Answer: c   LO: 14; factual, conceptual   page: 412

89. Which of the following is *not* a biological intervention that has been used to treat pedophilia?
   a. surgery on areas of the brain thought to control sexual behavior
   b. surgical castration of the penis
   c. use of antiandrogen drugs that reduce testosterone production
   d. use of drugs that are believed to reduce the sex drive.
   Answer: b   LO: 14; factual   page: 412

90. Which of the following is *true* concerning treatment of paraphilics?
   a. Insight-oriented therapies have been relatively successful in changing paraphilics' behavior.
   b. Behavior modification therapy can be successful if the paraphiliac is willing to change his behavior.
   c. Aversive therapy has proven particularly effective in eliminating paraphiliac behavior, even when the paraphiliac is not motivated to change.
   d. The best way to eliminate paraphiliac behavior appears to be long-term incarceration.
   Answer: b   LO: 14; factual, conceptual   page: 412

91. A person's perception of him- or herself as a male or female refers to _____, while the person's preference for sexual partners of the same or different sex refers to _____.
   a. gender identity; gender role
   b. gender role; sexual preference
   c. gender role; sexual preference
   d. gender identity; sexual orientation
   Answer: d   LO: 15; factual, conceptual   page: 413

Chapter 11

92. Richard believes he was born with the wrong sex genitalia. He believes that despite his male genitalia, he is a woman. Richard would be diagnosed with:
    a. gender identity disorder.
    b. sexual identity disorder.
    c. gender role disorder.
    d. sex role disorientation.
    Answer: a   LO: 15; applied   page: 413

93. Which of the following is *false* concerning gender identity disorder?
    a. Boys are more likely than girls to be brought by their parents for counseling for this disorder.
    b. The disorder, when seen in adulthood, is termed transsexualism.
    c. Gender identity disorder is closely linked with homosexuality.
    d. Unlike transvestites, when transsexuals dress in opposite sex clothing, it is not for purposes of sexual arousal.
    Answer: c   LO: 15, 17; factual, conceptual   pages: 413-414

94. Which of the following is *true* concerning gender identity disorder?
    a. Transsexuals consistently show hormonal abnormalities.
    b. Transsexuals consistently show a history of troubled upbringing.
    c. Gender identity disorder often develops in synchrony with alcohol and drug problems.
    d. Most transsexuals say that even as children they felt they were the wrong gender.
    Answer: d   LO: 15; factual, conceptual   page: 414

95. Which best describes the differences between transvestism and transsexualism?
    a. Transvestites believe they have been born with the wrong genitals, whereas transsexuals simply enjoy dressing as a member of the opposite sex.
    b. Transsexuals believe they have been born with the wrong genitals, whereas transvestites simply enjoy dressing as a member of the opposite sex.
    c. Transvestites are almost always homosexual, whereas transsexuals are almost always bisexual.
    d. Transvestites and transsexuals both believe they were born with the wrong genitals, but only transsexuals believe this strongly enough to request sex change operations.
    Answer: b   LO: 17; factual, conceptual   page: 414

96. Chris has been diagnosed with gender identity disorder and wishes to undergo a sex change operation. If the operation is performed, it is most likely to occur after Chris has:
    a. received a psychiatric diagnosis.
    b. had any other psychiatric diagnoses ruled out.
    c. lived for a period of time as a member of the opposite sex.
    d. convinced a psychiatrist that Chris is homosexual.
    Answer: c   LO: 16; factual   page: 415

Sexual Disorders

Essay Questions

97. Discuss the differences between the psychiatric and legal definitions of pedophilia and child sexual abuse. Examine the factors that may cause a person to become a pedophile, and the legal, biological, and psychological ways to deal with this disorder, considering also the effects on the victim. What do you believe is the best way to handle this type of behavior that would be to the most benefit of society.

    Discuss the differences in age of perpetrator and victim, as well as the differential required (5 years) for child sexual abuse; and explore how they are similar in terms of the behaviors exhibited (e.g., from self-exposure, to fondling, to intercourse and sodomy). Explore the early childhood experiences of the pedophile, including the possibility of having been the victim of childhood sexual abuse himself. Discuss the options of keeping a child molester removed from society, as well as castration and use of drugs to lower sexual urges, and the behavioral therapies (e.g., aversion therapy), and the poor prognosis for these treatments. There are multiple negative effects on the child, particularly (as is usually the case) when the perpetrator is someone known to the child. The student should present a thoughtful argument of how this type of behavior should be handled to the optimum benefit of society.

98. While many sexual dysfunctions result from biological factors, such as medical conditions and drug usage, many of them result from psychosocial factors. Describe four difficulties in relationships and two attitudes that can lead to sexual dysfunctions. How could a clinician treat these problems? Give specific examples of techniques a therapist could use to treat these problems.

    A proper answer should describe four relationship problems (e.g., unconcern with one's partner's sexual needs), and two attitudes (e.g., performance anxiety) that interfere with sexual functioning. Steps for treating these problems should then be described (e.g., sensate focus therapy or couples therapy). The best answer would provide specific solutions in therapy to the problems listed in response to the question, e.g., "Couples therapy can help couples resolve non-sex-related issues that interfere with their sexual functioning, a problem identified above."

99. Because you are taking the course in Abnormal Psychology, your roommate has asked you about why homosexuality is no longer considered a sexual disorder. Explain to your roommate the important differences between a gay relationship and those sexual behaviors that are considered paraphilias. List three arguments about why gay relationships should *not* be considered a paraphilia.

    This is partly a matter of opinion, but proper answers will include a clear line of logic and evidence (if available). An example answer would be, in brief: "Homosexuals do

-267-

Chapter 11

not take advantage of their partner's immaturity and do not threaten them as pedophiles do their victims. Pedophiles do not have their partner's consent, and their actions have demonstrably negative effects on their child victim, such as PTSD, conduct disorder, etc."

100. Some of the paraphilias appear to be rather innocuous and cause harm to no one. Discuss which paraphilias fall within this range, and then address the issue of whether you believe they should be categorized as psychological disorders and/or criminal offenses, using evidence from the chapter to support your position. Are there social or cultural factors that either have or have not been included in the chapter that would affect society's view of whether these are or are not psychological disorders and/or crimes?

Perhaps the most innocuous of the paraphilias is fetishism; another that is considerably more vivid but harms no one is transvestism. The students should discuss what these paraphilias are, and then how the particular behaviors do not involve inflicting harm on others and that fetishism is typically done in private. However, the student needs to address the fact that these disorders may co-occur with more extreme atypical sexual behaviors that may have victims. Societal attitudes and cross-cultural variations should be brought in here, much of which may come from outside sources (e.g., attitudes toward transvestism is extremely different in many Native American tribes).

101. Max and Morris have been friends since childhood. Both have married and they both have teenage children. After all their years of friendship, Max finally confides to Morris that he is a transvestite and has been hiding this from his wife for years because she was totally appalled when she once saw him cross-dressing in her clothes. In turn, Morris confides to Max that for as long as he can remember he has always believed he should be a girl, and he recently began seeing a therapist to help him decide whether he should have a sex change operation and suggests that Max should see this therapist as well. Discuss both transvestism and transsexualism, giving the diagnostic characteristics of each and the differences between them, and what might cause each of them. If you were the therapist treating both Max and Morris, what techniques would you use with each of them? How would you incorporate their families into the therapy?

The student needs to note that transvestism is literally "cross-dressing," or a man dressing in women's clothes, whereas transsexualism is feeling that you are the wrong sex (although they may also cross-dress). The former is possibly established through classical conditioning; the latter is probably biologically and socially based. Both men would probably benefit most from couples therapy with their respective spouses (and for Morris also family therapy to help his children deal with any changes in gender identity that he may choose to undergo). For Max, behavioral therapy could work, as well as possibly some interpersonal and skills training; however, if his wife is not

Sexual Disorders

turned off by the behavior, there may be no need to hide it. For Morris, he would have to undergo extensive counseling to deal with his gender identity issues, to determine how he wanted to proceed--either remain a male or become a female. In the latter case, he would have to dress and live as a woman for two years, then begin to undergo hormone treatments before having the surgery to remove his penis and construct a vagina. He would need to be prepared for the physical and emotional pain involved, as would his family--having one's father become one's "other mother" could be traumatizing.

102. Using what you learned in the chapter on sexual disorders, what would you say to a friend who has asked you how a person could decide when "kinky" sex is sick?

As noted in the text, judgments about what is or is not acceptable varies by culture and across historical contexts. The student should list sexual activities noted in table 11.3 in terms of the types of sexual practices that men and women find appealing, and comment on what are and are not "acceptable" versus "diagnosable" sexual practices in our culture, as delineated by DSM-IV.

Chapter 12   Substance Use Disorders

1. As defined in the text, a _____ is any natural or synthesized product that has psychoactive effects, i.e., it changes perceptions, thoughts, emotions, and behavior.
    a. drug
    b. substance
    c. hallucinogen
    d. medicine
    Answer: b   LO: 1; factual, conceptual   page: 422

2. From research stated in the text, which of the following is *true* concerning attitudes about use of psychoactive substances?
    a. It is more common for societies to view the use of these substances as a danger to public health and security than as a matter of individual choice.
    b. The United States has, throughout its history, been relatively consistent in its negative attitude toward substance use.
    c. Societies have little motivation to regulate the use of psychoactive substances since they produce high revenues.
    d. Psychoactive substances have been used for thousands of years, often in religious ceremonies and for medical purposes.
    Answer: d   LO: 1; factual, conceptual   pages: 422-423

3. Which of the following is *true* with respect to substance use or abuse in the United States?
    a. The prevalence of illegal use and abuse has increased substantially in the last four decades.
    b. The prevalence of illegal use and abuse has increased minimally in the last four decades.
    c. The prevalence of illegal use and abuse has remained relatively consistent over the last four decades.
    d. The prevalence of illegal use and abuse has decreased in the last four decades.
    Answer: a   LO: 2; factual   page: 423

4. Prevalence data on substance abuse in the United States suggest:
    a. about 10% of the population admitted to having tried an illegal substance at some time in their lives in the early 1960s.
    b. about 25% of the population admitted to having tried an illegal substance at some time in their lives in the mid-1990s.
    c. Most people who use illegal substances do so before age 20.
    d. NIDA (1995) found that 50% of young adults used an illegal substance by age 25.
    Answer: c   LO: 2; factual   page: 423

Chapter 12

5. In terms of addiction, which of the following is *true*?
   a. Most adolescents and young adults who experiment with drugs come to use them chronically.
   b. Some drugs, such as crack cocaine, have such powerful reinforcing effects on the brain that many people who try them become addicted.
   c. Some people have a greater vulnerability to becoming addicted psychologically, but this is not a physiologically based vulnerability.
   d. Some people have a greater vulnerability to becoming addicted physiologically, but this is not a psychologically based vulnerability.
   Answer: b   LO: 3; factual, conceptual   page: 423

6. Which of the following is *not* one of the substance-related conditions recognized by the DSM-IV?
   a. substance intoxication
   b. substance withdrawal
   c. substance abuse
   d. substance addiction
   Answer: d   LO: 3; factual   page: 423

7. Which of the following is *not* one of the categories delineated in the text for grouping psychoactive substances?
   a. central nervous system depressants
   b. central nervous system stimulants
   c. narcotics
   d. hallucinogens
   Answer: c   LO: 3; factual   pages: 423-424

8. Which of the following are nonrestricted substances for which the DSM-IV lists disorders?
   a. alcohol and amphetamines
   b. nicotine and caffeine
   c. nicotine and marijuana
   d. codeine and caffeine
   Answer: b   LO: 3; factual   page: 424

9. A set of behavioral and psychological changes that occur as a direct result of the physiological effects of a substance on the central nervous system is referred to as:
   a. intoxication.
   b. drug withdrawal.
   c. drug abuse.
   d. dependence.
   Answer: a   LO: 3; factual, conceptual   page: 425

Substance Use Disorders

10. Which of the following statements about substance intoxication and/or withdrawal is *true*?
    a. The end of substance intoxication is marked by the point at which the substance exits the bloodstream, which is when symptoms are no longer experienced.
    b. People who use a substance chronically experience the same symptoms as people who use it for the first time, except that chronic users experience slightly less intense symptoms of intoxication.
    c. Because chronic substance users have more of a substance in their body, they experience withdrawal symptoms that are identical to the symptoms of intoxication even after they stop using the substance.
    d. The symptoms of substance intoxication result from physiological effects of the substance on the central nervous system.
    Answer: d   LO: 3; factual, conceptual   page: 425

11. Jimmy has been diagnosed with substance intoxication. This means:
    a. he has ingested a sufficient amount of a substance to alter his or her cognitive abilities.
    b. the people in his social environment have condemned his drunken behavior.
    c. the behavioral and psychological changes he experiences are significantly maladaptive.
    d. he has ingested a substance that is considered illegal, or more than three ounces of alcohol.
    Answer: c   LO: 3; applied   page: 426

12. Substance withdrawal involves:
    a. a set of maladaptive physiological and behavioral symptoms that result when a person who has used a substance heavily for a prolonged period of time stops, or greatly reduces, use of the substance.
    b. a set of behavioral and psychological changes that occur as a direct result of the physiological effects of a substance on the central nervous system.
    c. a condition when a person's recurrent use of a substance results in significant harmful consequences.
    d. a condition when a person experiences less and less effect from the same dose of a substance and needs greater and greater amounts to achieve intoxication.
    Answer: a   LO: 3; factual, conceptual   page: 426

13. Which of the following is *not* included in the diagnostic criteria for substance abuse?
    a. use of the substance in situations in which it is physically hazardous to do so
    b. failure to meet important obligations at work, school, or home
    c. development of tolerance to the substance, or withdrawal symptoms when not used
    d. legal problems as a result of substance use
    Answer: c   LO: 3; factual   page: 426

Chapter 12

14. Which of the following is *false* concerning substance withdrawal?
    a. The symptoms of withdrawal can begin within a few hours after the person stops ingesting the substance.
    b. The symptoms of withdrawal from a given substance are typically the opposite of the symptoms of intoxication of that substance.
    c. The diagnosis of substance withdrawal is made whenever symptoms occur, even if those symptoms do not cause significant distress or impairment in daily functioning.
    d. Withdrawal symptoms may end within a few days to a few weeks, or may be present for weeks or months after a person stops using a substance.
    Answer: c   LO: 3; factual, conceptual   page: 426

15. When is a diagnosis of substance abuse warranted?
    a. when the problem has evolved into substance dependence
    b. when a person repeatedly has problems in at least one of the four diagnostic categories for at least 12 consecutive months
    c. when a person repeatedly has problems in at least two of the four diagnostic categories for at least 12 consecutive months
    d. when a person's use of a substance causes significant harm
    Answer: b   LO: 3; factual, conceptual   pages: 426-427

16. The term that is most closely associated with the common perception of addiction is:
    a. substance abuse.
    b. substance dependence.
    c. substance tolerance.
    d. substance withdrawal.
    Answer: b   LO: 3; factual, conceptual   page: 427

17. John began snorting cocaine about a year ago. He said the first high was the most astounding, exciting, mind-blowing experience he has ever had. Although he gets high every weekend, he has never been able to recapture that initial euphoria, and now he needs more and more of the drug to get anywhere close. John:
    a. has developed a tolerance to cocaine.
    b. has become physiologically dependent on cocaine.
    c. is addicted to cocaine.
    d. needs to find a better source since the first stuff was probably the purest.
    Answer: a   LO: 3; applied   page: 427

Substance Use Disorders

18. Which of the following is *true* concerning a diagnosis of substance dependence?
    a. It requires a compulsive use of the substance despite significant social, occupational, psychological, or medical problems resulting from its use.
    b. It requires physiological evidence of tolerance to or withdrawal from the drug.
    c. People who are dependent on a substance will do anything to get it, including prostitution or stealing.
    d. It requires both physiological and a psychological evidence of obsessive craving.
    Answer: a   LO: 3; factual, conceptual   page: 427

19. Which of the following substances has the lowest risk of tolerance?
    a. alcohol
    b. PCP
    c. stimulants
    d. nicotine
    Answer: b   LO: 4; factual   page: 427

20. Which of the following properties of substances and their administration do *not* increase the likelihood of abuse and dependence?
    a. substances that are snorted, smoked, or injected
    b. substances that act rapidly on the brain and nervous system
    c. substances whose effects are longer-lasting
    d. substances that are absorbed rapidly and efficiently into the bloodstream
    Answer: c   LO: 4; factual   page: 428

21. Which of the following methods of administering a drug is *least* likely to lead to overdose?
    a. injection
    b. snorting
    c. smoking
    d. in solution
    Answer: d   LO: 4; factual   page: 428

22. A loss of memory for recent and distant events resulting from alcohol use is known as:
    a. alcohol-induced dementia.
    b. delirium tremens.
    c. Korsakoff's psychosis.
    d. blackout.
    Answer: d   LO: 4; factual   page: 429

Chapter 12

23. Which of the following statements about cultural differences in alcohol disorders is *true*?
    a. Lower rates of alcohol problems in China and Taiwan are partly due to an enzyme that, when present, causes a flushed face and heart palpitations during alcohol ingestion in 50% of Asians.
    b. Mexican-Americans who immigrated to the United States have lower rates of alcohol problems than Mexican-Americans born in the United States.
    c. There are lower rates of alcohol problems in South Korea compared to other Asian countries partly due to the Confucian moral ethic, which discourages drunken behavior and views alcohol as appropriately used for ceremonies but inappropriate for personal indulgence.
    d. Native Americans have lower rates of alcohol problems than African-Americans and Hispanics partly due to cultural proscriptions against creating disharmony between a person and his or her spirit.
    Answer: b   LO: 4, 10; factual   page: 434

24. Which of the following is a *true* explanation for why rates of alcohol problems are higher among older people?
    a. Older people metabolize alcohol at a slower rate than younger people, which leads them to become intoxicated more quickly.
    b. Older people are more likely than younger people to conform to traditional gender roles; thus more older men drink alcohol excessively, which accounts for their higher rates.
    c. Older people have grown up under fewer prohibitions against alcohol use and abuse, since alcohol problems were much less common during their younger years.
    d. The rates of alcohol problems are actually lower, not higher, among older people.
    Answer: d   LO: 4; factual   pages: 435-436

25. Alcohol is considered a _____ because _____.
    a. stimulant; it makes people less inhibited in their behavior
    b. depressant; it has a dampening effect on the central nervous system.
    c. stimulant; it activates the brain
    d. stimulant; it activates the sex drive
    Answer: b   LO: 4; factual, conceptual   page: 429

26. Which of the following is *true* concerning the effects of alcohol?
    a. People whose behavior is not disinhibited by alcohol tend not to drink it.
    b. It has a physiological effect of improving sexual functioning.
    c. A sufficient amount of alcohol can help a person sleep better.
    d. In countries like France, where people drink alcohol with their meals, there are higher rates of alcohol related disorders than in the United States.
    Answer: a   LO: 4; factual   page: 429

Substance Use Disorders

27. How many glasses of wine can put a 100-lb woman over the legal limit of alcohol intoxication in those states where the legal limit is 0.08% blood level alcohol?
    a. 1
    b. 2
    c. 4
    d. 6
    Answer: b LO: 5; factual page: 430

28. Which of the following is *true* concerning the connection between the legal definition of intoxication and the psychiatric diagnosis?
    a. They are the same.
    b. They are almost identical.
    c. They are similar in all states, but the legal definition does differ according to state.
    d. The legal definition is much narrower.
    Answer: d LO: 5; factual page: 429

29. Of the following, which is the *most* common cause of alcohol-related deaths?
    a. automobile accidents
    b. respiratory paralysis
    c. interaction with other substances
    d. alcohol toxicosis
    Answer: a LO: 5, 6; factual pages: 429-430

30. Which of the following is not one of the stages of severe alcohol withdrawal symptoms?
    a. a hangover that is gone within several hours to a day
    b. symptoms of the "shakes," the "jitters," vomiting, and "seeing" or "hearing" things that disappear in a few days
    c. convulsive seizures, which begin between 12 hours and 3 days after cessation of drinking
    d. delirium tremens, or auditory, visual, and tactile hallucinations, terrifying dreams, sleep disturbances, hyperthermia, and irregular heartbeat
    Answer: a LO: 7; factual pages: 430-431

31. A diagnosis of _____ is appropriate when a person uses alcohol in dangerous situations, fails to meet important obligations, and has recurrent legal or social problems resulting from using alcohol.
    a. alcohol use
    b. alcohol abuse
    c. alcohol dependence
    d. alcohol tolerance.
    Answer: b LO: 8; factual, conceptual page: 431

Chapter 12

32. Alexander not only uses alcohol in dangerous situations and fails to meet his social, financial, and work obligations, but he also has developed a physiological tolerance to alcohol. He spends much of his time either intoxicated or in withdrawal and continues to drink despite the problems it causes. Alexander would be diagnosed as:
    a. an alcohol abuser.
    b. alcohol dependent.
    c. alcohol tolerant.
    d. chronically intoxicated.
    Answer: b   LO: 8; applied   page: 431

33. Which of the following is *not* one of the distinct patterns of drinking outlined in the text?
    a. drinking large amounts of alcohol every day and planning the day around drinking
    b. abstaining from drinking for long periods of time, then going on extended binges
    c. abstaining from drinking during the day or the work week, then drinking heavily during evenings or on weekends
    d. abstaining from drinking until 5:00 P.M., then promptly having a 5:00 drink, having another with dinner, and a "nightcap" before going to bed
    Answer: d   LO: 8; factual, conceptual   page: 432

34. Jimmy never admits he's drunk. Unless he loses his keys or someone takes them away, he'll get into the car and drive away, so long as he's still conscious. He's been fired from every job he ever had because he "calls in sick" several days a week. It doesn't take long for his bosses to understand that he has a drinking problem. He was married once, but his wife left him when she couldn't sober him up for a month. His whole life seems to be organized around his drinking, and now he's dying from cirrhosis. Sometimes his liver "turns off" and he hallucinates--he sees Dali-esque people jumping out of closed doors and slamming them, coming toward him and attacking him. He reeks so badly of alcohol and urine that his 10-year-old niece refuses to see him anymore. He no longer remembers her name, anyway. Jimmy has:
    a. alcohol psychosis.
    b. Wernicke's encephalopathy.
    c. alcohol-induced dementia.
    d. fetal alcohol syndrome.
    Answer: c   LO: 9; applied   page: 433

35. Alcohol-induced persisting amnestic disorder is a permanent cognitive disorder caused by damage to the central nervous system. It consists of two syndromes:
    a. Wernicke's encephalopathy and Korsakoff's psychosis.
    b. alcohol-induced dementia and alcohol psychosis.
    c. alcohol tolerance and alcohol dependence.
    d. Wernicke's encephalopathy and Tarasoff syndrome.
    Answer: a   LO: 9; factual   page: 433

Substance Use Disorders

36. An alcohol-related syndrome that involves mental confusion and disorientation and, in severe states, coma is:
    a. alcohol psychosis.
    b. Korsakoff's psychosis.
    c. Wernicke's encephalopathy.
    d. fetal alcohol syndrome.
    Answer: c   LO: 9; factual, conceptual   page: 433

37. A syndrome that involves a loss of memory for recent events and problems in recalling distant events is:
    a. alcohol dementia.
    b. Wernicke's encephalopathy.
    c. Korsakoff's psychosis.
    d. alcohol psychosis.
    Answer: c   LO: 9; factual, conceptual   page: 433

38. Sandra has been advised by her doctor not to drink alcohol when she is pregnant. Her doctor warned that consumption of alcohol by a pregnant woman may cause _____ in her child, which is characterized by retarded growth, facial abnormalities, central nervous system damage, mental retardation, motor abnormalities, tremors, hyperactivity, heart defects, skeletal anomalies, severe behavior problems, and an inability to learn from experience.
    a. Down syndrome
    b. fetal alcohol syndrome
    c. alcohol dementia
    d. Wernicke's encephalopathy
    Answer: b   LO: 9, 13; applied   page: 434

39. Higher rates of alcohol-related problems among _____ are tied to _____.
    a. Asian-Americans; lack of the enzyme acetaldehyde to process alcohol
    b. older African-American men; low socioeconomic status, being reared in single-parent homes, and low level of education
    c. Mexican-Americans born in the United States; assimilation into the dominant culture, which has caused adoption of dominant culture drinking patterns
    d. Native Americans; high poverty and unemployment, low education, and an overwhelming sense of helplessness and hopelessness
    Answer: d   LO: 10; factual, conceptual   pages: 434-435

Chapter 12

40. Which of the following is *not* a reason stated in the text for older people to be less likely to abuse alcohol?
    a. As people get older, there are changes in their sense of taste such that alcohol comes to taste extremely bitter, causing them to stop drinking.
    b. As people grow older, they become more mature in their choices and many choose not to drink alcohol excessively.
    c. People who have used alcohol excessively for many years may die from alcohol-related diseases before they reach old age.
    d. Slower liver metabolization rate of alcohol causes the elderly to become intoxicated faster and experience the negative effects of alcohol more severely and quickly.
    Answer: a   LO: 11; factual, conceptual   pages: 435-436

41. Which developmental pattern of barbiturate abuse and dependence is *most* likely to be seen among teenagers or young adults?
    a. While hospitalized for surgery, the drugs are prescribed for the individual who comes to depend on them.
    b. Due to the high stress of achieving an identity and handling conflict with their parents, teenagers or young adults obtain sedatives from their family physician and gradually increase their use as tolerance builds.
    c. Initially, the individual uses the drugs recreationally to produce a sense of euphoria, and this escalates into chronic use and physiological dependence.
    d. All of the above are common patterns for this age group.
    Answer: c   LO: 8; factual, conceptual   pages: 435-436

42. Which developmental pattern of barbiturate abuse and dependence is particularly seen among women?
    a. While hospitalized for surgery, the drugs are prescribed for the individual, who becomes to depend on them.
    b. To treat anxiety or insomnia, they initially obtain sedatives from their family physician and gradually increase their use as tolerance builds.
    c. Initially, they use the drugs recreationally to produce a sense of euphoria, and this escalates into chronic use and physiological dependence.
    d. The drugs are so common that initially a depressed woman will receive them from a friend and then go to several doctors for prescriptions.
    Answer: b   LO: 8; factual, conceptual   page: 437

43. The most common causes of death from overdosing on barbiturates are:
    a. respiratory arrest and cardiovascular collapse.
    b. destruction of the brain and shutting down of the central nervous system.
    c. hepatitis and lack of oxygen to the brain.
    d. hepatitis and respiratory arrest.
    Answer: a   LO: 12; factual   page: 437

Substance Use Disorders

44. Which of the following is *not* one of the harmful consequences described in the text that results from chronic use of inhalants?
    a. death due to depression of the respiratory and cardiovascular systems
    b. permanent damage to the central nervous system, including degeneration of the brain
    c. eczema and other skins disorders
    d. hepatitis, liver, and kidney disease
    Answer: c   LO: 12; factual   page: 437

45. The fact that cocaine _____ makes it _____.
    a. depresses the frontal lobe; more likely than other drugs to reduce the brain's censoring mechanisms, thereby leading to hypersexuality and rash behavior
    b. activates the central nervous center; more likely than other drugs to lead to agitated behavior and psychotic symptoms
    c. activates the sympathetic nervous system; more likely than other drugs to result in a heart attack or stroke
    d. activates the brain's pleasure centers; more likely than other drugs to result in patterns of abuse and dependence
    Answer: d   LO: 12; factual, conceptual   page: 439

46. Which of the following is *not* one of the reasons noted in the text that cocaine is such an insidiously addicting substance?
    a. The initial high is so outstandingly wonderful that people continue to take it, trying to recapture that feeling.
    b. Its short half-life means the effects wear off quickly, so a user must take frequent doses of the substance to maintain a high.
    c. Tolerance to cocaine can easily develop, so the user must obtain increasingly larger amounts in order to experience a high.
    d. Of all of the popular drugs, cocaine, coming as it does from coca leaves, is the most natural and thus the least likely to cause damage to the body.
    Answer: d   LO: 12; factual, conceptual   pages: 439-440

47. Which of the following is *not* discussed in the text to be a consequence of cocaine on an unborn fetus?
    a. cocaine addiction
    b. sudden infant death (SIDS)
    c. hyperirritability and low birth weight
    d. learning disabilities and neurological impairment
    Answer: a   LO: 12, 13; factual   page: 440

Chapter 12

48. Which of the following is *true* concerning prevalence and use of cocaine?
    a. One reason stated in the text for the decrease in cocaine use is its escalating cost.
    b. There has been a decline in use of cocaine among casual users, but chronic abusers and dependents have continued to use the substance.
    c. Because most women who use cocaine tend to be relatively wealthy, at least they are getting good prenatal care for their babies when they are pregnant.
    d. The placenta in pregnant women serves as a protective barrier for the fetus; thus, the unborn child is not at risk if the mother uses cocaine.
    Answer: b   LO: 12, 13; factual, conceptual   page: 440

49. Which pair of substances produce symptoms of euphoria, self-confidence, alertness, agitation, paranoia, and often frightening perceptual illusions?
    a. heroine and morphine
    b. cocaine and amphetamines
    c. alcohol and nicotine
    d. cocaine and marijuana
    Answer: b   LO: 4; factual   page: 440

50. Which statement is *true* concerning withdrawal from high-dose use of amphetamines?
    a. They may cause such severe depression that the person becomes suicidal.
    b. The user may have visual hallucinations during withdrawal.
    c. The user may suddenly die from cardiovascular excitation.
    d. With sudden withdrawal ("cold turkey"), the user may die from renal failure.
    Answer: a   LO: 12; factual, conceptual   page: 441

51. Which of the following substances are *most* similar to substances naturally occurring in the human body?
    a. opioids
    b. amphetamines
    c. cocaine
    d. cannabis
    Answer: a   LO: 4; factual   page: 441

52. Joe likened his "high" to an orgasm, with a tingling sensation a sense of warmth all over, and then feeling lethargic. He nodded off and had vivid ("wow") dreams. He was using:
    a. cocaine.
    b. marijuana.
    c. opioids.
    d. alcohol.
    Answer: c   LO: 4; factual   pages: 441-442

53. Severe intoxication with opioids can lead to all of the following *except*:
   a. euphoria.
   b. unconsciousness.
   c. seizures.
   d. death.
   Answer: a   LO: 4; factual   page: 442

54. Users of which of the following drugs are at the highest risk for developing HIV?
   a. PCP
   b. opioids
   c. amphetamines
   d. alcohol
   Answer: b   LO: 6, 12; conceptual   page: 442

55. The most obvious difference between the hallucinogens, PCP, and cannabis and other substances, such as alcohol, cocaine, and opioids, is that hallucinogens, PCP, and cannabis _____, whereas alcohol, cocaine, and opioids _____.
   a. cause hallucinations; do not
   b. produce perceptual changes; do not
   c. produce perceptual changes even in small doses; need large doses to produce the same types of changes
   d. can be made or grown in a person's own home; need special equipment to be produced
   Answer: c   LO: 4, 6, 12; factual   pages: 442-443

56. Which of the following are considered to be hallucinogens?
   a. LSD, phenylalkylamines, MDMA, and peyote
   b. cocaine and amphetamines
   c. heroin, morphine, and endorphins
   d. alcohol and cannabis
   Answer: a   LO: 4; factual   page: 442

57. Which of the following substances was popular (and legal) during the 1960s but resulted in highly publicized accounts of people inadvertently committing suicide because they believed they could fly, walk on water, or land on their feet when they jumped out of a high window?
   a. marijuana
   b. LSD
   c. opium
   d. PCP
   Answer: b   LO: 4, 6, 12; factual, conceptual   page: 443

Chapter 12

58. Which of the following groups of symptoms is *not* an indication of PCP intoxication?
    a. a sense of intoxication, euphoria or affective dulling, talkativeness, lack of concern, slowed reaction time, dizziness, twitching, and weakness
    b. disorganized thinking, distortions of body image, depersonalization, feelings of unreality, hostility, and violence
    c. increased clarity of thought, weight loss, paranoia, and suicidal ideation.
    d. amnesia and coma, profound pain reduction, seizures, severe respiratory problems, hypothermia, and hyperthermia.
    Answer: c   LO: 4, 6, 12; factual, conceptual   page: 443

59. The most widely used illicit substance(s) in the world is(are):
    a. inhalants.
    b. opioids.
    c. cannabis.
    d. cocaine.
    Answer: c   LO: 4, factual   page: 443

60. In terms of prevalence rates, which of the following is *true* concerning cannabis?
    a. Over half the U.S. population has tried marijuana at some time in their lives.
    b. Of those who have tried marijuana, 12% say they "didn't inhale."
    c. Of those who have tried marijuana, 10% of them currently use it monthly.
    d. Although its use continues to be illegal, 80% of people with glaucoma and 10% of those suffering from cancer are using marijuana to help with their medical problems.
    Answer: a   LO: 2; factual   page: 443

61. Cannabis is categorized as a hallucinogen because:
    a. it has been found to be equally as potent as LSD, PCP, and MDMA.
    b. at moderate to large doses users experience perceptual distortions, feelings of depersonalization, and paranoid thinking.
    c. the government wishes to keep it classified as an illegal substance and thus has categorized it as a hallucinogen.
    d. even a small dose can cause the user to have hallucinations and delusions that may be extremely frightening.
    Answer: b   LO: 4, 6; factual, conceptual   page: 444

62. Which of the following is *not* one of the health risks of cannabis use discussed in the text?
    a. chronic cough and sinusitis
    b. cancer
    c. bronchitis and emphysema
    d. suicide
    Answer: d   LO: 4, 6, 12; factual   page: 444

Substance Use Disorders

63. The irony of the health issues concerning cannabis is:
    a. on the one hand, smoking cannabis can cause cancer because of the high levels of carcinogens, but it has been useful in relieving nausea in cancer patients.
    b. that in its natural form, it is a potent source of vitamin C and high energy, but in its processed form, it produces lethargy.
    c. when cooked into brownies or other food products, it adds healthful nutrients, but when smoked it can cause respiratory problems and cancer.
    d. many cultures have used it as a medicinal herb, but in the United States its use is prohibited for medical purposes.
    Answer: a   LO: 4, 6, 12; factual, conceptual   page: 444

64. One of the most addictive substances in existence that is completely legal for adults and easily accessible for minors is:
    a. nicotine.
    b. cannabis.
    c. ethylene.
    d. steroids.
    Answer: a   LO: 4; factual   page: 444

65. In terms of prevalence rates concerning nicotine use, which of the following is *true*?
    a. Mortality rates for smokers are 80% greater than for nonsmokers.
    b. Of individuals who begin smoking in adolescence and continue into adulthood, 85% become regular, daily smokers.
    c. Over the last few decades, tobacco use has increased dramatically in the United States.
    d. In the United States, 55% of adults have smoked cigarettes at some time in their lives and 30% currently smoke.
    Answer: d   LO: 4, 6, 12; factual   page: 444

66. Which of the following statements about smoking is *false*?
    a. The rates of smoking have increased recently in developing countries.
    b. Nicotine operates on both the central and peripheral nervous systems and leads to suppression of the cardiovascular and respiratory systems.
    c. The babies of female smokers are smaller at birth.
    d. The smoke inhaled by the children of smokers contains more toxins than the smoke that the smoker actively inhales.
    Answer: b   LO: 4, 6, 12; factual   page: 444

Chapter 12

67. Whenever Arthur ran out of cigarettes, he turned from "Dr. Jekyll" to "Mr. Hyde." He became irritable, depressed, angry, anxious, and restless. He would have his children run out to the car to find "the longest butts." Soon after he lit the crumpled cigarette butt and inhaled the smoke he returned to his loving, fun, jovial self. This was a constant pattern of behavior for him. This would provide support for the position that
    a. nicotine is an addictive substance.
    b. cigarettes are only psychologically "addicting."
    c. second hand smoke does not harm children because his children could run.
    d. cigarette smoking can have a negative effect on personality.
    Answer: a   LO: 3, 4, 6, 12; applied   page: 445

68. With respect to quitting smoking, which of the following is *true*?
    a. Over 90% of people who smoke want to quit smoking.
    b. Most people who try to quit are able to do so by the first or at least the second time they try.
    c. Fewer than half the people who have ever smoked eventually stop smoking.
    d. Of those who have quit smoking, half of them claim to have had a desire for a cigarette within the past 12 hours.
    Answer: c   LO: 3, 6; factual, conceptual   page: 445

69. Which of the following is *not* one of the issues stated in the text concerning the debate over whether to regulate the sale of tobacco?
    a. personal freedom
    b. massive amounts of money
    c. lack of proof that it damages health
    d. maladaptiveness
    Answer: d   LO: 4; factual   pages: 445-446

70. The disease model of alcoholism:
    a. views alcoholics as weak, bad people, unable to control their impulses over drinking.
    b. views alcoholism as an incurable physical disease.
    c. says that alcoholism is a disease that can be controlled through use of proper medication.
    d. says that alcoholism is a disease that can be cured through genetic engineering.
    Answer: b   LO: 14; factual, conceptual   page: 446

71. Which of the following is a biological cause of cravings for a substance?
    a. neural sensitization in the mesolimbic dopamine system
    b. neural desensitization in the mesolimbic dopamine system
    c. increased levels of norepinephrine
    d. reduction in the body's natural level of endogenous opioids
    Answer: a   LO: 15; factual   page: 447

Substance Use Disorders

72. When the _____ system is activated by a psychoactive substance, the brain may try to balance this state of activation with mechanisms that have effects that are opposite of the psychoactive substance. These mechanisms are referred to as _____.
    a. sympathetic nervous; defense mechanisms
    b. parasympathetic nervous; opponent processes
    c. mesolimbic dopamine; defense mechanisms
    d. mesolimbic dopamine; opponent processes
    Answer: d   LO: 15; factual, conceptual   page: 447

73. Which of the following statements about alcohol is *true*?
    a. Family history studies have found higher rates of alcoholism among the offspring of depressed people than among the offspring of nondepressed people.
    b. Adolescents who are depressed are more likely to become alcoholics than adolescents who are not depressed.
    c. Family history studies have found higher rates of depression among the offspring of people with alcohol problems compared to people without alcohol problems.
    d. Alcohol-related disorders are more common in societies with few legal or cultural restrictions on alcohol use.
    Answer: c   LO: 16; factual, conceptual   page: 448

74. Which of the following statements about biological causes of alcoholism is *true*?
    a. No studies have suggested that alcoholism is heritable among females.
    b. The offspring of alcoholics may develop alcoholism themselves because they do not experience its effects as strongly when ingesting moderate doses of alcohol.
    c. The evidence for a genetic transmission of alcoholism is strong only for late-onset alcoholism.
    d. The daughters of alcoholics are four to five times more likely to develop alcoholism than the daughters of nonalcoholics.
    Answer: b   LO: 16; factual   page: 448

75. Which of the following is *true* concerning the role of genetics in alcoholism?
    a. The evidence for genetic transmission has been much more consistent for males than for females.
    b. At high doses of alcohol, sons of alcoholics are less intoxicated than the sons of non-alcoholics.
    c. There are many findings that support a strong link for neurological anomalies and alcoholism, but not for biochemical links.
    d. There are many findings that support a strong link for biochemical anomalies and alcoholism, but not for neurological links.
    Answer: a   LO: 16; factual   page: 448

Chapter 12

76. Which of the following is *not* a reason the text stated to view alcoholism as a form of depression?
    a. While children of alcoholics have higher rates of depression than children of nonalcoholics, the depression might arise from the stress of having an alcoholic parent, not from genetics.
    b. As a central nervous system depressant, alcohol can cause the classic symptoms of depression; thus, it's as likely that the symptoms may result from the alcohol itself.
    c. Depression among alcoholics usually disappears once they become abstinent, even without antidepressant treatment.
    d. The symptoms of alcoholism associated with depression are much milder, and if they are to be categorized at all, they would more properly be categorized as dysthymia.
    Answer: d   LO: 17; conceptual   page: 449

77. The highest rates of substance abuse and dependence are seen among:
    a. people facing severe chronic stress and an environment that supports substance use.
    b. teenagers who are attempting to define their identity.
    c. the elderly who are faced with loss of family, friends, and independence.
    d. people facing moderate stress and attractive media portrayal of substance use.
    Answer: a   LO: 18; factual   page: 450

78. One of the most powerful ways children learn alcohol-related behaviors is by:
    a. reading about them in books.
    b. seeing them on television.
    c. modeling their parents.
    d. hearing about them on radio.
    Answer: c   LO: 18; factual, conceptual   page: 451

79. The view that people's expectancies for the effects of alcohol and their beliefs about the appropriateness of using alcohol to cope with stress is a _____ theory of alcohol abuse.
    a. behavioral
    b. cognitive
    c. psychodynamic
    d. sociocultural
    Answer: b   LO: 18; factual, conceptual   page: 451

80. Cynthia has entered a substance abuse program. The first step the therapist will likely take for treating her for this substance abuse disorder is:
    a. psychotherapy.
    b. detoxification.
    c. providing emotional support.
    d. providing community support.
    Answer: b   LO: 19; applied   page: 451

Substance Use Disorders

81. Getting a person with a substance abuse disorder to stop using the substance and then allowing the substance to be eliminated from the body is called:
    a. withdrawal.
    b. substance elimination.
    c. detoxification.
    d. biological therapy.
    Answer: c LO: 19; factual page: 451

82. Disulfiram (Antabuse) has been show to:
    a. reduce alcohol consumption among animals.
    b. block the effects of heroin.
    c. make a person extremely sick if he or she takes even one drink.
    d. block the effects of alcohol.
    Answer: c LO: 19; factual page: 452

83. Naltrexone and naloxone have been used to reduce the reinforcing effects of:
    a. alcohol and heroin.
    b. heroin and cocaine.
    c. cocaine and alcohol.
    d. morphine and alcohol.
    Answer: a LO: 19; factual page: 452

84. The synthetic drug that is most often used to help a person withdraw from heroin is:
    a. endorphin.
    b. methadone.
    c. cocaine.
    d. morphine.
    Answer: b LO: 19; factual page: 452

85. Which of the following is *false* concerning methadone?
    a. It is a more potent but less addictive opioid that has been successful in helping heroin users become drug free.
    b. Heroin dependents on methadone maintenance programs are more likely to remain in treatment and less likely to relapse compared to those not on methadone.
    c. It helps reduce the negative withdrawal symptoms from heroin.
    d. Because methadone blocks the receptors for heroin, if an individual takes heroin while on methadone, she or he will not experience the intense psychological effects of the heroin.
    Answer: a LO: 19; factual, conceptual page: 452

Chapter 12

86. Which of the following is *false* concerning Alcoholics Anonymous (AA)?
    a. AA's intervention is based on the disease model of alcoholism.
    b. AA contends that the only way to control alcoholism is to abstain completely.
    c. AA prescribes 12 "steps" that alcoholics must take toward recovery.
    d. AA believes that by following the 12 steps and giving oneself up to a higher power, it is possible to be cured of alcoholism.
    Answer: d   LO: 20; factual, conceptual   pages: 452-453

87. Gerry got up and said, "Hi. I'm Gerry, and I'm a social drinker. . . . If you believe that, I have a bridge to sell you. I've been a drunk for 45 years, since I was 15 years old. You know what a drunk is? An alcoholic who's in denial. I'll always be an alcoholic, but I don't have to be a drunk." It sounds like Gerry is:
    a. in a business meeting.
    b. at an AA group.
    c. at an NA group.
    d. in group therapy.
    Answer: b   LO: 20; applied   pages: 452-454

88. Which of the following is *true* about AA?
    a. It emphasizes the alcoholic's powerlessness over alcohol and need for a higher power.
    b. It has extremely wide appeal that attracts any kind of alcoholic.
    c. There is a great deal of research indicating its effectiveness.
    d. It says that some alcoholics can limit their drinking instead of abstaining completely.
    Answer: a   LO: 20; factual, conceptual   page: 454

89. Dr. Cameron often uses a therapy for treating alcoholism based on a combination of classical and operant conditioning. Most likely she is using:
    a. covert sensitization.
    b. reinforcement therapy.
    c. aversive classical conditioning.
    d. classicoperant conditioning.
    Answer: c   LO: 21; applied   page: 455

90. A therapy in which the alcoholic uses imagery to create an association between thoughts of alcohol use and thoughts of highly unpleasant consequences of alcohol use is:
    a. systematic desensitization therapy.
    b. covert sensitization therapy.
    c. cue exposure and response prevention.
    d. mental imagery therapy.
    Answer: b   LO: 21; conceptual   page: 455

Substance Use Disorders

91. Edgar is in therapy for his alcoholism. His therapist is using a behavioral technique that involves having Edgar hold a glass with his favorite drink, smell it, place it to his lips, but refrain from drinking. This is known as:
    a. controlled drinking.
    b. covert sensitization.
    c. cue exposure and response prevention.
    d. abstinence violation therapy.
    Answer: c   LO: 21; applied   page: 455

92. Which of the following is *not* a step that is used in cognitively oriented treatments for alcohol abuse and dependency?
    a. help clients identify situations in which they are most likely to drink and lose control over drinking, as well as their expectancies that alcohol will help them cope better
    b. challenge clients' expectancies that alcohol helps them cope better by reviewing the negative effects of alcohol on their behavior
    c. help clients learn to anticipate and reduce stress, develop more adaptive ways of coping with stressful situations
    d. help clients learn to say "no" after one drink, despite social pressure to continue drinking
    Answer: d   LO: 22; conceptual   pages: 455-457

93. Which of the following is *false* concerning controlled drinking?
    a. People who have had many alcohol-related problems function better in their daily lives while on a controlled drinking program than they do with total abstinence.
    b. Some studies of the progression of alcoholism over time find that some alcoholics spontaneously develop a pattern of controlled social drinking on their own.
    c. Some studies have found that controlled drinking programs are at least as beneficial as abstinence programs.
    d. A study by Sobell and Sobell (1978) found that alcoholics in a controlled drinking program functioned well for a longer period of time in the year following treatment than did alcoholics in an abstinence program.
    Answer: a   LO: 22; factual, conceptual   page: 457

94. An approach to treating alcoholism that teaches alcoholics to view slips as temporary and emotionally caused, helps clients identify high-risk situations where they may drink, and helps them to avoid those situations or use effective coping strategies in them is a(n):
    a. aversive therapy program.
    b. relapse prevention program.
    c. guided imagery program.
    d. abstinence violation program.
    Answer: b   LO: 22; factual, conceptual   page: 457

Chapter 12

95. Approximately _____% of people who are dependent on alcohol seek treatment, and approximately _____% recovery on their own.
    a. 1; 10
    b. 5; 25
    c. 10; 35
    d. 10; 40
    Answer: d   LO: 22; factual   page: 457

96. Which of the following statements about gender differences in substance abuse is *false*?
    a. Women are more likely than men to participate in their partner's substance abuse treatment.
    b. Women may be less prone to alcoholism than men because more alcohol enters their bloodstream when they drink.
    c. Women are more likely than men to expect alcohol to interfere with their ability to cope with difficult situations.
    d. Women substance abusers are more difficult to treat because they are most frequently also diagnosed with antisocial personality disorder.
    Answer: d   LO: 23; factual, conceptual   pages: 458-459

97. Which country considers substance addiction to be a medical problem and, therefore, has physicians treat its addicts?
    a. China
    b. Holland
    c. Great Britain
    d. Switzerland
    Answer: c   LO: 24; factual, conceptual   page: 459

98. What is the relationship between the harshness of the penalties for drug use and the level of drug problems?
    a. Countries with harsh penalties have significantly fewer problems with substance abuse.
    b. Countries with moderate penalties have significantly fewer problems with substance abuse.
    c. Countries with near-legalization attitudes have significantly fewer problems with substance abuse.
    d. No one method clearly works the best.
    Answer: d   LO: 24; factual, conceptual   pages: 459-460

Substance Use Disorders

99. Which of the following is *false* concerning the Alcohol Skills Training Programs (ASTPs) currently being used on college campuses?
    a. Evaluations have shown that there is a decrease in alcohol consumption.
    b. Evaluations have shown that the programs have helped students learn the importance of having a designated driver who remains sober.
    c. Evaluations have shown that there is an increase in social skills for resisting alcohol abuse.
    d. Although ASTP was designed for a group format, its positive results could also been seen if it were presented in written form as a self-help manual.
    Answer: b   LO: 24; factual, conceptual   page: 464

Essay Questions

100. Your roommate knows you're learning about substance abuse, so she's come to you for advice. When she was 2 years old, her father died in an automobile accident while driving under the influence of alcohol. She has also noticed that there are several other family members who have problems with alcohol or other illicit substances, particularly cocaine. She is confused about whether she is going to become an alcoholic or addicted to other drugs and wants to know about the biological, psychological, and social factors that might interact to produce and maintain substance abuse behavior. Explain these to her and identify specific processes at each level, and illustrate how they interact to produce and maintain addictive behaviors, particularly for alcohol and cocaine dependence. With respect to cocaine, what specific aspects of the substance make it especially addictive?

A proper answer should identify specific biological factors (e.g., activation of the mesolimbic dopamine system), psychological factors (e.g., the expectation that cocaine will help one cope or become a better person), and social factors (e.g., an environment of chronic stress that also supports substance abuse), and describe how each type of factor may increase the likelihood of alcohol and cocaine abuse and dependence. The aspects of cocaine that make it an addictive substance (e.g., incomparable euphoria, short half-life) should also be discussed.

Chapter 12

101. How does the philosophy of Alcoholics Anonymous compare with the controlled drinking perspective? Describe both positions and the similarities and differences between them. What evidence supports each position? What information would a clinician need in order to determine which treatment would work best for an alcoholic?

    A proper answer should summarize the disease model of alcoholism and controlled drinking perspectives, as well as the evidence for the effectiveness of each (e.g., research has shown that controlled drinking programs are at least as beneficial, if not more beneficial, than programs that promote total abstinence). The 12-step program of AA should be outlined here as well. The information needed by a clinician (e.g., a client's past history of attempts to control his or her drinking) should also be identified.

102. The text outlines a strategy for "promoting responsible alcohol use in young adults." Your friend, who works at the Student Health Services, sees students come in hung-over and dealing with other alcohol and drug problems on a daily basis. This friend has asked for your help in developing a program to help alleviate this problem. To do this, you need to outline the background for the Alcohol Skills Training Program (ASTP), including the rationale for the intervention, the format of the program, the skills taught, and evaluations of ASTP. Then consider the suggestions in the text for students to reduce their drinking, and explain how they would or would not be effective for you, personally, as well as for the students your friend is seeing at the Student Health Services.

    The student should address the prevalence of drinking among young adults, generally, and college students particularly (73 to 98% drink alcohol) and the reasons for drinking (easy access, peer pressure), together with the concomitant problems of drinking (accidents, death, illegal activities, etc.) form the backdrop for needing ASTP. Educational programs on health consequences and preaching abstinence have not been effective, and thus a program that focuses on risks of excess and payoffs of moderation was designed. The student should address the format of teaching self-awareness, attitudes, alternatives, etc. The evaluations have been positive. The student should then consider the eight suggestions in the text to reduce their drinking, and discuss how they would or would not be effective for the student.

103. Psychoactive substances have been used by people in different societies perhaps since *homo sapiens* first evolved. In what contexts have they been used? Specifically, who has used them (explain how use has been general or restricted to certain people/groups)? How have attitudes toward use of psychoactive substances changed over time and over cultures?

    The history of drugs should be presented in terms of how they have been used for medicinal purposes for at least thousands of years (although there is archeological evidence that they have been used much farther back than stated in the text), and for

Substance Use Disorders

religious ceremonies, for nutrition (coca leaves are high in vitamin C) and energy. They have, however, also been used for recreation and escape, and these behaviors are often frowned upon. The student should discuss Andean chewing of coca leaves, early use of cocaine in Europe and the United States, etc., and the various attitudes within the various contexts outlined in the text.

104. Margaret married Ronald after knowing him for a month. Her husband had died a year before, and she was lonesome and found Ronald to be intelligent and good company. Shortly after the marriage, however, Margaret realized that Ronald had a pattern of starting a fight with her right before he was going to get paid. He would then take his paycheck and go off to drink with his friends. He would come back a few days later, sober and apologetic, and she would take him in. After a few of these episodes, Margaret started to sense a pattern and would try to avoid escalating into an argument, but Ronald would continue to push until the inevitable happened. One time it became so heated that Ronald pushed Margaret and threatened her with a gun, and she called the police and had him arrested. She still let him come back, though. She finally confronted him with the fact that he was an alcoholic, which he vehemently denied. In fact, they went to his doctor together and the doctor asked her, "Does he fall down on his face?" and Margaret said "No, but when he's drunk he can't walk very straight and loses control of his behavior." The doctor said, "Well, if he's not falling down, he's not an alcoholic." Discuss the issues involved here in determining whether Ronald does or does not have a problem with alcohol abuse and dependence, what factors contribute to his behavior (whether or not an alcohol problem), and what you believe would be the most effective way to handle this situation (a) from Margaret's perspective, and (b) from the point of view of a therapist who would work with Ronald for the behavior leading to his battering arrest.

Despite the doctor's denial, Ronald clearly has a problem with alcohol abuse and alcohol dependence. The binging pattern should be discussed, and the fact that Margaret continues to let him come back, which positively reinforces his behavior. If Margaret wishes to remain with him, she'll need to explore AA and Al-Anon and learn how not to reinforce his behaviors. A therapist working with Ronald would probably either direct him (them) to AA or try to work with Ronald on establishing controlled drinking. However, considering his binging behavior, total abstinence might be more in order. Behavioral treatments (e.g., aversive classical conditioning), and cognitive therapies that would help Ronald understand his drinking behavior, deal with stressful situations, cope with his anxiety and anger, and say "No thanks" need to be addressed, as does the issue of relapse, which is to be expected and should be seen as a temporary slip, not a failure.

Chapter 13 Personality, Behavior, and the Body

1. Which of the following is *not* a primary concern of health psychologists?
    a. the role of personality factors, coping styles, and stress on the development and progress of physical disease
    b. whether changing the way a person perceives the world can influence the course of a physical disease
    c. whether diseases can be prevented by adopting healthy lifestyles and attitudes
    d. the role of genetics in the development and progress of physical disease
    Answer: d   LO: 1; factual, conceptual   page: 468

2. Which of the following is *true* concerning the mind-body question?
    a. Historically and cross-culturally, the predominant and accepted view has been that the mind and body work together and influence each other.
    b. In Eastern medicine, there has consistently been an emphasis on the importance of a positive mental state and psychological balance for physical well being.
    c. The mind-body question is a relatively new debate that has its origins in the modern biological theories of mental illness.
    d. In Western medicine, technological advances in identifying and treating the physical causes of disease have supported reliance on the mind-body connection.
    Answer: b   LO: 1; factual, conceptual   page: 468

3. Which of the following is *not* one of the three predominant models of mind-body interaction in health psychology?
    a. the direct effects model
    b. the interactive model
    c. the separationist model
    d. the indirect effects model
    Answer: c   LO: 1; factual   pages: 468-469

4. The indirect effects model suggests that:
    a. psychological factors can only cause or exacerbate physical illness in people who already have a biological vulnerability to an illness or a mild form of the illness.
    b. psychological factors influence the development and progress of physical illness by affecting people's health-related behaviors.
    c. physiological factors can only indirectly affect cognitive and emotional functioning.
    d. psychological factors influence the development and progress of physical illness by causing physiological changes that lead to or exacerbate disease.
    Answer: b   LO: 1; factual, conceptual   page: 469

Chapter 13

5. The mind-body model that believes that prolonged stress or a maladaptive personality style will contribute to disease only in people who already have a biological vulnerability to the disease or who have already developed a mild form of the disease is the _____ model.
   a. direct effects
   b. interactive
   c. reactive
   d. indirect
   Answer: b   LO: 1; factual, conceptual   page: 469

6. The mind-body model that suggests that psychological factors have an impact on disease by influencing the types of health-promoting behaviors they engage in is the _____ model.
   a. direct effect
   b. interactive effect
   c. lifestyles effect
   d. indirect effect
   Answer: d   LO: 1; factual, conceptual   page: 469

7. Mark went to see a doctor at Student Health Services and complained of migraine headaches and a terrible rash all over his body. The doctor started asking Mark about the kinds of stress he had been experiencing lately, the kinds of things Mark finds to be stressful, and how he handles his stress. She also asked if Mark had been feeling depressed lately or was having a hard time getting his studying done. The model for the effects of psychological factors on disease that the doctor was using is the _____ model.
   a. direct effect
   b. interactive effect
   c. lifestyles effect
   d. indirect effect
   Answer: a   LO: 1; applied   page: 468-469

8. Cynthia got the worst flu she ever experienced. In fact, it was so severe she was worried she might catch pneumonia, so she went to the Student Health Center. The doctor there asked Cynthia whether there was a history in her family for lung problems, such as pneumonia, pleurisy, asthma, or emphysema, and he also asked whether Cynthia had been under any extraordinary stress lately. The doctor explained to Cynthia that she should be particularly concerned about a predisposition to pneumonia if this has been common in her family, and she should try to schedule her classes so she has plenty of time to rest and relax. This doctor is looking at the _____ model for the effects of psychological factors on disease.
   a. direct effect
   b. interactive effect
   c. lifestyles effect
   d. indirect effect
   Answer: b   LO: 1; applied   page: 469

Personality, Behavior, and the Body

9. Tiffany was brought to the Health Center by her roommate. Dr. Bradley asks her about recent events in her life and how she handles them. Tiffany tells the doctor that after she broke up with her boyfriend, she became extremely depressed. Dr. Bradley then asked Tiffany about her health habits since this happened, and Tiffany said she was so upset she had stopped eating healthy foods, started eating junk foods, and began smoking. She has now had a bronchial cough that keeps her (and her roommate) up all night. Which model for the effects of psychological factors on disease would this characterize?
   a. direct effect
   b. interactive effect
   c. lifestyles effect
   d. indirect effect
   Answer: d   LO: 1; applied   page: 469

10. Which of the following are the two factors that are the major focus of health psychology?
    a. stress and coping styles
    b. coping styles and personality styles
    c. stress and personality styles
    d. coping styles and adaptability
    Answer: c   LO: 2; factual   page: 469

11. Which of the following is not one of the characteristics or events that are identified as contributing to stress?
    a. controllability
    b. enjoyability
    c. predictability
    d. extent of threat
    Answer: b   LO: 2; factual   page: 469

12. In Selye's (1978) research, animals exposed to uncontrollable stressors experienced all of the following *except*:
    a. enlarged lymph nodes.
    b. stomach ulcers.
    c. suppressed lymphocytes.
    d. enlarged adrenal glands.
    Answer: a   LO: 2; factual   page: 472

Chapter 13

13. Which of the following events is most stressful, according to the text?
    a. Losing one's home and belongings in an earthquake that also leaves you injured and confined to a wheelchair for life.
    b. Losing your job when the CEO of your company finally agrees, after several months of negotiations, to sell the company, which forces you to move to another area to find a job.
    c. Finding out that your child has phenylketonuria (PKU), a childhood disease that can cause mental retardation and death unless your child is fed a diet devoid of phenylalanine.
    d. Finding your spouse in bed with another man or woman the day after you revealed your own extramarital affair.
    Answer: a   LO: 2; conceptual   pages: 470-471

14. Dr. Suzanne C. Thompson has done research with stroke patients and their caregivers to assess the factors involved in whether these patients improve. Considering the characteristics of events identified as contributing to stress and affecting the stress-health interaction, which of the following might be expected to predict their improvement?
    a. how much the stroke patients like their doctors
    b. the quality of care provided by the caregiver
    c. the amount of control the patient believes he or she has over daily activities in his or her life
    d. the amount of education the patient and/or the caregiver have had
    Answer: c   LO: 2; factual, conceptual   pages: 469-470

15. Suzanne C. Thompson and Shirlynn Spacapan (1989) ran an experiment in which half of the participants were told that they could turn off the shock they would get if they chose to do so, although they did not know when to expect the shock. The other participants were only told that they would get shock, although they did not know when and they were not given the option to turn it off. The participants who were told they could turn off the shock (although none of them tried) registered lower levels of stress than the other group. Which characteristic of events having an impact on stress were Thompson and Spacapan studying?
    a. autonomy
    b. predictability
    c. challenge
    d. controllability
    Answer: d   LO: 2; applied   pages: 469-470

Personality, Behavior, and the Body

16. The safety signal hypothesis asserts that:
    a. knowing when a negative event will occur makes it less stressful because it is more predictable and we can prepare for it better.
    b. uncontrollable events are more stressful than controllable events.
    c. negative events are more likely than positive events to be stressful and negatively affect physical and mental health.
    d. even positive life events can be stressful and negatively affect a person's health.
    Answer: a   LO: 3; conceptual   page: 470

17. Irving Janis has found that prior to surgery:
    a. allowing patients to talk about their fears improved postoperative recovery.
    b. providing patients with information about what to expect improved postoperative recovery.
    c. allowing patients to talk about their fears impaired postoperative recovery.
    d. providing patients with information about what to expect impaired postoperative recovery.
    Answer: b   LO: 2; factual   page: 470-471

18. Which statement is *true* about the interaction of predictability, control, and challenge?
    a. By having a sense of predictability and control, a person will be able to avoid feeling stressed when faced with a challenging situation.
    b. Even events that are controllable and predictable may be stressful if they challenge the limits of our capabilities.
    c. Positive changes in our life, particularly if they are anticipated and desired, produce little if any stress, even though they produce new challenges.
    d. In reality, positive changes in our lives produce greater perceptions of stress because we purposely open ourselves to new challenges, and thus it is our responsibility.
    Answer: b   LO: 2, 4; factual, conceptual   pages: 469-471

19. Which of the following does *not* occur physiologically when the body faces a stressor?
    a. The liver releases extra sugar (glucose) to help fuel muscles.
    b. The spleen releases more red blood cells to help carry oxygen.
    c. Saliva and mucus dry up, increasing the size of air passages to the lungs.
    d. Metabolism decreases in order to delay digestion.
    Answer: d   LO: 5; factual   page: 472

20. The response that activates bodily systems to enable them to deal with stress is the:
    a. fight-or-flight.
    b. physiological.
    c. stress.
    d. adaptation.
    Answer: a   LO: 5; factual   page: 472

Chapter 13

21. The physiological responses that have evolved to help humans overcome threatening situations:
    a. are, in fact, highly adaptive in virtually all situations a person may encounter.
    b. can severely damage the body if the stressor is chronic and the person cannot confront or remove the stressor.
    c. reduce rates of heart disease and hypertension, which is why we live longer than our ancestors.
    d. have been shown to reduce destruction of our immune systems, as evidenced by the fact that we live longer than our ancestors.
    Answer: b   LO: 5; factual, conceptual   page: 472

22. The physiological changes that occur during the fight-or-flight response result primarily from activation of the _____ and _____.
    a. the limbic system; the adrenal-cortical system
    b. the hypothalamus; the limbic system
    c. the sympathetic nervous system; the adrenal-cortical system
    d. the limbic system; the hippocampus
    Answer: c   LO: 6; factual   page: 472

23. The sympathetic nervous system and the adrenal-cortical system are controlled by the:
    a. hippocampus.
    b. adrenal-cortical system.
    c. hypothalamus.
    d. sympathetic nervous system.
    Answer: c   LO: 6; factual   page: 472

24. Which of the following statements about coronary heart disease (CHD) is *true*?
    a. CHD occurs when blood in the vessels puts excessive pressure on vessel walls.
    b. CHD is typically a short-lived condition because it is so fatal.
    c. Myocardial infarctions typically precede angina pectoris.
    d. CHD is the leading cause of death among women.
    Answer: d   LO: 7; factual   pages: 472-473

25. Which of the following is *not* a psychosocial risk factor for CHD?
    a. gender
    b. high-risk jobs
    c. religion
    d. immigrant status
    Answer: c   LO: 7; factual, conceptual   pages: 472-473

Personality, Behavior, and the Body

26. What is the relationship between work environment and CHD?
    a. People whose jobs are highly demanding and who have high levels of responsibility and control over operations are at highest risk of CHD.
    b. People whose jobs make few demands on their intellectual or physical abilities are at highest risk of CHD because these jobs tend to be boring and tedious.
    c. People whose jobs are highly demanding have little control over their work environment are at highest risk of CHD.
    d. People whose jobs are not demanding but do offer individual autonomy and control are at high risk for CHD because of the responsibility involved.
    Answer: c	LO: 7; factual, conceptual	pages: 472-473

27. The condition in which the supply of blood through the vessels is excessive, putting pressure on the vessel walls is:
    a. hypertension.
    b. CHD.
    c. arterial dysfunction.
    d. arterial blockage.
    Answer: a	LO: 8; factual	page: 473

28. Essential hypertension is:
    a. a form of hypertension in which genetics appear to play a role.
    b. a form of hypertension that can be traced to a specific organic cause, such as kidney dysfunction.
    c. a form of hypertension not typically found in African Americans.
    d. a form of hypertension in which the causes are unknown.
    Answer: d	LO: 8; factual	page: 473

29. The research on hypertension tends to show that:
    a. it is largely genetically based, with almost 90% of cases being traced to family history.
    b. there are very low rates of hypertension among African-Americans, perhaps because of their high incidence of sickle cell anemia.
    c. only about 10% of cases can be traced to genetics or specific organic causes.
    d. it is an indicator of lowered physiological reactivity to stress.
    Answer: c	LO: 8; factual	pages: 473-474

30. Which of the following statements about the effects of stress on physical health is *false*?
    a. Consistent evidence shows stress increases vulnerability to cancer and increases the progression of existing cancer.
    b. Biochemicals released as part of the fight-or-flight response increase lymphocytes.
    c. There is consistent evidence that stress contributes to the progression of AIDS.
    d. All of the above are false.
    Answer: d	LO: 6, 7, 8, 9; factual, conceptual	pages: 473-474

Chapter 13

31. In the research done on the effects of stress on disease, the factor that determines the impact of the stressor on the immune system functioning appears to be:
    a. perception or appraisal of stress, not the presence of the stressor.
    b. presence of stressor, not the perception or appraisal of the stress.
    c. actual impact of the stress, not the presence of the stressor.
    d. intensity of the stress, not the presence of the stressor.
    Answer: a   LO: 9; factual, conceptual   page: 475

32. The National Commission on Sleep Disorders Research (1993) has estimated that at least _____ of American adults have chronic sleep disturbances.
    a. one-quarter
    b. one-third
    c. one-half
    d. two-thirds
    Answer: b   LO: 10; factual   page: 476

33. The National Commission on Sleep Disorders Research (1993) has estimated that at least one-third of American adults have:
    a. chronic sleep disturbances.
    b. chronic disruption of their dream-state sleep.
    c. insomnia.
    d. hyposomnia.
    Answer: a   LO: 10; factual   page: 476

34. The research on sleep indicates that:
    a. the older we get, the more sleep we need.
    b. people who sleep fewer than 8 hours a night are healthier than those who sleep longer.
    c. each year, 300,000 automobile accidents are sleep related.
    d. some of the most serious disasters in modern history were caused by sleepy people.
    Answer: d   LO: 10; factual   page: 476

35. Which of the following is *not* a psychological effect of sleep deprivation?
    a. cognitive impairment
    b. emotional lability
    c. perceptual distortions
    d. placidity
    Answer: d   LO: 10; factual   pages: 476-477

Personality, Behavior, and the Body

36. Chapter 13 addresses the effects that our personality and behavior have on our body. It noted that certain behaviors can lead to deficits in learning and decision making, causing people to experience irritability and mild hallucinations. In that context, which of the following would be an effective treatment for the problem?
    a. biofeedback
    b. increased sleep
    c. guided mastery techniques
    d. cognitive therapy
    Answer: b　　　　LO: 10; factual, conceptual　　　　page: 477

37. Sleep experts suggest:
    a. if you don't get enough sleep one night, you should try to make up for it by sleeping longer the next night.
    b. a nap of between 15 to 30 minutes may be necessary for many people to restore them to optimal functioning.
    c. you should avoid taking naps during the day since naps will interfere with getting a good night's sleep.
    d. you should avoid taking naps during the day since naps can make you groggy.
    Answer: b　　　　LO: 10; factual, conceptual　　　　page: 477

38. A person's habitual way of explaining events is referred to as that person's:
    a. coping style.
    b. explanatory style.
    c. attitude style.
    d. habitual style.
    Answer: b　　　　LO: 11; factual, conceptual　　　　page: 477

39. As noted in chapter 13, people with a pessimistic explanatory style:
    a. are not as likely to make medical visits.
    b. have suppressed immune and autonomic nervous system functioning.
    c. are less likely to maintain a proper diet, get enough sleep, and exercise.
    d. endure more stress because they view more events as controllable.
    Answer: c　　　　LO: 11; factual, conceptual　　　　pages: 477-478

Chapter 13

40. Which of the following is *true* concerning the effects of pessimism on health?
   a. Pessimistic people tend to have a more realistic view of life than optimists; thus, they are more cautious and take better care of their health.
   b. Pessimistic people are more likely to develop physical illnesses than optimists, since they appraise more events as stressful and thus experience more stress.
   c. Researchers have not been able to find any substantial health differences between pessimists and optimists.
   d. A pessimistic outlook can help a person live longer and healthier because it necessitates developing better coping skills.
   Answer: b   LO: 11; factual, conceptual   page: 478

41. Some days Teri's friends want to call her "Chicken Little," because she almost literally says "The sky is falling." Whatever happens, she interprets in the worst way possible. She stresses out about all of her classes and "knows" she's going to fail them all, even though she's actually a good student. After an exam, she does the "Monday night quarter backing," thinking about all the answers she got wrong. If someone comes up behind her just to say hello, she jumps about a mile. Teri appears to be a(n):
   a. Type A personality.
   b. optimist.
   c. pessimist.
   d. stress carrier.
   Answer: c   LO: 11; applied   page: 478

42. The specific findings in this chapter that link a pessimistic explanatory style to poorer health support the:
   a. direct effects model and indirect effects model.
   b. interactive model.
   c. direct effects model and interactive model.
   d. indirect effects model and interactive model.
   Answer: a   LO: 11; factual, conceptual   page: 478

43. Findings linking hypertension to psychological factors support the:
   a. interactive model and direct effects model.
   b. direct effects model.
   c. indirect effects model.
   d. interactive model and indirect effects model.
   Answer: a   LO: 11; factual, conceptual   page: 478

Personality, Behavior, and the Body

44. According to the more current research, which of the following personality styles most strongly predicts coronary heart disease?
    a. Type A personality
    b. competitiveness
    c. hostility
    d. time urgency
    Answer: c   LO: 12; factual   page: 479

45. Bernadette has high blood pressure. She has noticed that certain environmental stimuli, such as the low, pounding bass of her neighbors' stereos, cause her a great deal of physiological arousal that she finds particularly distressing. She tries to use cognitive coping techniques to view the neighbors and their noise in a more positive light but has not been successful. She sometimes calls the police or goes into the yard and screams, however, this increases her anxiety and feelings of hostility toward them. In addition to the stress brought on by the neighbors' music and insensitivity, Bernadette's health may be jeopardized by her:
    a. attempts to get her neighbors to keep quiet.
    b. feelings of hostility.
    c. inability to change the way she thinks about the music.
    d. neighbors' lack of consideration.
    Answer: b   LO: 12; applied   page: 479

46. Which of the following is *most* likely to experience coronary heart disease?
    a. Arthur is an amiable fellow who speaks "loud and fast," he is always in a hurry, always trying to meet deadlines, and trying to get 20 things done at once.
    b. Max is an angry person who shouts at his subordinates and holds grudges against people he perceives to be his enemies (and they are "everywhere").
    c. Burt bets on everything (even on if the sun will come up tomorrow), whatever you've done, he's done it more successfully, and whatever you have, his is better.
    d. Reginald likes to take it easy and relax; he gets his work done in a timely, but not rushed manner; and he rarely seems to get upset.
    Answer: b   LO: 12; applied   pages: 479-481

47. Which of the following statements about Type A personality is *true*?
    a. Only men with Type A personalities are at increased risk for heart attacks.
    b. Type A behavior may be partly adaptive, because Type A people have a decreased vulnerability to depression.
    c. People with Type A personalities may experience more adverse health effects due to a decreased release of catecholamines (norepinephrine and dopamine) during times of stress.
    d. Type A men are more likely to evidence heightened physiological reactivity to stress than women, but these results differ as a function of task.
    Answer: d   LO: 12; factual   pages: 480-481

Chapter 13

48. Which of the following is *least likely* to be a mechanism by which Type A characteristics, hostility, and other negative emotions leads to coronary heart disease?
    a. over arousal of the sympathetic nervous system
    b. frequent rise and fall of catecholamines in response to stress
    c. engaging in unhealthy behaviors, such as smoking and heavy drinking
    d. engaging in stereotypical sex-role behaviors
    Answer: d   LO: 13, 14; factual, conceptual   pages: 479-481

49. Most recent research on Type A personality has shown that:
    a. children whose parents repeatedly urge them to try harder and perform better but do not give concrete criteria to determine their success are especially vulnerable to CHD.
    b. men who model their fathers' behavior and women who model their mothers' behavior are equally as likely to succumb to CHD.
    c. the behavior patterns of Type A personality are so entrenched that it is more stressful to try to change them than it is to live with them.
    d. contrary to previous beliefs, it is not only the hostility factor, but also the sense of time urgency and the need for perfection that lead to CHD.
    Answer: a   LO: 12, 13; factual, conceptual   page: 481

50. Which gender difference is likely to be found with regard to Type A personality?
    a. While men are more likely to be classified as Type A, women who are Type A are more likely to exhibit the hostility component related to CHD.
    b. Men are more likely to carry the risk factors for CHD or smoking and hypertension, but women are more likely to have high cholesterol.
    c. Data collected within the past 5 years indicated that men now have only a slightly higher incidence of heart attacks than women.
    d. When female stereotyped tasks are used to induce stress, gender differences in physiological reactivity (and thus risk to CHD) are not found.
    Answer: d   LO: 14; factual, conceptual   page: 481

51. People with a repressive coping style:
    a. do not recognize or admit their own negative emotions but are aware that they evidence chronic autonomic arousal.
    b. have higher base levels of cortisol, a hormone released in response to stress.
    c. do not recognize or admit that they evidence chronic autonomic arousal but are aware they evidence negative emotions that they repress in order to avoid them.
    d. have lower base levels of cortisol, a hormone released by the immune system to fight disease.
    Answer: b   LO: 15; factual   page: 481

Personality, Behavior, and the Body

52. People who tend to "bottle up their feelings" and not express their negative emotions have a(n) _____ coping style.
    a. oppressive
    b. guilt-laden
    c. repressive
    d. restrained
    Answer: c   LO: 15; factual, conceptual   page: 481

53. Which of the following is *not* one of the reasons noted in the text that may cause a repressive coping style to be harmful to your health?
    a. You are unaware of when there is a problem, so you may wait until it's too late to deal with it.
    b. Chronic physiological arousal can cause damage to the immune system and cardiovascular systems.
    c. Repressors have no outlet for their negative emotions, so they can't let go of them.
    d. It take a lot of unconscious psychological and physiological work to constantly repress your emotions.
    Answer: a   LO: 15; factual, conceptual   page: 481

54. Which of the following has been shown to predict hypertension?
    a. John Henryism
    b. Type A personality
    c. a pessimistic explanatory style
    d. sleep deprivation
    Answer: a   LO: 16; factual   pages: 481-482

55. As related in the text, John Henry was:
    a. a runaway slave who died trying to reach freedom through the Underground Railroad.
    b. a prominent pioneer in the study of hypertension among African Americans.
    c. a steel-driving African-American man who outperformed a steam drill in drilling through a mountain but then dropped dead after the contest.
    d. the first African-American Senator who, after being sworn in, died of a heart attack.
    Answer: c   LO: 16; factual, conceptual   page: 482

56. The term that refers to a pattern of active coping with stressors involving trying harder and harder against overwhelming obstacles, particularly noted to lead to hypertension in African-American men is:
    a. John Henryism.
    b. persistence.
    c. chronic resolution.
    d. hypertensive style.
    Answer: a   LO: 16; factual, conceptual   pages: 481-482

Chapter 13

57. Lamar, a 24-year-old African American, is working his way through college. He got out of the Army, enrolled in an engineering program, and has two jobs. He uses his salary from one to pay for rent, food, and school expenses; he uses the other to support his mother and grandmother. He's worked hard since he was a child because he had to buy his own shoes and school supplies since Mama barely got enough from his father to support Grandma and "the kids." Lamar barely sleeps and occasionally dozes off in class, even though he's really interested. Recently, he went to the Health Center. They took his blood pressure and said it was 187/101. Which would be an appropriate term to describe Lamar's condition?
    a. persistence
    b. John Henryism
    c. chronic resolution
    d. hypertensive style
    Answer: b   LO: 16; applied   pages: 481-482

58. Which of the following is suggested by the text as a strategy for coping with negative emotions that appears to help people physically and emotionally?
    a. understanding the stressors in one's life
    b. seeking emotional support from others
    c. getting one's mind off of the stress
    d. removing the source of the stress
    Answer: b   LO: 17; factual, conceptual   page: 482

59. Research by Levy et al. (1990) showed which of the following with respect to social support?
    a. There were no significant physiological differences between cancer patients who did or did not seek social support, but those who did had more positive psychological measures.
    b. One study by Levy et al. found no significant physiological differences, but another found that 6 months after surgery the cancer patients who sought social support were healthier than those who did not.
    c. Women who had just received surgery for breast cancer, who actively sought social support from others, had higher natural killer cell activity.
    d. Women who had recently undergone surgery for breast cancer, who were placed into support groups, had lower rates of recurrence for their cancer.
    Answer: c   LO: 17; factual, conceptual   pages: 482-483

Personality, Behavior, and the Body

60. With respect to the benefits of social support for illness:
    a. having many friends and family members around is almost always beneficial since those who are supportive help reduce stress, and those who are critical help us cope.
    b. persons who have a high degree of conflict in their social networks tend to show poorer physical and emotional health following a major stressor.
    c. support groups for women believed to have terminal cancer have actually helped the women go into remission as compared with women with similar cancers who were not in support groups.
    d. it is not the quality of the support that is important, it is the number of people we have around us for support.
    Answer: b   LO: 17; factual, conceptual   pages: 482-483

61. Therapies designed to improve people's health are typically focused on:
    a. understanding the roots of the problems and learning how to cope with stress.
    b. learning and practicing new health-related skills and challenging negative cognitions.
    c. learning how to cope with stress and learning and practicing new health-related skills.
    d. learning and practicing new health-related skills and developing a high-quality support system.
    Answer: b   LO: 18; factual   page: 483

62. _____ techniques provide people with explicit information about how to enact health-related behaviors and opportunities to enact those behaviors in increasingly challenging situations.
    a. Guided imagery
    b. Guided mastery
    c. Cognitive restructuring
    d. Skills training
    Answer: b   LO: 18; factual, conceptual   page: 483

63. The text noted that guided mastery techniques are especially effective treatments for:
    a. hypertension.
    b. migraine headaches.
    c. coronary heart disease.
    d. reducing risky sexual behavior.
    Answer: d   LO: 18; factual   pages: 483-484

Chapter 13

64. The goals of guided mastery techniques are:
   a. to increase people's skills at and their self-efficacy to use health enhancing behaviors.
   b. to help people understand the physical and psychological underpinnings of illness.
   c. to help people visualize what being healthy entails and visualize themselves doing those behaviors.
   d. to teach people how to teach health enacting behaviors to others in order to reach more people.
   Answer: a　　　　　LO: 18; factual, conceptual　　　　　page: 483

65. Sheldon went to the doctor because he was having chest pains that also extended down his left arm. He thought he had carpal tunnel syndrome from working on his computer, but the doctor told him it was a mild heart attack, and he would have to stop smoking, cut back on fatty foods, and begin walking a mile a day. Sheldon "knew" his doctor was hiding the truth from him, that changing his lifestyle would be a futile effort, and that, in fact, his death was imminent. In terms of cognitive therapy, Sheldon was:
   a. overreacting.
   b. catastrophizing.
   c. using an effective strategy, "the worst possible case scenario."
   d. malingering.
   Answer: b　　　　　LO: 18; applied　　　　　pages: 484-485

66. The first step a psychologist might take with a patient who catastrophizes her illness is to:
   a. try to comfort her and assure her that it's not as bad she thinks.
   b. challenge her beliefs and get her to understand that it is not as bad as she thinks.
   c. educate her about the illness, including its prevalence, treatments for it, and typical prognoses.
   d. ask that she bring in her medical records, so the therapist has a better idea how serious the medical problem really is.
   Answer: c　　　　　LO: 18; factual, conceptual　　　　　page: 484

67. Much of the catastrophizing that patients do about their illnesses stems from:
   a. superstition, because if they believe it's not bad they may be "jinxing" their chances for recovery.
   b. a habitual way of looking at the world and expecting the worse to happen.
   c. not having heard what their physician said because they were in a highly aroused state.
   d. misunderstanding what they have been told about their illness by their physician.
   Answer: d　　　　　LO: 18; factual, conceptual　　　　　page: 484

Personality, Behavior, and the Body

68. In a controlled study with patients suffering from irritable bowel syndrome that assessed the effectiveness of challenging patients' catastrophizing cognitions about their illness (Greene & Blanchard, 1994) compared with patients who reported their symptoms on a weekly basis:
    a. there was significant improvement in symptoms for the patients receiving cognitive therapy as compared with those who merely reported symptoms.
    b. the patients whose beliefs were challenged got worse, possibly because they became upset that the therapist was not sensitive to their distress.
    c. the placebo (reporting) group actually experienced greater relief after 8 weeks than the patients in therapy.
    d. no statistically significant differences were found between patients in the two groups.
    Answer: a   LO: 18; factual   page: 485

69. Which of the following has been shown to be an effective treatment for both Type A personality and irritable bowel syndrome?
    a. guided mastery technique
    b. cognitive therapy
    c. biofeedback
    d. support groups
    Answer: b   LO: 18; factual   page: 485

70. The goal of biofeedback is to:
    a. let a machine cure stress-related illnesses electronically.
    b. detect signs of bodily dysfunction and control the body independently of the machine.
    c. learn to relax by listening to tones that go up and down depending on level of anxiety.
    d. detect how the body produces pain so the pain can ultimately be eliminated.
    Answer: b   LO: 18; factual, conceptual   page: 485

71. Which of the following statements about biofeedback is *true*?
    a. Consistent evidence has shown that biofeedback relieves migraine headaches by altering a person's body temperature.
    b. Biofeedback is a treatment in which a machine identifies and deliberately raises a person's body temperature to a safe but elevated level to help the body fight infection.
    c. Biofeedback is more effective than standard relaxation techniques for reducing headaches, pain, and hypertension.
    d. Biofeedback has been successful in reducing tension-related headaches.
    Answer: d   LO: 18; factual   page: 485

Chapter 13

72. Anita complained to Dr. David about headaches, tension, irritability, and stress. Her blood pressure is high even on medication. As Anita relates the sources of stress in her life and the fact that even thinking about certain things get her "all tensed up," Dr. David decides to try a way to teach her to teach her body to relax. He hooks her up to a machine and instructs her to listen to the tones, watch the digital lights, and focus on getting the tone low and the lights toward the bottom of the monitor. She's told to do "whatever it takes," whether it's breathing slowly, imagining lying on a warm beach in Hawaii, or thinking: "down, down, down." What type of therapy is Dr. David using with Anita?
   a. cognitive restructuring
   b. biofeedback
   c. relaxation therapy
   d. behavioral therapy
   Answer: b   LO: 18; applied   pages: 485-486

73. One advantage of relaxation over biofeedback is that relaxation:
   a. is easier for the therapist to monitor objectively.
   b. is less invasive in terms of interfering with bodily functions.
   c. is more effective for reducing headaches and hypertension.
   d. requires more training; thus, the individual receives more support from the therapist.
   Answer: c   LO: 18; factual   page: 486

74. Which of the following is *not* an element of time management described in the chapter?
   a. scheduling specific times to accomplish urgent activities
   b. breaking large tasks into smaller tasks
   c. distinguishing between distal goals and proximal goals
   d. rewarding yourself
   Answer: a   LO: 18; factual, conceptual   pages: 486-488

75. The first step of time management is determining:
   a. which activities are most urgent.
   b. which activities can be put off for a while.
   c. what activities are worth your time and what activities are not.
   d. how much time you have to get things done.
   Answer: c   LO: 18; factual   page: 487

76. Which of the following is *false* about urgent activities?
   a. Activities labeled as urgent are extremely important activities.
   b. Activities labeled as urgent are activities that need to be done immediately.
   c. Activities labeled as urgent can often be postponed.
   d. Activities are often labeled as urgent when we want to avoid doing something else.
   Answer: a   LO: 18; conceptual   page: 487

Personality, Behavior, and the Body

77. Deciding what activities are important involves:
    a. assessing what needs to be done.
    b. deciding one's goals and values.
    c. evaluating what others, such as family and friends, find important.
    d. listing all the things that need to be done and then prioritizing them.
    Answer: b   LO: 18; conceptual   page: 487

78. Breaking large activities into smaller ones necessitates having:
    a. distal goals and proximal goals.
    b. ideas and energy.
    c. plans and ideas.
    d. creative ideas and follow-through.
    Answer: a   LO: 18; factual, conceptual   page: 487

79. As noted in the text, the final step in time management involves:
    a. evaluating whether goals have been accomplished.
    b. getting feedback on the outcome of your activities.
    c. learning from what you've done.
    d. rewarding yourself for accomplishing goals.
    Answer: d   LO: 18; factual, conceptual   page: 488

80. A study by Freidman et al. (1985) to help men decrease Type A behavior had men in the treatment group:
    a. become more open in expressing their feelings, which sometimes meant yelling.
    b. use waiting time to reflect on things they usually don't have time to think about.
    c. think about the fact that if they do not reduce their Type A behavior patterns, they are likely to have another heart attack.
    d. understand their beliefs about success so that they can consistently do quality work to reduce their stress.
    Answer: b   LO: 19; factual, conceptual   pages: 488-489

81. A follow-up on the study by Friedman et al. (1985) to help men decrease Type A behavior found that four and a half years later:
    a. the experimental group had reverted back to their Type A pattern, and no significant differences between experimental and control groups were evident.
    b. men in the experimental group had intensified their Type A behaviors and had significantly more heart attacks then those in the control group.
    c. men in the control group had spontaneously reduced their Type A behaviors and had a nonsignificant trend toward fewer heart attacks.
    d. men in the experimental group were only half as likely as control subjects to have had another heart attack.
    Answer: d   LO: 19; factual, conceptual   pages: 488-489

Chapter 13

82. From a biopsychosocial perspective, the field of health psychology is based on the notion that:
    a. research must be directed at understanding which is the most potent force: biology, psychology, or environment.
    b. the mind, the body, and the environment are intimately connected.
    c. a child is born with a predetermined genetic plan, which will unfold in the context of the environment and thus affects our psychological underpinnings.
    d. the more we know about physical health, the more it will inform our understanding of psychological health around the world.
    Answer: b   LO: 19; factual, conceptual   page: 489

83. Psychological and social factors affect the body's physiology:
    a. directly and indirectly.
    b. interactively.
    c. indirectly.
    d. directly.
    Answer: a   LO: 19; factual, conceptual   page: 489-490

84. Psychological and social factors lead people to:
    a. engage in health-promoting or health-impairing behaviors.
    b. remember that each has an effect on the other.
    c. consider their habits, such as smoking.
    d. engage in behaviors that promote good health
    Answer: a   LO: 19; factual, conceptual   page: 489-490

85. Health psychologists make the assumption that our biology, psychology, and social environment have _____ influences on each other.
    a. characteristics
    b. bilateral
    c. reciprocal
    d. competing
    Answer: c   LO: 19; factual, conceptual   page: 489

86. Which of the following is *not* one of the suggestions made in the text for reducing stress?
    a. self-monitoring
    b. challenge cognitions that contribute to stress
    c. use the "worst case scenario"
    d. worry less about what might happen
    Answer: d   LO: 19; factual, conceptual   page: 491

Personality, Behavior, and the Body

87. A critical element of time management suggested for helping college students reduce stress is:
    a. take time for deep breathing exercises.
    b. scheduling.
    c. attend all your classes.
    d. make time for sleep.
    Answer: b LO: 19; factual page: 491

88. One of the hardest but most rewarding activities that students need to work into their schedule is:
    a. classes.
    b. work.
    c. leisure.
    d. eating.
    Answer: c LO: 19; factual page: 491

Essay Questions

89. You are arguing with a medical student friend about the importance of the mind and its effects on physical health. "It's a matter of biology," says your friend. "Disease strikes and the body becomes ill. Why would the mind make a difference?" Argue against this view by illustrating how psychological factors contribute to coronary heart disease, hypertension, and immune system dysfunction. For each condition, explain how psychological factors are thought to affect the body (directly, indirectly, or interactively) and cite experimental evidence to support your view. Finally, give one evidence-supported example of how changing or altering certain psychological factors may lead to positive effects on physical health.

A proper answer illustrates how psychological factors may contribute to the three health conditions listed (e.g., by explaining the hostility element of Type A personality and its link with coronary heart disease). The link between psychological factors and the body should be explained (e.g., people with Type A personality show greater physiological arousal in anticipation of stressors and in the early stages of dealing with a stressor, which increases blood pressure and risk of CHD). Specific evidence should be cited (e.g., a study that interviewed 3,000 healthy men in a deliberately annoying way found those rated as Type A had twice as many heart attacks or other forms of CHD as Type B men). A psychosocial intervention should be described (e.g., cognitive therapy for Type A personality), and evidence of its effectiveness should be summarized (e.g., a study comparing cognitive-behavioral therapy to no therapy in 1,000 men who had experienced a heart attack found that subjects in the treatment group were only half as likely as controls to have experienced another heart attack four and a half years later).

Chapter 13

90. How do dispositional pessimism, repressive coping, and John Henryism affect physical health? Explain each of these psychological factors, and describe the mechanisms by which they negatively affect health.

    A proper answer should explain how pessimism, a repressive coping style, and John Henryism affect physical health (e.g., repressive coping is associated with poorer immune system functioning, which increases the risk of physical disease), and describe the mechanisms by which they negatively affect health (e.g., people with a repressive coping style have high base levels of cortisol and greater autonomic arousal during challenging tasks).

91. Jason recently had a stroke that affected the speech areas of his brain and left him with partial paralysis on the right side of his body. He is in therapy to regain his speech and to overcome the paralysis. His wife, Joanne, has been his helpmate for the past 30 years and enjoys caring for Jason. In fact, she has always taken control of many of the family tasks, and the therapists have begun to work with her on how to release as much control as possible, so Jason increasingly takes on more responsibility for his own recovery. Remembering that the text has indicated that even events that are controllable and predictable may be stressful if they challenge the limits of our capabilities, discuss all of the factors that you believe would be relevant to Jason's continued improvement toward maximal functioning in light of his current condition.

    Here the student needs to address the issues of predictability and control, which might include understanding exactly what it is that has happened to his brain and the course the rehabilitation might take, as well as having control over as many areas of his life as possible (or, at least, having the *perception* that he has control). Further, the student needs to discuss how to make the "challenge" achievable--the types of cognitive and behavioral techniques that can be used to accompany the physical rehabilitation that he is receiving, and his wife needs to understand the importance of empowering Jason to gain increasing control over his life as he improves (and that in large part his improvement will have much to do with achieving a sense of predictability, control, and the ability to meet the challenges).

Personality, Behavior, and the Body

92. Canadian cross-cultural psychologist, John Berry (1996), has conducted extensive research on the psychological influences of acculturation and how (as well as whether) people are able to adapt to new or conflicting cultural settings. One of the ideas he discusses is that of marginalization, where an individual does not fit into his or her own culture or into the dominant culture where she or he resides. One consequence of marginalization is a high suicide rate among these individuals. Considering issues of health psychology, what stress factors would be relevant in terms of such a person's mental and physical well-being? Which of the three models discussed in the text (direct, indirect, interactive) do you believe is most relevant to this problem? Provide evidence for that belief. What behavioral patterns (in addition to high risk for suicide) might indicate that a person is feeling marginalized? What steps might be taken to assist such a person to reduce the stress factors in her or his life? As a society, what steps might we be able to take to eliminate, or at least diminish, marginalization for our citizens?

The student will need to discuss the stress factors that affect mental and physical health. First, there are the issues of controllability, predictability, challenge, and self-esteem that need to be addressed as they relate to stress and being involved in a social group. The issue of support system is critical here. The student should choose one of the three models and show how it applies (e.g., the direct model could apply because the marginalized person may have a psychological make-up that predisposes her or him to stress-related illnesses; indirect could address the fact that a marginalized person is likely to engage in unhealthy activities, such as alcohol and/or drug abuse). Indicators of marginalization could be personal withdrawal and isolation, alcoholism, etc. The student should suggest ways to intervene that help a person to connect with his or her own roots and/or aspects of the dominant culture that can become meaningful and supportive. Then, the student should discuss an appropriate intervention design to help people generally to identify with what is meaningful and valuable to be appreciated in their culture of origin and what is useful and valuable to be adopted from the dominant culture. It is important to note that marginalization can occur either because the individual rejects *or is rejected by* both cultures; thus, a plan must be implemented to deal with both possibilities.

93. Dissociative identity disorder (DID) is a fascinating disorder that underscores the mind-body connection. Persons with DID have totally distinct personalities, many of which have no knowledge of the others, and most of which will have amnesia for the periods of time when they are not "out." In terms of the mind-body question, perhaps what is most fascinating is that each personality will have its own behavioral and physiological patterns. For example, the personalities can have different brain wave patterns (as seen in EEGs), different handwriting, different visual acuity, and different allergies (a caution to anyone prescribing medications to someone with DID). While DID may, in itself, be a coping mechanism that allowed the person to "survive," each personality will have different styles of coping as well. From this description, explore this disorder in terms of health psychology, looking at both the

Chapter 13

healthy, survival issues and the maladaptive components of DID that may have a negative impact on the person's health. How would the three models used to explain the mind-body relationship help to understand DID? How might a therapist work with a client who has DID to ensure that person's optimal health?

The student needs to address how the mind and body influence each other to such an extent that not only does our biological predisposition affect our behavior, health, and emotional well being, but also that our psychological make-up will affect our health. As that psychological component changes, so may physiological components. The student should look at the processes by which this occurs, such as exploring the fight-or-flight response and the physiological changes that take place. Also, coping styles need to be addressed here as they influence our health. The three models should each be addressed in terms of the effect that psychological factors have directly on physiology and disease; how they may interact with pre-existing biological vulnerability to predict disease; and how the lifestyles of the various personalities may influence the body. The student may want to suggest referring the client to a therapist who specializes in DID; however, the student should be sure to discuss some of the more effective treatments, such as guided mastery techniques, biofeedback, and cognitive therapy, and time management--having a person with DID keep track of time would be a critically important way to have the various alters (personalities) communicate with each other. Because the different personalities will have different reactions to drugs, drug therapy would probably be a treatment to avoid.

Chapter 14   The Cognitive Disorders: Dementia, Delirium, and Amnesia

1. _____ is characterized by the gradual and usually permanent decline of intellectual functioning.
   a. Senility
   b. Dementia
   c. Delirium
   d. Amnesia
   Answer: b   LO: 2; factual, conceptual   page: 494

2. What is the most common cognitive disorder?
   a. dementia
   b. amnesia
   c. delirium
   d. dissociation
   Answer: a   LO: 1; factual   page: 494

3. Which of the following is *not* a recognized classification of cognitive disorders?
   a. dementia
   b. delirium
   c. senility
   d. amnesia
   Answer: c   LO: 2; factual   page: 494

4. A disorder characterized by impairments in cognition caused by a medical condition or by substance intoxication or withdrawal is:
   a. dementia.
   b. delirium.
   c. senility.
   d. amnesia.
   Answer: d   LO: 2; factual, conceptual   page: 494

5. By definition, a cognitive disorder cannot be caused by:
   a. medical diseases.
   b. substance intoxication.
   c. infections.
   d. psychiatric disorders.
   Answer: d   LO: 1; factual   page: 494

Chapter 14

6. The cognitive disorders were formerly referred to as:
    a. thought disorders.
    b. organic brain disorders.
    c. amnestic disorders.
    d. senility.
    Answer: b   LO: 1; factual   page: 494

7. The label of _____ for cognitive disorders was discontinued in DSM-IV.
    a. senility
    b. cognitive impairment
    c. organic brain disorders
    d. dementia
    Answer: c   LO: 1; factual, conceptual   page: 494

8. Use of the label organic brain disorders was discontinued in DSM-IV because:
    a. the label is too vague.
    b. the disorders are more severe than that label implies.
    c. it implies that other disorders are not caused by biological factors.
    d. that term is not restricted to physiological disorders.
    Answer: c   LO: 1; factual, conceptual   page: 494

9. Cognitive disorders are diagnosed when cognitive impairments appear to be the result:
    a. of a nonpsychiatric medical disease or substance intoxication or withdrawal.
    b. of a psychiatric disorder, such as schizophrenia or depression.
    c. of either a nonpsychiatric medical disease or a psychiatric disorder, such as schizophrenia or depression.
    d. primarily of substance intoxication or withdrawal.
    Answer: a   LO: 2; factual   page: 494

10. Which of the following is *true* concerning dementia?
    a. It generally has a sudden onset.
    b. It is most commonly psychogenic.
    c. It is typically irreversible.
    d. It is a synonym for "insane."
    Answer: c   LO: 3; conceptual   page: 496

Cognitive Disorders

11. Which of the following deficits do not occur in dementia?
    a. memory deficit
    b. alogia
    c. apraxia
    d. aphasia
    Answer: b   LO: 4; factual   pages: 496-497

12. The most prominent cognitive deficiency in dementia is:
    a. memory deficit.
    b. speech deficit.
    c. irrational thought processes.
    d. illogical thought processes.
    Answer: a   LO: 4; factual   page: 496

13. Which of the following symptoms must be present for a diagnosis of dementia?
    a. persistent illogical thought processes
    b. inability to repeat words coherently
    c. memory deficit
    d. All of the above are required for a diagnosis of dementia.
    Answer: c   LO: 4; factual   page: 496

14. The difference between "normal" memory lapses and dementia is that:
    a. in dementia, the memory does not return spontaneously and may not respond to memory cues.
    b. in dementia, the person is much more greatly troubled by the memory lapses.
    c. with normal memory lapses, the person is much more troubled than is someone with dementia.
    d. people with normal memory loss tend to ask that a question be repeated, while a person with dementia will not.
    Answer: a   LO: 4; factual, conceptual   page: 496

15. The progression of memory loss in dementia is such that:
    a. short-term memory deficits appear prior to long-term memory deficits.
    b. long-term memory deficits appear prior to short-term memory deficits.
    c. short-term memory deficits and long-term memory deficits begin around the same time.
    d. whether short-term or long-term memory deficits begins first depends on the individual.
    Answer: a   LO: 4; factual, conceptual   page: 496

Chapter 14

16. The term for the deterioration of language that is seen in dementia is:
    a. alogia.
    b. apraxia.
    c. aphasia.
    d. agnosia.
    Answer: c   LO: 4; factual   page: 496

17. Janet has her Ph.D. in psychology and has taught at a prestigious Ivy League college for 25 years. Her research papers have been published in all of the cognitive psychology journals, and she has had a particular interest in dementia because of the devastating effects it has had on her family. Her husband, Carl, has recently noticed that Janet seems to have problems remembering things, over and above the possibly well-warranted "absent-minded professor" stereotype that his wife has always fit so well. He is noticing that she "loses words" and is either vague or uses a description--so that, rather than asking for a glass, she might ask for "that thing that holds the water." This is indicative of:
    a. agnosia.
    b. apraxia.
    c. aphasia.
    d. alogia.
    Answer: c   LO: 4; applied   page: 496

18. The advanced form of language loss in which people repeat exactly what they heard is:
    a. aphasia.
    b. echolalia.
    c. palilalia.
    d. agnosia.
    Answer: b   LO: 4; factual, conceptual   page: 497

19. When people simply repeat sounds or words over and over it is:
    a. agnosia.
    b. palilalia.
    c. echolalia.
    d. aphasia.
    Answer: b   LO: 4; factual, conceptual   page: 497

Cognitive Disorders

20. An impaired ability to execute common actions, such as waving good-bye or tying one's shoes is referred to as:
    a. aphasia.
    b. agnosia.
    c. apraxia.
    d. alogia.
    Answer: c   LO: 4; factual, conceptual   page: 497

21. Apraxia is caused by:
    a. problems in motor functioning.
    b. problems in sensory functioning.
    c. problems in comprehending what action is required.
    d. None of the above.
    Answer: d   LO: 4; factual   page: 497

22. Which of the following is a term that refers to an inability to recognize objects or people that is present in dementia?
    a. apraxia
    b. alogia
    c. agnosia
    d. aphasia
    Answer: c   LO: 4; factual, conceptual   page: 497

23. The ability to plan, initiate, monitor, and stop complex behaviors is referred to as
    a. cognitive processing.
    b. executive functioning.
    c. cortical functioning.
    d. frontal lobe processing.
    Answer: b   LO: 4; factual, conceptual   page: 497

24. Deficits in executive functioning would not produce marked impairments in:
    a. planning.
    b. behavioral inhibition.
    c. abstract thinking.
    d. All of the above would be impaired.
    Answer: d   LO: 4; factual, conceptual   page: 497

Chapter 14

25. Which of the following are *not* likely behaviors of someone with dementia?
    a. shoplifting, exhibitionism, and wandering into traffic
    b. failure to recognize or admit their cognitive deficits
    c. a belief that others are conspiring against them
    d. putting their affairs in order (e.g., updating their will) before it's "too late."
    Answer: d   LO: 5; factual, conceptual   page: 497

26. Approximately _____% of people _____ are afflicted with Alzheimers.
    a. 1 to 2; over 65
    b. 1 to 2; over 80
    c. 2 to 4; over 65
    d. 2 to 4; over 80
    Answer: c   LO: 6, 7; factual   pages: 497-498

27. The most common cause of dementia is due to:
    a. head injury.
    b. Alzheimer's disease.
    c. cerebrovascular disease.
    d. HIV.
    Answer: b   LO: 7; factual   page: 498

28. In light of the fact that approximately _____% of people over 80 have some form of dementia, it is apparent that severe cognitive decline _____.
    a. 5; is a serious problem of aging
    b. 20; is a serious problem of aging
    c. 5; is not an inevitable part of aging
    d. 20; is not an inevitable part of aging
    Answer: d   LO: 6; factual, conceptual   page: 497-498

29. From the media attention directed at Alzheimers disease, it appears that the prevalence of this disease is on the rise. One explanation for this is that:
    a. Alzheimers was previously called "senility," and now we know more about it so we can recognize it more accurately.
    b. because people are living longer than in previous decades, they are more likely to develop such diseases as Alzheimers that do not show up until old age.
    c. modern advances in technology have polluted not only the atmosphere, but our food supply as well, and over time that makes us vulnerable to diseases like Alzheimers.
    d. the heavy demands made on us intellectually and socially have a negative effect on our physiology, and one result is Alzheimers.
    Answer: b   LO: 7; factual, conceptual   page: 498

Cognitive Disorders

30. Florence was at her grandson, Eddy's, wedding in California. It was a warm, sunny day, and she was wearing a brand new dress for the occasion. She was talking to her grandniece, Anita, saying, "I'm not sure I'm going to stay here for my grandson's wedding. Do you know my grandson, Eddy? He's a good boy, but I think my daughter doesn't want me to stay here that long. She's trying to get me to go home. She thinks I'm too much trouble." During the same conversation, she had asked Anita several times, "How's your father?" to which the younger woman had replied the first two times, "Aunty, my father died 10 years ago." Which of the following might we suspect that Florence has?
    a. Korsakoff's syndrome
    b. retrograde amnesia
    c. agnosia
    d. Alzheimer's disease
    Answer: d   LO: 7; applied   page: 498

31. Approximately ____% of all dementias are due to _____.
    a. 10; Alzheimers
    b. 50; Alzheimers
    c. 10; brain injury
    d. 50; Parkinson's
    Answer: b   LO: 7; factual   page: 498

32. The typical caregiver for an Alzheimer's patient is:
    a. the wife, daughter, or daughter-in-law of the patient.
    b. husband, son, or son-in-law of the patient.
    c. the patient's spouse.
    d. a medical facility designed to deal with these patients.
    Answer: a   LO: 8; factual   pages: 498-499

33. The term for the group that is caught between caring for their young children and their elderly parents is the:
    a. intermediate generation.
    b. intermediary generation.
    c. sandwich generation.
    d. nuclear generation.
    Answer: c   LO: 8; factual   page: 499

Chapter 14

34. Which of the following is *not* a problem of persons who are caregivers of Alzheimer's patients presented in the text?
    a. They show higher rates of depression and anxiety than controls.
    b. They show higher rates of physical illness than controls.
    c. They are at high risk for resorting to elder abuse.
    d. They find their role fulfilling and satisfying.
    Answer: d   LO: 8; factual, conceptual   page: 499

35. Support groups for caregivers of Alzheimer's patients focus on:
    a. problem-solving skills for managing the patient at home.
    b. allowing caregivers a forum for venting their negative feelings.
    c. helping them view their situation in a more positive, self-fulfilling light.
    d. providing some respite for the caregivers from the demands of their situation.
    Answer: a   LO: 8; factual, conceptual   page: 499

36. Neurofibrillary tangles are most often found in the:
    a. limbic system.
    b. hypothalamus.
    c. hippocampus.
    d. thalamus.
    Answer: c   LO: 9; factual   page: 499

37. Plaques and cell death in Alzheimer's disease occur primarily in the:
    a. cerebellum.
    b. caudate nucleus.
    c. hypothalamus.
    d. cerebral cortex.
    Answer: d   LO: 9; factual   page: 499

38. Which of the following is *not* one of the primary neurological signs of Alzheimer's?
    a. neurofibrillary tangles
    b. plaques
    c. shrinking of ventricles
    d. loss of dendrites
    Answer: c   LO: 9; factual   page: 499

Cognitive Disorders

39. Alzheimer's disease is definitively diagnosed:
    a. after assessment with memory tests and review of neuroimaging techniques.
    b. after the patient has died and a brain autopsy can be performed.
    c. by assessing the patient's history and current functioning and looking at the patient's family history.
    d. after reviewing the patient's PET scans, MRIs, and CT scans.
    Answer: b   LO: 9; factual   page: 500

40. The most promising lines of research concerning the causes of Alzheimers focus on:
    a. viral infections.
    b. genetic transmission.
    c. exposure to toxic levels of aluminum.
    d. head trauma.
    Answer: b   LO: 10; factual   page: 502

41. Gene abnormalities on which of the following chromosomes are associated with an increased risk of late-onset Alzheimer's disease?
    a. 4
    b. 14
    c. 18
    d. 19
    Answer: d   LO: 10; factual   page: 502

42. Gene abnormalities on which of the following chromosomes is responsible for a protein on the membrane of cells known as S182 and may be responsible for up to 80% of early-onset Alzheimer's disease?
    a. 4
    b. 14
    c. 18
    d. 21
    Answer: b   LO: 10; factual   page: 502

43. Which of the following conditions is thought to share its genetic basis on a chromosome with Alzheimer's disease?
    a. Parkinson's disease.
    b. Down syndrome.
    c. Huntington's disease.
    d. Phenylketonuria (PKU).
    Answer: b   LO: 10; factual   page: 502

Chapter 14

44. Which of the following is *true* concerning a potential link between Alzheimer's and Down syndrome?
    a. People with Down syndrome are more likely than people in the general population to develop late-onset Alzheimers.
    b. People with Down syndrome are more likely than people in the general population to develop early-onset Alzheimers.
    c. People with Down syndrome are less likely than people in the general population to develop late-onset Alzheimers.
    d. While researchers are looking for a link, so far no significant evidence has been found to support such a connection.
    Answer: a   LO: 10; factual   page: 502

45. A person who has symptoms or laboratory evidence of cerebrovascular disease, and who demonstrates signs of dementia, would be diagnosed with:
    a. Alzheimer's disease.
    b. Down syndrome.
    c. vascular dementia.
    d. senility.
    Answer: c   LO: 11; factual   page: 503

46. A stroke is:
    a. sudden damage to an area of the brain due to blockage of blood flow or hemorrhage.
    b. damage to the brain caused by cessation of oxygen flow for over 30 seconds.
    c. a sudden shock a person experiences that causes brain cells to deteriorate rapidly.
    d. loss of brain cells caused by a person not using certain areas or functions of the brain.
    Answer: a   LO: 11; factual   page: 503

47. Max was a millionaire. He never finished high school but had an innate ability to understand and manipulate figures, and he built several investment companies. One day, while driving home from his office, he blacked out and hit a tree. He suffered a minor concussion and a few cuts and bruises but had no serious injuries. He was back at work two days later. Over the next few months, however, he seemed to have increasing memory loss and sometimes would appear not to "be there" when his wife or children were speaking to him. A neurological examination confirmed that he had been suffering from a series of little strokes, that left him with
    a. Alzheimer's disease.
    b. vascular dementia.
    c. Parkinson's disease.
    d. traumatic brain dementia.
    Answer: b   LO: 11; applied   page: 503

Cognitive Disorders

48. The most common cause of closed head injuries is:
    a. sports injuries.
    b. blows to the head (during a violent assault).
    c. motor vehicle accidents.
    d. gunshot wounds.
    Answer: c   LO: 12; factual   page: 504

49. Which of the following is *not* a symptom of frontal lobe injury?
    a. disorderliness, suspiciousness, and anxiousness
    b. apathy and lack of concern for others
    c. risk taking and poor impulse control
    d. disorientation and memory loss
    Answer: d   LO: 12; factual   page: 504

50. Which of the following is *not* one of the medical conditions commonly thought to lead to dementia?
    a. Parkinson's disease
    b. HIV
    c. Huntington's disease
    d. neurologia
    Answer: d   LO: 13; factual   pages: 504-505

51. Of the following medical conditions associated with dementia, which is *least likely* to occur?
    a. HIV
    b. Huntington's chorea
    c. Parkinson's disease
    d. vascular dementia
    Answer: b   LO: 13; factual   page: 505

52. Epidemiological studies of HIV-associated dementia indicate that:
    a. it is extremely rare.
    b. it is inevitable.
    c. there is a narrow range (7 to 15%) of HIV-infected persons who develop dementia.
    d. there is a wide range (7 to 66%) of HIV-infected persons who develop dementia.
    Answer: d   LO: 13; factual   page: 505

Chapter 14

53. Parkinson's disease results from the death of neurons that produce:
   a. serotonin.
   b. acetylcholine.
   c. dopamine.
   d. amyloid protein.
   Answer: c   LO: 14; factual   page: 505

54. Mild neurocognitive disorder consists of cognitive deficits and mild impairments in social/occupational functioning as a result of which of the following medical conditions?
   a. Parkinson's disease
   b. Huntington's disease
   c. HIV
   d. Pick's disorder
   Answer: c   LO: 13; factual   page: 505

55. In 1996, scientists reported that thousands of British cows had died of "mad cow disease," a fatal brain infection. According to our text, people who died from eating the meat of these infected cows may have developed:
   a. Pick's disorder.
   b. dementia.
   c. Creutzfeldt-Jakob disease.
   d. HIV infection.
   Answer: c   LO: 13; factual   page: 505

56. A single dominant gene on which of the following chromosomes leads to Huntington's disease?
   a. 4
   b. 14
   c. 18
   d. 21
   Answer: a   LO: 13; factual   page: 505

57. Which of the following is *false* concerning the connection between dementia and chronic heavy use of alcohol and other drugs?
   a. Once the dementia sets in, there is a rapid progression to total dementia.
   b. It is often irreversible.
   c. It may be slowed with nutritional supplements.
   d. As many as 10% of chronic alcohol abusers may develop dementia.
   Answer: a   LO: 14; factual   page: 505

Cognitive Disorders

58. A disease that is characterized by tremors, muscle rigidity, the inability to initiate movement, and possibly dementia in its later stages is:
    a. Alzheimer's.
    b. Korsakoff syndrome.
    c. Parkinson's.
    d. multi-infarct dementia.
    Answer: c   LO: 14; factual   page: 505

59. People with Alzheimer's disease have reduced levels of _____ in their brains.
    a. acetylcholine
    b. ApoE4
    c. amyloid protein
    d. dopamine
    Answer: a   LO: 15; factual   page: 505

60. With respect to treatment of dementia, which of the following is *true*?
    a. Some Alzheimer's patients show improvement in cognitive functioning when given drugs that increase levels of dopamine in their brains.
    b. Some Parkinson's patients show improvement in cognitive functioning when given drugs that increase levels of acetylcholine in their brains.
    c. While the drugs that reduce dementia in Parkinson's patients may not work for all of these patients, for the patients who are helped this is a relatively permanent reversal.
    d. For both Alzheimers and Parkinson's patients, the drugs, if they do work at all, have only temporary effects.
    Answer: d   LO: 15; factual   pages: 505-506

61. Which of the following is *not* a treatment currently used for dementia?
    a. antidepressant and antianxiety drugs for emotional symptoms
    b. antipsychotic drugs to control hallucinations and delusions
    c. behavioral therapies for controlling emotional lability
    d. All of these are currently being used.
    Answer: d   LO: 15; factual   pages: 505-506

62. When discussing cognitive disorders, _____ involves an acute, usually transient, disorientation and memory loss.
    a. anterograde amnesia
    b. retrograde amnesia
    c. dementia
    d. delirium
    Answer: d   LO: 2; factual, conceptual   page: 506

Chapter 14

63. Which of the following is *not* a symptom of delirium?
    a. disorientation
    b. hearing voices in one's head
    c. recent memory loss
    d. clouding of consciousness
    Answer: b   LO: 16; factual   page: 506

64. *Sundowning* is a term used to indicate that:
    a. a person with dementia improves at night.
    b. a person with dementia is in the late stages and may be expected to die soon.
    c. symptoms of delirium worsen at night.
    d. symptoms of delirium improve at night.
    Answer: c   LO: 16; factual   page: 506

65. Typically, the first sign of delirium to appear is:
    a. disorientation as to time.
    b. disorientation as to place.
    c. inability to recognize familiar people.
    d. loss of remote memory.
    Answer: a   LO: 16; factual   page: 506

66. Alan is brought into the emergency department of County General Hospital presenting with symptoms of sudden disorientation and memory loss. He can't recognize his wife, who became alarmed when they were shopping at a mall and he started saying bizarre things and had no idea where he was. Even now he does not know that he is in a hospital, nor can he say what day it is or if it is night or day. Alan appears to be suffering from:
    a. dementia.
    b. delirium.
    c. psychosis.
    d. Korsakoff's syndrome.
    Answer: b   LO: 16; applied   pages: 506-507

67. Which of the following substances is *least expected* to induce delirium?
    a. alcohol
    b. muscle relaxants
    c. SSRIs
    d. corticosteroids
    Answer: c   LO: 17; factual   page: 507

Cognitive Disorders

68. Which type of disorientation is *not* one of the requisite symptoms for a diagnosis of delirium?
    a. time
    b. place
    c. person
    d. objects
    Answer: d   LO: 16; factual   page: 507

69. It is important to monitor delirious persons because:
    a. delirium quickly progresses into psychotic conditions.
    b. they are likely to have a serious if not fatal accident.
    c. delirium can cause more serious brain damage.
    d. their disorientation can lead to permanent amnesia.
    Answer: b   LO: 17; factual, conceptual   page: 508

70. Which of the following is *not* one of the possible causes of delirium discussed in the text?
    a. medical, surgical, chemical, or neurological problems
    b. stroke, congestive heart failure, infectious disease
    c. a maladaptive coping style that leads to psychogenic problems
    d. drug intoxication or withdrawal, or medications and toxic substances
    Answer: c   LO: 17; factual   pages: 507-508

71. The syndrome known as ICU/CCU psychosis is:
    a. a form of mental illness due to excess medication when a patient is in intensive care.
    b. an experience of hospitalized patients in which they hear noises from machines they believe to be human voices, see walls quiver, or hallucinate that someone is tapping them on the shoulder.
    c. a syndrome that patients often experience after prolonged surgery due to extended use of anesthesia that affects the ability of their brain to process information in a realistic manner.
    d. a form of schizophrenia that develops after surgery due to chemical changes in the patient's brain due to the combination of general anesthetic and trauma.
    Answer: b   LO: 17; factual, conceptual   page: 507

72. Men are at increased risk for _____, whereas women are at increased risk for _____.
    a. Alzheimer's disease; Huntington's disease
    b. cardiovascular disease; cerebrovascular disease
    c. dementia; delirium
    d. delirium; dementia
    Answer: d   LO: 17; factual   page: 507

Chapter 14

73. Which of the following is *most likely* to develop delirium?
    a. 85-year-old Samuel, who 5 years ago was diagnosed with Parkinson's disease.
    b. 87-year-old Sarah, whose husband died 5 years ago.
    c. 28-year-old Sandy, who suffered from auditory hallucinations during her 3-year siege with depression.
    d. 25-year-old Sean, who was recently had head trauma after a motor cycle accident.
    Answer: a   LO: 17; applied   page: 507

74. Which of the following is *true* concerning the effects of delirium?
    a. The elderly have a lower mortality than younger people from delirium because as soon as it is noticed physicians will adjust medication, since that is the primary problem.
    b. Between 15 and 40% of delirious hospital patients die within one month as compared with half that rate for nondelirious patients.
    c. Approximately 12% of nursing home residents have been reported to be delirious.
    d. Of all the iatrogenic disorders brought on by medication interactions, delirium is the most easily recognized and treated.
    Answer: b   LO: 17; factual   page: 507

75. Which of the following is *not* one of the treatments presented in the text for delirium?
    a. use of restraints
    b. use of psychotropic medications
    c. a quiet, isolated environment
    d. placing clocks, calendar, and photographs in the patient's room
    Answer: c   LO: 18; factual   page: 508

76. The disorder in which only memory is affected is:
    a. amnesia.
    b. alogia.
    c. dementia.
    d. delirium.
    Answer: a   LO: 19; factual   page: 509

77. The person with _____ amnesia is impaired in ability to learn new information; the person with _____ amnesia is impaired in ability to recall previously learned information.
    a. present; past
    b. retrograde; anterograde
    c. anterograde; retrograde
    d. proactive; retroactive
    Answer: b   LO: 19; factual   page: 509

Cognitive Disorders

78. It is more common for people with amnesia to forget:
    a. numbers than names.
    b. recent events than past events.
    c. past events than recent events.
    d. faces than names.
    Answer: b   LO: 19; factual   page: 509

79. Korsakoff's syndrome is an amnestic disorder caused by damage to the:
    a. cerebral cortex.
    b. hypothalamus.
    c. hippocampus.
    d. thalamus.
    Answer: d   LO: 20; factual   page: 509

80. Korsakoff's syndrome is associated with a deficiency of:
    a. thiamine.
    b. beta-carotenes.
    c. calcium.
    d. nitrogen.
    Answer: a   LO: 20; factual   page: 509

81. Korsakoff's syndrome is associated with:
    a. a genetic defect on chromosome 21.
    b. chronic and heavy alcohol abuse.
    c. excessive dopamine.
    d. insufficient serotonin.
    Answer: b   LO: 20; factual   page: 509

82. The first step in treating amnestic disorders is:
    a. stabilizing the environment to keep it as familiar as possible.
    b. providing adequate nutrition.
    c. removing conditions contributing to the amnesia.
    d. attending to accompanying health conditions.
    Answer: c   LO: 21; factual   page: 510

Chapter 14

83. Which of the following is suggested in the text as appropriate for the amnestic person's environment?
    a. quiet music
    b. burning incense
    c. calendars and photographs
    d. audiotapes with self-affirming subliminal messages
    Answer: c   LO: 21; factual   page: 510

84. African Americans are at increased risk for _____, whereas European Americans are at increased risk for _____ .
    a. Alzheimer's disease; Huntington's disease
    b. vascular dementia; Parkinson's disease
    c. Parkinson's disease; vascular dementia
    d. Huntington's disease; delirium
    Answer: b   LO: 22; factual   page: 510

85. Having a low education level is *not* associated with:
    a. poorer scores on the Mini-Mental State Examination.
    b. greater decline in language skills associated with dementia.
    c. greater brain deterioration associated with dementia.
    d. higher rates of dementia.
    Answer: b   LO: 22; factual   pages: 510-511

86. With respect to the interaction of gender with language skills:
    a. women typically have higher language skills than men and show fewer language deficits than men when both are diagnosed with dementia.
    b. women typically have higher language skills than men, but both exhibit similar types of language deficit when diagnosed with dementia.
    c. women typically have higher language skills than men but show greater language deficits than men when both are diagnosed with dementia.
    d. due to greater bilateralization of language between the hemispheres for women, they are less likely than men to exhibit language decrements in the event of dementia.
    Answer: c   LO: 22; factual, conceptual   page: 510

Cognitive Disorders

87. The text suggests that African Americans may have higher rates of _____ than European Americans because _____.
    a. delirium; they lack health insurance and thus do not receive early medical care for serious illnesses
    b. Alzheimer's disease; they lack health insurance and thus do not receive early medical care to slow the progression
    c. Alzheimer's disease; genetic factors leading to Alzheimer's may be more prevalent among African Americans
    d. Parkinson's disease; genetic factors leading to Parkinsonism may be more prevalent among African Americans
    Answer: a   LO: 22; factual   page: 510

88. Neuroimaging studies demonstrate:
    a. more dramatic brain deterioration among people with higher levels of education than for those with less education.
    b. no significant differences in the brain tissue of highly educated versus poorly educated persons.
    c. greater brain deterioration associated with dementia for people with less education than for those with more education.
    d. Research is not yet sufficiently sophisticated to compare differences in brain deterioration as they relate to level of education.
    Answer: c   LO: 22; factual   page: 511

89. You bring your ailing father for assessment because he has been having a problem remembering things that has begun to interfere with his life, and you are concerned about his welfare. He is asked questions such as, "What year is this?" "What season is this?" "What state do you live in?" "I'm going to name three objects, and I want you to say them after me, okay? An apple, an orange, and a lemon. Can you repeat them?" It is most likely that your father is taking:
    a. an intelligence test.
    b. the Mini-Mental State Examination.
    c. the Minnesota Multiphasic Personality Inventory.
    d. the Bender-Gestalt Neuromotor Assessment.
    Answer: b   LO: 22; applied   pages: 510-511

Chapter 14

90. Max is an 82-year-old man whose behavior is becoming an increasing embarrassment to his family. He is constantly accusing them of attempting to poison him because he knows they want to take over the automobile empire he has built over the past 50 years. He yells at his sons and his grandsons constantly, and his daughter-in-law in whose home he lives, has given her husband an ultimatum that either the older man goes, or she goes. Most recently, Max took off all of his clothes and ran through the streets of the downtown section, then stopped in at the local convenience store and shoplifted candy that he never eats. What might we suggest about Max's behavior in his earlier years?
    a. He was probably a really nice man who took care of his wife and children.
    b. It is not unlikely that he exhibited paranoid behaviors, as well as irritability and impulsivity.
    c. He probably suffered from paranoid personality disorder as a younger man.
    d. There is no way to know from this scenario what his previous behavior was like.
    Answer: b   LO: 23; applied   page: 511

91. The symptoms of paranoia, irritability, and impulsivity seen in the early stages of dementia
    a. are more noticeable in persons who were easy-going and affable before developing dementia.
    b. probably will not develop in persons who had well-established behavior patterns that exhibited control over impulsive behaviors.
    c. show little correlation to personality prior to onset of dementia.
    d. may be especially pronounced in people who were somewhat paranoid, hostile, or impulsive before developing dementia.
    Answer: d   LO: 23; factual, conceptual   page: 511

92. In the case of persons who are easily confused or forgetful, their cognitive deficits:
    a. can become increasingly severe if family members expect too much of them.
    b. will not be affected by the behavior of people around him or her because they do not interact with their environment.
    c. will improve when the people around them make many demands on them to behave in an acceptable way.
    d. will improve when the people around them do not acknowledge these cognitive problems.
    Answer: a   LO: 23; factual, conceptual   page: 512

Cognitive Disorders

93. Rose (83) is concerned about her younger sister, Dorothy (81). Others, too, have noticed that Dorothy's memory is becoming a health problem, since she has trouble remembering when to take her medications, which resulted in an unsuccessful outcome from her cataract surgery. Her niece, Myrna, recently commented that lately Dorothy will ask the same question over several times but suspects it may be a hearing problem. Dorothy has raised five children, who all have college educations and are successful in their own creative endeavors, but she, herself has never been intellectually inclined. She lives alone, but spends a lot of time with her children, sister, nieces and nephews, and friends. For years she has been described as an "ostrich," who "sticks her head in the sand" and doesn't pay attention to problems, including her own health. Which of the following is *unlikely* to be true?
    a. Because of the memory deficit, and Dorothy's lack of intellectual activity, it would be appropriate to have her evaluated for Alzheimer's or vascular dementia.
    b. Despite her involvement with family and friends, it is possible that as an elderly woman with an apparent hearing problem, Dorothy may be experiencing depression.
    c. Since Dorothy has managed to raise a family of successful offspring and is able to care for herself, the only problem is lack of sufficient social stimulation.
    d. Her apparent memory deficit and hearing impairment, and her inability to attend to her daily health needs would make it imperative for Dorothy to be fully evaluated for possible cognitive disorder, as well as for her other medical problems.

    Answer: c   LO: 2; applied   pages: 511-512

Chapter 14

Essay Questions

94. Your best friend's grandmother has been diagnosed with Alzheimer's disease and your friend asks you what you know about this disease. Describe the symptoms and causes of Alzheimer's disease for your friend, then identify and discuss five of the cognitive abilities that are impaired. Also explain to your friend the changes in the brain that accompany Alzheimer's disease, and summarize the evidence that genetics contribute to the development of this disease.

    A proper answer should discuss the symptoms and causes of Alzheimer's disease by identifying and discussing five cognitive abilities that are impaired by the disease (e.g., loss of executive functioning), the changes in the brain that accompany the disease (e.g., plaques, cortical cell death), and summarize the evidence for a genetic contribution to the disease (e.g., chromosomes 14, 19, and 21 have been associated with Alzheimer's disease).

95. What symptoms must a person display to receive a diagnosis of delirium? What is the typical progression of symptoms in delirium? How should people with delirium be treated?

    A proper answer should discuss the symptoms evident in delirium (e.g., episodes of disorientation) and describe the typical progression of these symptoms (e.g., the symptoms begin with disorientation to time, then place, etc.). The ways in which people with delirium should be treated should also be described (e.g., people should be treated quickly in order to prevent brain damage).

96. Your roommate's mother is caring for her mother-in-law, who has dementia. Your roommate is concerned about whether "Mom" can handle this and has asked for your opinion. From your Abnormal Psychology class, you know that caregivers of persons with dementia are at high risk for stress related illnesses, as well as for becoming abusive of the elders in their care. Enlighten your friend on the issue of who is most likely to become the caregiver of an elder with dementia, then discuss the issue of elder abuse in terms of how it begins, how to avoid it, and how, as a caregiver, your roommate's mother can take care of herself as well as her mother-in-law.

Cognitive Disorders

97. Which of the disorders discussed in this chapter is/are avoidable? Describe the disorder(s) in terms of symptoms and causes, and how to avoid the problems inherent in the disorder(s).

The prime candidate for discussion here is amnesia resulting from Korsakoff's syndrome. The student should discuss the symptoms of Korsakoff's, its relationship to alcoholism and ways to avoid the negative cognitive consequences of alcohol abuse.

98. Current research is being conducted by the National Institutes of Health on Alzheimer's disease. Particularly interesting is the study being conducted by David Snowdon from the University of Kentucky who is studying nuns at a teaching order in Mankato, Minnesota (The Sisters of Notre Dame). These 678 participants ranged in age from 75 to 103 when the study began, and the average age was 85; upon their deaths, they are all donating their brains to NIH for continuing research. Among the participants are some biological sisters, who provide an interesting subsample in terms of genetic studies on Alzheimers. What Snowdon and his colleagues have found is that the nuns who demonstrated more complex use of language and more idea density (how many ideas in relation to the number of words used) when they first took their vows (approximately at age 19-20), the less likely they were to exhibit the decrements incident to Alzheimer's. The research is not necessarily finding that these nuns do not have the disease, but that it has less of a negative impact on their cognitive abilities. Present evidence from the text that would help to explain these findings. How can this research be used to help mitigate the devastating effects of this disease?

The student needs to discuss what we know about the brain in terms of Alzheimer's, and the areas that are affected (e.g., the plaques and neurofibrillary tangles, loss of dendrites, etc.); the student also must discuss the evidence on genetic transmission. Then the relationship between keeping mentally/intellectually active and the manifestation of symptoms is important to discuss here. In terms of determining whether the sisters do or do not have Alzheimer's, this cannot be done until they die, since the only definitive diagnosis can be made from examining the brains on autopsy. However, since there appears to be a clear connection between keeping mentally active and not manifesting the symptoms as early or as devastatingly, the student should come up with some plan for keeping people mentally active from a young age continuously into old age.

Chapter 15   The Research Endeavor

1. Which of the following is *true* concerning stories on dramatic research studies that make the headlines in newspapers?
    a. They provide detailed information of the research.
    b. They present the results in a simplified, clear-cut, often misleading manner.
    c. While the information they present is not usually in depth, it is usually accurate.
    d. They provide sufficient information for the lay public to understand the complex issues involved in the research.
    Answer: b   LO: 1; factual   page: 518

2. Which of the following is *not* one of the special challenges that researchers interested in abnormal behavior face?
    a. Abnormal behaviors and feelings are extremely difficult to measure accurately.
    b. Researchers often must rely on self-reports to gather information, and these may be distorted.
    c. Observer assessments of a target person may be biased or lack sufficient information.
    d. While we may manipulate and control the variables of interest in our research with humans, we have to be especially careful to be ethical in doing so.
    Answer: d   LO: 1; conceptual   page: 518

3. Which of the following is a challenge discussed in the text that is inherent in psychological research?
    a. People's thoughts, feelings, and behaviors change over time.
    b. Because researchers have developed highly sensitive measurement instruments, they often have too much data to analyze.
    c. The measurement instruments that researchers have developed are so sensitive that the results they get may actually be an artifact of the measure rather than a true reflection of abnormality.
    d. Since there are multiple factors that influence behavior, researchers have to control for each of them in order to determine how much contribution is being made by the factor of interest.
    Answer: a   LO: 1; factual, conceptual   page: 518

4. Researchers attempt to overcome many of the challenges of researching abnormality is by using:
    a. nonhuman subjects.
    b. the multimethod approach.
    c. only well-tested theories.
    d. the most accurate measures possible.
    Answer: b   LO: 1; factual   page: 518

Chapter 15

5. Theories are:
   a. broad and abstract.
   b. easy to test directly.
   c. subsets of hypotheses.
   d. the end product of what we learn after we conduct an experiment.
   Answer: a   LO: 1; factual, conceptual   page: 518

6. An hypothesis is:
   a. a broad and abstract idea.
   b. a testable statement of what you expect to happen in a research study.
   c. the end product of what we learn after we conduct an experiment.
   d. a foundation we use for explaining some phenomenon.
   Answer: b   LO: 2; factual, conceptual   page: 519

7. The question, "What kind of evidence supports the theory that stress causes depression?" is a:
   a. testable theory.
   b. testable hypothesis.
   c. way to generate a testable hypothesis.
   d. testable model.
   Answer: c   LO: 2; factual, conceptual   page: 519

8. The statement, "People who have recently experienced stress are more likely to be depressed than people who have not," is:
   a. a theory.
   b. an hypothesis.
   c. a null hypothesis.
   d. a model of behavior.
   Answer: b   LO: 2; factual, conceptual   page: 519

9. Which of the following is correct regarding theories and hypotheses?
   a. A theory is a broad statement from which an hypothesis is derived.
   b. An hypothesis is a broad statement from which a theory is derived.
   c. Both the "theory" and the "hypothesis" are derived from the null hypothesis.
   d. The null hypothesis suggests a cause-and-effect relationship, that if you manipulate one variable, it will have an effect on another variable.
   Answer: a   LO: 2; factual, conceptual   page: 519

The Research Endeavor

10. The alternative to the hypothesis is the:
    a. theory.
    b. null hypothesis.
    c. antithesis.
    d. synthesis.
    Answer: b   LO: 2; factual   page: 519

11. Which of the following is *true* concerning the relationship among theory, hypothesis, and null hypothesis?
    a. Evidence that supports the hypothesis proves that the theory from which the hypothesis originated is correct.
    b. Evidence that supports the hypothesis may suggest that the methods used to test the theory were faulty.
    c. Evidence that supports the null hypothesis suggests that the theory from which it originated is false.
    d. Evidence that supports the null hypothesis suggests that the theory from which the null hypothesis originated is correct.
    Answer: c   LO: 2; factual, conceptual   page: 519

12. If a null hypothesis is supported, it means:
    a. the theory that generated the primary hypothesis is correct.
    b. there may not have been any support for the accuracy of the hypothesis.
    c. the theory that generated the primary hypothesis is incorrect.
    d. the researcher must either reject the theory or totally redesign the study.
    Answer: b   LO: 2; factual, conceptual   page: 519

13. Which of the following statements is *false*?
    a. No single study can definitively prove a hypothesis is correct.
    b. Results that are not statistically significant support the null hypothesis.
    c. Results that support the null hypothesis disprove the primary hypothesis.
    d. Variables must be defined before being operationalized.
    Answer: c   LO: 2; factual, conceptual   page: 519

14. A variable is:
    a. a factor or characteristic that can vary within an individual.
    b. a factor or characteristic that can vary between individuals.
    c. something of interest in research that changes.
    d. something that can harm the research design because it changes unpredictably.
    Answer: c   LO: 3; factual, conceptual   page: 519

Chapter 15

15. The factor that the researcher is trying to predict is the:
    a. independent variable.
    b. dependent variable.
    c. null hypothesis.
    d. unknown x.
    Answer: bLO: 3; factualpage: 519

16. The factor the researcher manipulates in order to investigate its effect on another factor is the:
    a. independent variable.
    b. dependent variable.
    c. null hypothesis.
    d. unknown x.
    Answer: aLO: 3; factualpage: 519

17. Professor Rosenfield wants to know if making exams an enjoyable experience will result in her students performing better on their exams. She has four sections of Introductory Psychology and randomly assigns two of them to an experimental condition in which students eat homemade chocolate chip cookies while they take the exam; the other two classes do not get cookies. (Prior to the intervention she had determined that all classes had achieved approximately the same grades on their midterms.) In this experiment, the independent variable is:
    a. eating chocolate chip cookies during the final exam.
    b. how well the students perform on their final exam.
    c. the belief that students will perform better on exams if the exams are enjoyable.
    d. the belief that students will perform better on their final exam if they eat chocolate chip cookies during an exam.
    Answer: aLO: 3; appliedpage: 519

18. Professor Rosenfield wants to know if making exams an enjoyable experience will result in her students performing better on their exams. She has four sections of Introductory Psychology and randomly assigns two of them to an experimental condition in which students are given homemade chocolate chip cookies (that she has baked) while they take the final exam; the other two classes do not get cookies. (Prior to this intervention she has already determined that all four classes have been achieving approximately the same grades on their midterms.) In this experiment, the dependent variable is:
    a. eating chocolate chip cookies during the final exam.
    b. how well the students perform on their final exam.
    c. the belief that students will perform better on exams if the exams are enjoyable.
    d. the belief that students will perform better on their final exam if they eat chocolate chip cookies during an exam.
    Answer: bLO: 3; appliedpage: 519

The Research Endeavor

19. Which of the following rankings of terms from most general to most specific (reading from left to right) is accurate?
    a. theory-->hypothesis-->operationalization
    b. operationalization-->theory-->hypothesis
    c. hypothesis-->operationalization-->theory
    d. theory-->operationalization-->hypothesis

    Answer: a   LO: 2, 4; factual, conceptual   pages: 519-520

20. Researchers examined the influence of panic patients' beliefs about the controllability of their panic symptoms on their actual experience of panic in the laboratory. Two groups of panic patients were asked to wear breathing masks through which they inhaled air enriched slightly with carbon monoxide. They were told that inhaling carbon monoxide could induce a panic attack. One group was told they could not control the amount of carbon monoxide they received; the other group was told they could control the amount by turning a knob. Actually, neither group had any control over the amount of carbon monoxide they inhaled. Eighty percent of the patients who believed they had no control over the carbon monoxide experienced a panic attack, but only 20% of the patients who believed they could control the carbon monoxide had an attack even though both groups inhaled the same amount of carbon monoxide. These results strongly suggest that beliefs about the uncontrollability of panic symptoms play a role in panic attacks (Sanderson, Rapee, & Barlow, 1989). In this study, panic patients' control beliefs were the:
    a. placebo.
    b. independent variable.
    c. null hypothesis.
    d. dependent variable.

    Answer: b   LO: 3; applied   page: 519

21. To study variables, they must be clearly defined and:
    a. ranked as to importance.
    b. operationalized.
    c. manipulated.
    d. measured.

    Answer: b   LO: 4; factual, conceptual   page: 520

22. A clear, specific explanation of the way in which a variable of interest will be measured or manipulated in a study is referred to as:
    a. generalization.
    b. hypothesization.
    c. delineation.
    d. operationalization.

    Answer: d   LO: 4; factual, conceptual   page: 520

Chapter 15

23. How a researcher operationalizes a variable will be most influenced by:
    a. how other researchers have operationalized that variable.
    b. what the researcher expects will be the outcome of the study.
    c. the researcher's definition of the variable.
    d. whether that form of operationalization was effective in previous research.
    Answer: c   LO: 4; factual, conceptual   page: 520

24. Which of the following is *not* one of the steps in operationalizing a variable?
    a. developing the hypothesis
    b. deciding exactly what aspect of the variable you will focus on
    c. devising a way to measure your variable
    d. devising some way to manipulate the variable
    Answer: a   LO: 4; factual, conceptual   page: 520

25. A researcher is interested in looking at qualities of a large group of people. However, it is impractical, if not impossible, to work with that entire large group. Thus, a smaller group is selected to participate from the larger group. The larger group is called the _____, and the smaller group is called the _____.
    a. sample; population
    b. population; sample
    c. general sample; random sample
    d. representative group; specific group
    Answer: b   LO: 6; factual, conceptual   page: 522

26. In order to avoid bias, a sample should be _____ the population of interest.
    a. similar to
    b. specific to
    c. representative of
    d. taken from
    Answer: c   LO: 6; factual, conceptual   page: 522

27. When we do research, we want to be able to say that our results can be applied to the entire population from which we took our sample. That is, we want our sample to be _____, so our results can be _____.
    a. representative; generalized
    b. random; applied
    c. random; generalized
    d. representative; applied
    Answer: a   LO: 6; factual, conceptual   page: 522

The Research Endeavor

28. When we compare two groups (e.g., experimental and control) in research, we specifically want to know what impact the independent variable has on the dependent variable. Therefore, we try to keep the two groups as similar as possible except for the independent variable, so if we see a difference in terms of the dependent variable, we will be confident about the cause-and-effect relationship. Thus, in the example of looking at the effects of stress on depression, we would try to _____ the two groups on any _____ variable (that is, on any variable other than stress) that we think might influence level of depression.
    a. align; extraneous
    b. control; extraneous
    c. match; third
    d. align; extraneous
    Answer: c   LO: 7; factual, conceptual, applied   page: 522

29. Which would be the best way to recruit a representative sample for a study on bereavement?
    a. Placing an advertisement in the newspaper, a researcher is able to reach an extremely large readership, and thus will be able to select a representative sample from people who respond to the ad.
    b. It would be unethical to contact relatives of a person who died within the last year because they are still grieving and the researcher would be intruding on their grief.
    c. Men are more greatly affected by the loss of their spouse than women are, and therefore, men would be more likely to participate in a study of bereavement.
    d. By using public records of recent deaths and contacting the relatives of all people who died within the last year, we would be less likely to generate a biased sample than we would if we relied upon responses to newspaper ads.
    Answer: d   LO: 6; factual, conceptual   page: 522

30. Statistical tests of differences between the experimental and comparison groups determine:
    a. if the difference occurred by chance or is unlikely to have occurred by chance.
    b. which of the two groups had more inconsistency in participants' scores.
    c. the scores that each group got in order to decide which one is higher.
    d. what the scores mean for each of the groups.
    Answer: a   LO: 8; factual   page: 523

31. To determine if differences between an experimental and a comparison group are unlikely to have occurred if the null hypothesis were true, we would use statistics to see if the groups are:
    a. the same.
    b. significantly different.
    c. similar.
    d. changed.
    Answer: b   LO: 8; factual   page: 523

Chapter 15

32. Which of the following would be used to determine whether there was a statistically significant difference between the experimental and comparison group?
    a. a t-test
    b. a continuum
    c. a prospective test
    d. a predictor variable
    Answer: a   LO: 8; factual   page: 523

33. Which of the following is an advantage of cross-sectional studies?
    a. They allow the researcher to match groups on all third variables.
    b. They consistently provide valuable information.
    c. They are relatively easy to conduct.
    d. They provide a format that makes it easy to understand cause and effect relationships.
    Answer: c   LO: 5; factual, conceptual   page: 524

34. Which of the following is a disadvantage of cross-sectional studies?
    a. They are complicated to design and to interpret.
    b. They are confounded by cohort effects.
    c. Vital information can be missed if observations are not made at the right time.
    d. They tend to be expensive and time consuming.
    Answer: c   LO: 5; factual, conceptual   page: 524

35. Many stressful events reported by depressed people may be a consequence of the depression rather than its cause. For example, the symptoms of depression may cause stress by impairing interpersonal skills and concentration at work and causing insomnia. Also, comparing two groups is not always a helpful way to test a theory about the relationship between stress and depression. This demonstrates the problem of cross-sectional studies with regard to:
    a. missing valuable information because of when the data were gathered.
    b. the effect of third variables.
    c. the complicated design of cross-sectional studies.
    d. teasing apart cause and effect.
    Answer: d   LO: 5; factual, conceptual   pages: 524-525

36. A study that follows people for an extended period of time rather than just assessing them at one point in time is a _____ study.
    a. correlational
    b. longitudinal
    c. cross-sectional
    d. sequential
    Answer: b   LO: 5; factual   page: 525

The Research Endeavor

37. A study in which the researcher obtains assessments of two groups *before* a stressor happens, then reassesses the two groups *after* the stressor happens is a _____ study.
    a. pre-test/post-test
    b. cross-sectional
    c. longitudinal
    d. prospective longitudinal
    Answer: d   LO: 5; factual   page: 525

38. Which of the following is *true* concerning the advantages of prospective longitudinal studies over cross-sectional studies?
    a. Researchers can determine whether there are differences between the groups of interest both before and after the crucial event so they are more confident when they actually find differences between the groups.
    b. Longitudinal studies are less expensive to run than cross-sectional studies.
    c. Because the researcher is constantly assessing the subjects, it is possible to collect a wealth of valuable information.
    d. It is easier to predict when events of interest to the researcher might occur when they get to know the subjects over time, and thus they can plan when to collect data.
    Answer: a   LO: 5; factual, conceptual   page: 526

39. A _____ study is designed merely to observe the relationship between two variables.
    a. cross-sectional
    b. correlational
    c. longitudinal
    d. experimental
    Answer: b   LO: 5; factual, conceptual   page: 527

40. When both variables of interest in a correlational study change in the same direction, this is a _____ correlation.
    a. positive
    b. negative
    c. primary
    d. secondary
    Answer: a   LO: 5; factual, conceptual   page: 527

41. Professor Rosenfield has observed that the longer she lectures, the more yawns she notices from her students. While it may not be something she wants to see, it is nonetheless a:
    a. good correlation.
    b. definite correlation.
    c. positive correlation.
    d. beneficial correlation.
    Answer: c   LO: 5; factual, conceptual, applied   page: 527

Chapter 15

42. When comparing police records with ice cream sales, we might well notice that as ice cream sales go up, so do violent assaults. This would be an example of a(n):
    a. negative correlation.
    b. positive correlation.
    c. cross-sectional study.
    d. archival study.
    Answer: b   LO: 5; factual, conceptual, applied   page: 527

43. It was an interesting revelation for Susan when she realized that the less time she spent partying, the better her grades were. This would be a(n) _____ correlation.
    a. interesting
    b. zero
    c. positive
    d. negative
    Answer: d   LO: 5; factual, conceptual, applied   page: 527

44. If two variables show no pattern of changing at the same time, whether in the same or the opposite direction, we would call it a _____ correlation.
    a. zero
    b. positive
    c. negative
    d. nonexistent
    Answer: a   LO: 5; factual, conceptual   page: 527

45. The major disadvantage of correlational studies is:
    a. it is difficult to know exactly what the variables are.
    b. they do not tell us about cause-effect relationships.
    c. they often have ethical problems to overcome.
    d. they do not provide enough data to make the research meaningful.
    Answer: b   LO: 5; factual, conceptual   page: 528

46. According to the text, the hallmark of experimental studies is:
    a. manipulation.
    b. use of the scientific method.
    c. control.
    d. ease of assessment.
    Answer: c   LO: 5; factual   page: 529

47. Which of the following is the goal of human laboratory studies?
    a. to induce the conditions that you theorize will lead to your outcome of interest
    b. to reduce conditions leading to the outcome of interest so as to reduce that outcome
    c. to see how a change in one variable relates to change in another variable
    d. to be able to generalize our findings from the laboratory to an entire population
    Answer: a   LO: 5; factual, conceptual   page: 529

48. In the human laboratory study of the effects of stress on depression, stress is operationalized as exposing subjects to unsolvable anagrams. The researchers _____ stress.
    a. observe and record
    b. manipulate and record
    c. observe and measure
    d. manipulate and measure
    Answer: d   LO: 5; factual, conceptual, applied   page: 529

49. Which of the following is the goal of therapy outcome studies?
    a. to induce the conditions that you theorize will lead to your outcome of interest
    b. to reduce conditions leading to the outcome of interest so as to reduce that outcome
    c. to see how a change in one variable relates to change in another variable
    d. to be able to generalize our findings from the laboratory to an entire population
    Answer: b   LO: 5; factual, conceptual   page: 531

50. A _____ group is a group in which subjects have all the same experiences as the group of main interest in the study, except that they do not receive the key manipulation.
    a. experimental
    b. control
    c. blind
    d. intervention
    Answer: b   LO: 9; factual   page: 529

51. The _____ group is the group of main interest in the study, which receives the key manipulation.
    a. experimental
    b. control
    c. blind
    d. intervention
    Answer: a   LO: 9; factual   page: 529

Chapter 15

52. Researchers examined the influence of panic patients' beliefs about the controllability of their panic symptoms on their actual experience of panic in the laboratory. Two groups of panic patients were asked to wear breathing masks through which they inhaled air enriched slightly with carbon monoxide. They were told that inhaling carbon monoxide could induce a panic attack. One group was told they could not control the amount of carbon monoxide they received; the other group was told they could control the amount by turning a knob. Actually, neither group had any control over the amount of carbon monoxide they inhaled. Eighty percent of the patients who believed they had no control over the carbon monoxide experienced a panic attack, but only 20% of the patients who believed they could control the carbon monoxide had an attack even though both groups inhaled the same amount of carbon monoxide. These results strongly suggest that beliefs about the uncontrollability of panic symptoms play a role in panic attacks (Sanderson, Rapee, & Barlow, 1989). This study is:
    a. cross-sectional.
    b. longitudinal.
    c. correlational.
    d. experimental.
    Answer: d   LO: 9; applied   pages: 529-530

53. Researchers examined the influence of panic patients' beliefs about the controllability of their panic symptoms on their actual experience of panic in the laboratory. Two groups of panic patients were asked to wear breathing masks through which they inhaled air enriched slightly with carbon monoxide. They were told that inhaling carbon monoxide could induce a panic attack. One group was told they could not control the amount of carbon monoxide they received; the other group was told they could control the amount by turning a knob. Actually, neither group had any control over the amount of carbon monoxide they inhaled. Eighty percent of the patients who believed they had no control over the carbon monoxide experienced a panic attack, but only 20% of the patients who believed they could control the carbon monoxide had an attack even though both groups inhaled the same amount of carbon monoxide. These results strongly suggest that beliefs about the uncontrollability of panic symptoms play a role in panic attacks (Sanderson, Rapee, & Barlow, 1989). The primary limitation of this type of study would be:
    a. that fact that it cannot establish causality.
    b. its generalizability.
    c. its lack of a proper control group.
    d. its demand effects.
    Answer: b   LO: 6, 9; applied   pages: 530-531

The Research Endeavor

54. Dr. Rose is interested how early discipline and punishment affect the child's later behavior as an adult. She designs a research study to survey a population of prisoners and a population of physicians. Since her key focus is on the effects of early discipline and punishment on later development, she will need to ask questions about the respondents' memories as they relate to these factors. However, if she *only* asks about these elements, respondents may not be completely honest with their answers since they would probably guess at her hypothesis and try to conform their answers to that hypothesis. This is a problem of _____, and Dr. Rose will attempt to overcome this problem by using _____ to obscure the real purpose of the study.
    a. demand characteristics; filler measures
    b. demand characteristics; a cover story
    c. subjective bias; filler measures
    d. social acceptability; filler measures
    Answer: a   LO: 5, 9; applied   page: 529

55. When a subject guesses the researcher's hypothesis and tries to conform their behavior according to that hypothesis, it is referred to as:
    a. second-guessing the researcher.
    b. social acceptability.
    c. demand characteristics.
    d. subjective bias.
    Answer: c   LO: 9; factual   page: 529

56. Which of the following types of studies, if done correctly, can establish causal relationships?
    a. animal studies
    b. longitudinal studies
    c. cross-sectional studies
    d. therapy outcome studies
    Answer: d   LO: 9; applied   page: 531

57. Professor Field suspects that females get higher grades and are more likely to graduate, given the same basic curriculum in all women's colleges than they do in coeducational institutions. She decides to study this. Assuming she studies populations of college women who are already enrolled in the college of their choice, it would be difficult for her to achieve:
    a. random selection.
    b. random assignment.
    c. experimental design.
    d. generalizability.
    Answer: b   LO: 5, 9; applied   page: 530

Chapter 15

58. Professor Field hypothesizes that a way to increase student success (defined by completing classes enrolled in with a minimum of a B or better and graduating on schedule) is to decrease student tuition for each B a student receives and to increase it further for each A received. She believes that if she were to offer this to all students on campus, it would be the most serious students (those who already get As and Bs) who would respond. Thus, she asks the Director of Admissions to have the computer generate a list of 25% of entering freshman class, whom Dr. Field will approach to participate in this experiment. In that way, she will later be able to compare those students participating with students who were not in the selected group. Since the only criterion input into the computer is that the students be freshman, this way of getting her sample is called:
    a. random assignment.
    b. random selection.
    c. self-selection.
    d. computer selection.
    Answer: b   LO: 5, 9; applied   page: 530

59. Dr. Flores has done research on depression in urban and rural populations and has a particular interest in groups affected by HIV or AIDS. He wants to compare the coping style of persons who are infected with coping styles of persons not infected and then connect those coping styles with incidence of depression. Which of the following would be impossible for Dr. Flores to achieve for purposes of this study?
    a. random selection
    b. random assignment
    c. experimental design
    d. generalizability
    Answer: b   LO: 5, 9; applied   page: 530

60. To minimize differences between the experimental and control groups and control for third variables, it will be necessary to:
    a. assign our subjects either to the experimental or the control group.
    b. poll the subjects to be sure they don't suspect what the underlying hypothesis is.
    c. be sure that our subjects are all alike in every way other than the key variables.
    d. keep the experimenters who interact with the subjects from knowing which condition the subjects are in.
    Answer: d   LO: 5, 9; factual, conceptual   page: 530

61. The primary limitation of human laboratory studies is:
    a. control.
    b. utility.
    c. generalizability.
    d. objectivity.
    Answer: c   LO: 5, 9; factual, conceptual   page: 530

62. Which of the following is *not* an advantage of human laboratory studies?
    a. The researcher has more control over variables.
    b. Participants can be randomly assigned to groups.
    c. Their results can be easily generalized to the "real world."
    d. Appropriate control groups can be created to rule out alternative explanations of important findings.
    Answer: c   LO: 5, 9, 10; factual, conceptual   page: 531

63. Human laboratory studies often elicit criticisms about ethics, particularly in terms of the potential harm to the participants and the subtle coercion applied for them to continue even if they are uncomfortable with the experimental procedures. Which of the following is one of the processes recommended to be used with participants after any potentially upsetting experiment?
    a. brief therapy
    b. process debriefing
    c. reminding them of the voluntary nature of participation
    d. providing them with a written report of the research findings
    Answer: b   LO: 10; factual, conceptual   page: 531

64. An important role of the Human Subjects Committees at colleges and universities is to:
    a. ensure that the benefits of the study substantially outweigh any risks to participants.
    b. ensure that all experiments are practical in terms of financial and human resources.
    c. oversee all research to be sure that faculty who conduct research follow through in writing their results so their findings can be used.
    d. be sure that all students have an equal opportunity to participate in research as a part of their general education requirements.
    Answer: a   LO: 10; factual, conceptual   page: 531

65. Which of the following is an advantage of therapy outcome studies?
    a. They provide help to people in distress while conducting research.
    b. Their results can easily be applied to real-world therapeutic settings.
    c. They are able to offer interventions to all of the people who participate.
    d. Because they are experimental studies, they easily lend themselves to teasing out the specific aspect of therapy that led to reduced psychopathology.
    Answer: a   LO: 5, 9, 10; factual, conceptual   page: 532

Chapter 15

66. An ethical consideration arises in therapy outcome studies because:
    a. we need a control group for comparison purposes, which means that there is a matched group of persons with a psychological disorder who are not being treated.
    b. often the intervention that is used in these studies create iatrogenic conditions in that the participants wind up in a worse condition that they were before the study.
    c. while we are using our intervention on the participants, they are not receiving the intervention they would ordinarily receive from their own therapists.
    d. the first rule of healing is, "Do not harm," and since our intervention is as yet untested, we do not know if we are doing any harm.
    Answer: a   LO: 5, 9, 10; factual, conceptual   page: 532

67. Wait list control groups are used in:
    a. human laboratory studies.
    b. cross-sectional studies.
    c. therapy outcome studies.
    d. longitudinal studies.
    Answer: c   LO: 9; factual, conceptual   page: 533

68. Subjects who agree to participate in therapy outcome studies, but who do not receive the intervention when the experimental group does, but instead have their names put on a roster to receive the intervention after the study is completed, are referred to as the:
    a. control group.
    b. placebo control group.
    c. roster control group.
    d. wait list control group.
    Answer: d   LO: 9; factual, conceptual   page: 533

69. The type of control group that is used most often in studying the effectiveness of drugs is the:
    a. wait list control group.
    b. placebo control group.
    c. participant control group.
    d. pretense control group.
    Answer: b   LO: 9; factual, conceptual   page: 533

70. Which of the following is *false* concerning psychological placebo control groups?
    a. By interacting with a warm, caring therapist, even participants in the placebo control group are likely to improve.
    b. Psychological placebo interventions are effective with moderately distressed people.
    c. It is nearly impossible to construct a true psychological placebo.
    d. Placebo control groups overcome ethical concerns since participants are helped.
    Answer: d   LO: 9, 10; factual, conceptual   page: 533

The Research Endeavor

71. Rose was participating in research on osteoporosis. Before she began the research, she was told that half of the participants would receive the drug that was being tested and half would receive a "sugar pill." Those who received the sugar pill were in the _____ group.
    a. wait list control
    b. placebo control
    c. clinical control
    d. double-blind control
    Answer: b   LO: 5, 9; applied   page: 533

72. Rose was participating in research on osteoporosis. Before she began the research, she was told that half of the participants would receive the drug that was being tested, and half would receive a "sugar pill." However, in addition to the participants not knowing whether they got the real drug or the sugar pill, the experimenter who gave the pills to the participants did not know either. This is an example of a _____ experiment.
    a. controlled
    b. drug
    c. clinical
    d. double-blind
    Answer: d   LO: 5, 9; applied   page: 533

73. One of the primary reasons for conducting animal studies is:
    a. ethical limitations with human studies.
    b. the results are easily generalizable to humans.
    c. that since animals aren't likely to succumb to demand characteristics, we are able to gain more information from working with animals than with humans.
    d. animals are easier to care for than human participants.
    Answer: a   LO: 5, 10; factual   page: 534

74. Which of the following is *not* a problem researchers encounter with animal studies?
    a. ethical issues
    b. issues of generalizability
    c. control over the experiment
    d. effects of the experiment and confinement on the animals
    Answer: c   LO: 5, 10; factual, conceptual   pages: 534-536

75. The in-depth study of single individuals is referred to as:
    a. an interview.
    b. a single case study.
    c. a clinical setting.
    d. limited study.
    Answer: b   LO: 5; factual   page: 536

Chapter 15

76. Sigmund Freud wrote about the sessions he had with his patients and built his theories on what he learned from treating them. What form of data collection did Freud use?
   a. clinical studies
   b. longitudinal studies
   c. single case studies
   d. therapy outcome studies
   Answer: c   LO: 5; applied   page: 536

77. Which of the following is an advantage of the single case study?
   a. Because the researcher has direct contact with the participant and other persons who know the participant, the information is highly objective.
   b. Despite problems that may be unique to each individual, there are certain underlying processes that we share in common; thus, the findings are, to a large extent, generalizable.
   c. The researcher comes to know the participant very well and thus has a clear, unbiased understanding of the underlying issues involved.
   d. Case studies help therapists see how the events in a person's life may affect his or her behavior.
   Answer: d   LO: 5; factual, conceptual   page: 537

78. Which of the following are used to prevent demand effects?
   a. wait list control groups.
   b. double-blind experiments.
   c. placebo control groups.
   d. process debriefing.
   Answer: b   LO: 8; factual   page: 533

79. Lack of generalizability is a primary criticism of all of the following types of studies *except*:
   a. human laboratory studies.
   b. animal studies.
   c. longitudinal studies.
   d. case studies.
   Answer: c   LO: 5, 9; factual, conceptual   page: 538

80. Which of the following is *true* concerning case studies?
   a. They are rich in the information they provide.
   b. They are highly generalizable to other populations.
   c. Case studies provide a clear, objective view, particularly of psychopathology.
   d. They help researchers to find cause-and-effect relationships for mental health.
   Answer: a   LO: 5; factual, conceptual   page: 538

The Research Endeavor

81. Lack of generalizability is a primary criticism of:
    a. human laboratory studies.
    b. animal studies.
    c. therapy outcome studies.
    d. case studies.
    Answer: d   LO: 5; factual, conceptual   page: 538

82. The primary reason that single case studies are not used in scientific research are that they:
    a. are too clinical.
    b. lack objectivity and generalizability.
    c. are too personal and thus risk breaking confidentiality.
    d. present too many ethical concerns.
    Answer: b   LO: 5; factual   page: 538

83. Ethical controversy surrounds all of the following research methods *except*:
    a. animal studies.
    b. case studies.
    c. therapy outcome studies.
    d. human laboratory studies.
    Answer: b   LO: 5, 10; factual, conceptual   page: 538

84. Laura Carstensen (1995) theorized that older people are more choosy than younger people about whom they want to interact with because their time on earth is short, and they want to maximize the emotional quality of their remaining time. Thus, they focus on close family and friends, rather than on people they don't know as well. To test her theory, Carstensen conducted several studies using different methodologies. This demonstrates use of the:
    a. multimethod approach.
    b. experimental approach.
    c. longitudinal approach.
    d. cross-sectional approach.
    Answer: a   LO: 1, 11; factual, conceptual   page: 539

85. One of the major challenges in cross-cultural research in abnormal psychology that was discussed in the text involves:
    a. lack of meaningful, or at least interpretable, data to be collected from other cultures.
    b. gaining trust from the groups we want to investigate so they will let us conduct our research.
    c. a group's lack of sophistication with psychological research makes it difficult to get information from group members.
    d. to gain the trust of another group, the researcher must become absorbed into the group, and then loses objectivity about the research.
    Answer: b   LO: 12; factual, conceptual   page: 541

Chapter 15

86. Which of the following is *not* a challenge presented in the text concerning cross-cultural research in abnormal psychology?
    a. applying theories or concepts developed in one culture to another culture
    b. translating assessment tools into different languages without changing their meaning
    c. understanding cultural or gender differences in people's responses to the social demands of interacting with a researcher that may affect the researcher's conclusions
    d. a rich array of information to be obtained and analyzed in order to assess the similarities and differences among cultures.
    Answer: d   LO: 12; factual, conceptual   pages: 541-543

87. The research of Harold Stevenson with children in the primary grades in Japan (Stevenson, Chen, & Lee, 1993) found that:
    a. there is such great pressure for children to excel academically that they were considerably more anxious and depressed than American children.
    b. children in Japan were no more anxious or depressed than children in the United States, however, American children enjoyed school more.
    c. Japanese children were no more anxious or depressed than American children but were more advanced in many educational domains than American children.
    d. American children were less stressed than Japanese children, but Japanese children were more advanced in many educational domains than American children.
    Answer: c   LO: 12; factual, conceptual   pages: 542-543

88. One outcome of Stevenson's research comparing Japanese and American children has been:
    a. a change in teaching methodologies in the United States.
    b. a reduction of pressure to perform on Japanese children.
    c. to motivate researchers to search for ways that American culture motivates children to achieve and supports them emotionally.
    d. to motivate researchers to search for ways that Japanese culture motivates children to achieve and supports them emotionally.
    Answer: d   LO: 12; factual   page: 543

89. Stevenson (e.g., Stevenson, Chen, & Lee, 1993) found that young children in Japan achieve more in specific academic domains but are no more anxious than American children. Stigler (1991) research with high school children found that they suffer from pressure to perform. This would suggest that:
    a. Stevenson's findings are incorrect.
    b. Stigler's findings are incorrect.
    c. there is a need for incorporating a multimethod approach that addresses children of all ages in these cultures.
    d. the testing instruments used in either Stevenson's or Stigler's research were not accurate measures of the variables studied.
    Answer: c   LO: 12; factual, conceptual   pages: 542-543

90. When researchers assume that abnormality is the result of a combination of person variables and situation variables, this would be termed a(n) _____ approach.
   a. interactionist
   b. trait
   c. integrational
   d. bilateral
   Answer: a   LO: factual, conceptual   page: 543

91. If the overlap between the scores of two groups is _____, and the difference between the average scores of the groups is _____, the two groups may be said to be significantly different.
   a. reasonably small; reasonably large
   b. reasonably large; reasonably small
   c. extremely small; extremely large
   d. extremely large, extremely small
   Answer: a   LO: 8; factual, conceptual   page: 523

92. The text shows a portion of a scale designed to measure happiness and depression, but the scale was imbedded in others scales to obscure the purpose of the study. This is done to eliminate the problem of:
   a. generalizability.
   b. demand characteristics.
   c. social acceptability.
   d. objectivity.
   Answer: b   LO: factual, conceptual   page: 530

93. The abstract section of a professional paper is:
   a. the researcher's conclusions after conducting the research and analyzing the results.
   b. a summary of previous literature that has been done prior to the research in question.
   c. a short description of other purpose, design, and results of the study.
   d. a conceptual idea about the research that may follow logically from previous research.
   Answer: c   LO: factual, conceptual   page: 546

94. Implications of the research discussed in a professional paper would be found in the ____ section.
   a. abstract
   b. literature review
   c. results
   d. discussion
   Answer: d   LO: factual   page: 547

Chapter 15

95. Harvey is researching the effects of ethnic identity on self-esteem. When following the APA guidelines to write up his results, which of the following will *not* be the title of a section heading?
   a. Abstract
   b. Analysis of Data
   c. Methods
   d. Discussion

   Answer: b   LO: applied   pages: 546-547

Essay Questions

96. Explain how you would design a study to test the theory that physical fitness improves mental health. What specific hypothesis can you derive from this theory? Based on this hypothesis, define your variables of interest and operationalize them. What are your dependent and independent variables? What experimental design would you use to test your hypothesis, and why? What results would you expect? What would be the limitations of your experiment?

   A proper answer would design a study to test the theory mentioned and accurately apply the terms in the chapter. For example, we can derive the hypothesis that people who exercise should be less likely than people who do not exercise to have symptoms of distress (e.g., depression and anxiety). We could define depression and anxiety as DSM-IV diagnoses, and perform a cross-sectional study comparing people who engage in physical exercise at least three times a week for 30 minutes with people who do not exercise at this level (which serves as the independent variable). We might use a cross-sectional study for its ease. We would expect to find higher rates of depression and anxiety among people who do not exercise. However, this study would not be able to establish causality; the subjects who do not exercise may not exercise *because* they are depressed or anxious, for example (and thus, they are not depressed or anxious because they do not exercise). Also, the study would represent only an isolated slice of time and would be vulnerable to third-variable explanations.

The Research Endeavor

97. What are four difficulties inherent in psychological research? What are five challenges faced specifically in cross-cultural research?

A proper answer would explain the difficulties inherent in psychological research (e.g., most forms of abnormality have multiple causes) and would describe the numerous difficulties inherent in cross-cultural research (e.g., translating assessment tools).

98. Catherine Cameron (1996) conducted research with 46 women who were sexually abused as children. Half of her sample had an extended period of time into adulthood when they experienced total amnesia for the abuse (the amnesia ranged from 15 to 54 years); the other half always remembered the abuse. All of the women had been in therapy to deal with the abuse and the residual effects that it had on their lives (those who had experienced amnesia for the abuse all sought therapy *after* remembering it). Dr. Cameron learned that the women who had amnesia were younger at the time the abuse was taking place (or first took place) and that it was more severe than for the group that did not have amnesia. She first contacted all of the women through their therapists, then by survey questionnaire, then by follow-up interviews. She reinterviewed the women at two times after the initial data collection to assess their later functioning (the last interviews took place 9 years after initial contact). What type of research techniques has Dr. Cameron used, and what research design has been employed? What hypotheses might be evident from this research? What are the most prominent variables that are addressed in this study? What third variables would you be concerned might interfere with this research? What limitations might you expect from this study?

The student ***should not*** say this is a therapy outcome study. It is not. Dr. Cameron used survey questionnaires and interviews in this longitudinal research. Because all of the women were in therapy at the time of initial contact, the student may suggest that case studies could have been used as well. The most evident hypotheses are that age and severity of abuse could be expected to predict amnesia (repression) for the traumatic events; additionally, Dr. Cameron predicted that the women with amnesia would demonstrate more maladaptive behaviors, although this was not found. One example of a third variable might be SES (although all of the women were from upper SES, intact families); a problem that she did suggest is that the instruments she used for measuring behavioral outcomes was not sufficiently sensitive to detect significant differences between the groups. One limitation of the study might be self-selection, since participation was voluntary and the women who participated (and continued with the research--six dropped out) may be very different from those who chose not to participate.

Chapter 15

99. "Dear Abby" once reported (December 28, 1992) that Dr. Christian Barnaard, the noted cardiologist who began the now common heart transplants, talked about why he does not use primates as heart donors. He had two males chimpanzees who lived in separate cages next to each other. He used one as a donor. "When we put him to sleep in preparation for the operation," he chattered and cried incessantly. . . [and] when we removed the body to the operating room, the other chimp wept bitterly and was inconsolable for days. The incident made a deep impression on me. I vowed never again to experiment with such sensitive creatures." Discuss the type of research being conducted here, the strengths and weaknesses of that research, and the ethical issues involved.

Obviously, this involved an animal study, addressing the utility of transplanting a chimpanzee heart into a human being. One strength of animal studies is that they have led to breakthrough treatments (especially in the medical field) for saving human lives; a major weakness deals with generalizability. Is what we learn from conducting research with nonhuman animals transferrable (generalizable) to humans (much of it is not; in the case of animal-to-human heart transplants, these have not been successful)? The big issues here, however, are ethical. The student should address cruelty to animals, and the ethical issue of balancing benefit to humanity versus the potential harm to the animal participants.

100. A classic film, *A Clockwork Orange* (1971) (based on the book of the same name) brought up the issue of taking a totally psychopathic adolescent and using behavioral techniques such as aversion therapy to turn him into a law-abiding citizen, and then, because of ethical "second-thoughts," counter-conditioning him back to his original psychopathic behavior. Discuss the type of research study this would entail; explain what the dependent, independent, and third variables would be; operationalize the dependent and independent variables; state your hypothesis(es); and state the limitations you would find on this type of study. Then discuss the ethical issues involved.

This would be a single-subject human laboratory experiment (although you might entertain other ideas), employing behavioral techniques such as aversion therapy (e.g., shocking him for unacceptable behaviors, ideas). One independent variable would be the aversion therapy (operationalized as administration of shock given when. . .); the dependent variable would be his behavior (operationalized, for example, as thinking about harming someone); and third variables might include environmental support received for antisocial behaviors. An hypothesis might be that by shocking the subject each time he had a socially unacceptable thought, he would stop thinking about performing socially unacceptable acts. A major ethical issue (not set out in APA guidelines) concerns drastic change of a person's behavior to turn the person into someone totally different from his or her original self. Other issues should be addressed as well, particularly the fact that they returned him to his previous antisocial personality.

Chapter 16   Society and Mental Health

1. Mental health professionals are often involved in legal situations where they are asked to assist in making judgments about appropriate actions to take. In that regard:
   a. they have access to a body of research literature that provides objective information on which judgment is best in each situation.
   b. they have consistent guidelines on the appropriate action to take in thousands of different scenarios.
   c. while the research might tell them what is likely to be the right action to take, it does not indicate what is definitely the right thing to do.
   d. the regulations are so explicit in terms of the appropriate action for different cases that they make it relatively simple to apply them to individual cases.
   Answer: c   LO: 1; factual, conceptual   page: 550

2. Which of the following is an important limitation on the ability of psychological research to inform legal decisions discussed in the text?
   a. Predictions made from research literature are probabilistic and can only tell us what is likely to occur, not what will definitely occur.
   b. Because psychology is a relatively new science, and forensic psychology is newer still, there is not yet a sufficient body of literature to guide these decisions.
   c. The courts and the legal system place little faith in psychologists and their understanding of human behavior and thus give their testimony little weight.
   d. Psychology and the legal system have such completely different ways of approaching behavior that they are unable to communicate effectively with each other.
   Answer: a   LO: 1; factual, conceptual   page: 550

3. The term *mentally ill* is often avoided (particularly in our text) because it:
   a. is an outdated term.
   b. is too limited in its scope of psychological disorders.
   c. takes too negative a view of psychological disorders.
   d. indicates that the only way to treat the problems is with drugs.
   Answer: b   LO: 1; factual, conceptual   page: 551

4. Justin was held in a mental health facility against his will. Such an action is called:
   a. unjust imprisonment.
   b. criminal incarceration.
   c. civil incarceration.
   d. civil commitment.
   Answer: d   LO: 1; applied   page: 551

Chapter 16

5. Which of the following is *true* concerning competency proceedings?
   a. They are held to determine whether the accused understand what is happening to them and are able to participate in their own defense.
   b. While they often receive a lot of media attention, they do not actually take place very frequently.
   c. The court considers the mental health professional's opinion in making a judgment, but other testimony often takes precedence if it is contrary to that opinion.
   d. Persons with long histories of psychiatric problems are as likely to be referred for competency evaluations as persons having acute episodes during commission of the crime.
   Answer: a   LO: 3; factual, conceptual   page: 551

6. Which of the following is *false* concerning the judgments of mental health professionals in the legal process?
   a. They are often asked to make judgments about a person's competency to stand trial.
   b. They are often asked to make judgments about a person's sanity at the time the crime was committed.
   c. Their recommendations tend to be the critical element in determining the decision of a judge or jury.
   d. They make recommendations to the court, but they do not make the final decision.
   Answer: c   LO: 2; factual, conceptual   pages: 551-552

7. Which of the following statements is *false*?
   a. Most people found not guilty by reason of insanity have a diagnosis of schizophrenia.
   b. People who are competent to stand trial and have no current diagnosis of a mental disorder can still be found not guilty by reason of insanity.
   c. The majority of people referred for competency evaluations have been accused of violent crimes.
   d. Low scores on cognitive tests that measure abilities important for following legal proceedings are the most common determinant of judgments of incompetence to stand trial.
   Answer: d   LO: 2, 3; factual   page: 552

8. Which of the following is *not* a typical characteristic of persons who are most likely to be referred for competency evaluations?
   a. previous psychiatric history
   b. lower level of education
   c. unsuccessful marriages
   d. poor
   Answer: c   LO: 3; factual   page: 552

Society and Mental Health

9. The term *insanity* is a:
   a. psychological term.
   b. legal term.
   c. medical term.
   d. psychiatric term.
   Answer: b   LO: 4; factual   page: 552

10. Dennis was found to be so mentally incapacitated at the time he murdered his wife that it was determined he could not conform to the rules of society. Consequently, he was found:
    a. criminally insane.
    b. mentally incompetent.
    c. not guilty by reason of insanity.
    d. guilty by reason of insanity.
    Answer: c   LO: 4; applied   pages: 552-553

11. Which of the following is *true* when comparing public perceptions of the insanity defense with actual use and results?
    a. The public believes that over one-third of all felony indictments result in an insanity plea, compared with an actual 1% of defendants doing so.
    b. The public believes that half of all insanity pleas result in a verdict of "not guilty by reason of insanity," when in fact it is only 25%.
    c. The public believes that 10% of persons found "not guilty by reason of insanity" are sent to a mental hospital, when in fact 75% of those defendants are institutionalized.
    d. The public believes that 26% of persons found "not guilty by reason of insanity" are actually set free, when in fact it is only 3%.
    Answer: a   LO: 4; factual   pages: 552-553

12. Fred was sent to a mental institution after a finding of "not guilty by reason of insanity." If his stay there is the average length of institutionalization, Fred will be institutionalized for:
    a. 6 months.
    b. 1 year.
    c. 3 years.
    d. 10 years.
    Answer: c   LO: 4; applied   page: 552

13. Elvira was found "not guilty by reason of insanity" after murdering her husband. If she is institutionalized the average length of time considering her crime, she will be there for:
    a. 1 year.
    b. 3 years.
    c. 6 years.
    d. 35 years.
    Answer: c   LO: 4; applied   page: 552

Chapter 16

14. Which of the following is *not* one of the rules used to evaluate a defendant's plea that he or she should be found not guilty by reason of insanity?
    a. the M'Naghten Rule
    b. the Uncontrollable Impulse Rule
    c. the Durham Rule
    d. the ALI Rule
    Answer: b   LO: b; factual   pages: 553-555

15. The court determined that Charles could not be held responsible for his crime because he did not know that his actions were wrong. The governing rule in such a case is the:
    a. M'Naghten Rule.
    b. Uncontrollable Impulse Rule.
    c. Durham Rule.
    d. ALI Rule.
    Answer: a   LO: 5; applied   page: 553

16. The condition most commonly referred to as a "disease of the mind" is:
    a. severe depression.
    b. psychosis.
    c. alcoholism.
    d. post-traumatic stress disorder.
    Answer: b   LO: 5; factual   page: 554

17. Which of the following is *not* a holding of the M'Naghten Rule?
    a. A person must be able to discern right from wrong to be held guilty of a crime.
    b. A person must be unable to assist in his or her own defense to be held not guilty by reason of insanity.
    c. A person must have been suffering from a "disease of the mind" at the time of the crime to be held not guilty by reason of insanity.
    d. A person must not know the nature and quality of the act he or she was doing to be held not guilty by reason of insanity.
    Answer: c   LO: 5; factual   page: 554

18. The major problem in interpreting M'Naghten has been:
    a. to be accurate in deciding when a defendant is unable to assist in his or her own defense.
    b. to define exactly what is meant by saying the defendant did not know the nature and quality of what he or she was doing.
    c. to define precisely what the term *insanity* means.
    d. to define clearly and consistently what disorders constitute diseases of the mind.
    Answer: d   LO: 5; factual, conceptual   page: 554

Society and Mental Health

19. The rule that broadened the insanity defense to include acts of passion is the:
    a. Durham Rule.
    b. ALI rule.
    c. irresistible impulse rule.
    d. American Psychiatric Association's definition of insanity.
    Answer: c   LO: 5; factual   page: 554

20. The notion of "diminished capacity" is most closely aligned with which rule?
    a. M'Naghten
    b. Durham
    c. irresistible impulse
    d. ALI
    Answer: c   LO: 6; factual   page: 554

21. The notion of "diminished capacity" refers to being:
    a. mentally ill (or legally insane) at the time the crime was committed.
    b. mentally retarded or otherwise incapable of understanding the law.
    c. under the influence of alcohol or other drugs.
    d. incapable of resisting the impulse to commit the crime.
    Answer: d   LO: 5; factual, conceptual   page: 554

22. The rule that allows the insanity defense for crimes that were the "product of mental disease or mental defect" that further broadened the criteria for the legal defense of insanity is:
    a. M'Naghten.
    b. diminished capacity.
    c. Durham.
    d. the American Psychiatric Association's definition of insanity.
    Answer: c   LO: 5, 6; factual   page: 554

23. The ruling in *Durham v. United States* (1954):
    a. established the irresistible impulse rule.
    b. established that temporary insanity created by voluntary use of alcohol or drugs did not qualify a defendant for acquittal by reason of insanity.
    c. established the duty of clinicians to protect others from their clients.
    d. established that the insanity defense could be used for any crimes that were the product of mental disease or mental defect.
    Answer: d   LO: 5, 6; factual   pages: 554-555

Chapter 16

24. The rule that holds that a person is not responsible for a crime if that crime is the result of mental defect, or if, during commission of the crime, the person lacked the capacity to understand the act was criminally wrong or to conform his or her conduct "to the requirements of the law," is the _____ Rule.
    a. ALI
    b. Durham
    c. Diminished Capacity
    d. M'Naghten
    Answer: a   LO: 5, 6; factual, conceptual   page: 555

25. Under which of the following legal principles could a person be found not guilty by reason of insanity even if he or she knows the act being performed is wrong (i.e., criminal)?
    a. the irresistible impulse rule
    b. the Durham Rule and the irresistible impulse rule
    c. the irresistible impulse rule and the American Psychiatric Association's definition of insanity.
    d. the M'Naghten Rule and the Durham Rule
    Answer: b   LO: 5, 6; factual   pages: 554-555

26. The introduction of the _____ broadened the criteria for the legal definition of insanity.
    a. American Psychiatric Association's definition of insanity
    b. M'Naghten Rule
    c. ALI Rule
    d. diminished capacity rule
    Answer: c   LO: 5, 6; factual   page: 555

27. The introduction of the _____ narrowed the criteria for the legal definition of insanity.
    a. Durham Rule
    b. irresistible impulse rule
    c. ALI Rule
    d. American Psychiatric Association's definition of insanity
    Answer: d   LO: 5, 6; factual   page: 555

28. The ruling in *Barrett v. United States* (1977):
    a. established that a person could not be involuntarily committed if he or she could survive with the help of able and willing family or friends.
    b. established the irresistible impulse rule.
    c. established that the insanity defense could be used for any crimes that were the product of mental disease or mental defect.
    d. established that temporary insanity created by voluntary use of alcohol or drugs did not qualify a defendant for acquittal by reason of insanity.
    Answer: d   LO: 7; factual   page: 555

29. Which of the following is *true* concerning the American Law Institute's ALI Rule?
    a. The rule is narrower than the M'Naghten Rule since it requires the defendant to have an appreciation of the criminality of the criminal act.
    b. The ALI Rule is more restrictive than the Durham Rule because it requires some lack of appreciation of the criminality of one's act.
    c. The ALI Rule is broader than the Durham Rule because it requires only the presence of a mental disorder.
    d. The ALI Rule allowed defense attorneys to argue that a defendant's history of antisocial conduct was evidence of the presence of mental disease or defect.
    Answer: b   LO: 5, 6; factual   page: 555

30. Which case so enraged the American public with a verdict of "not guilty by reason of insanity" that it led to further reappraisal of the use of the insanity defense?
    a. the assassination of John Lennon by Mark David Chapman
    b. the murder of Sharon Tate by Charles Manson's "family"
    c. the attempted assassination of Ronald Reagan by John Hinckley
    d. the assassination of John F. Kennedy by Lee Harvey Oswald
    Answer: c   LO: 5, 6; factual   page: 555

31. Which of the following legal principles specifically indicates that "mental disease or defect" does not include an abnormality manifested only by repeated criminal or antisocial conduct?
    a. the M'Naghten rule
    b. the Durham rule
    c. the ALI rule
    d. the American Psychiatric Association's definition of insanity
    Answer: c   LO: 5, 6; factual, conceptual   page: 555

32. The Insanity Defense Reform Act of 1984 adopted which definition of insanity?
    a. the American Psychiatric Association's definition
    b. the American Law Institute's definition
    c. the American Psychological Association's definition
    d. the American Bar Association's definition
    Answer: a   LO: 5, 6; factual   page: 555

33. As a result of _____, for a plea of not guilty by reason of insanity, most states began requiring the defense to prove that the defendant was insane at the time of the crime, as opposed to requiring the prosecution to prove that the defendant was sane.
    a. *Durham v. United States* (1954)
    b. The Insanity Defense Reform Act of 1984
    c. *Wyatt v. Stickney* (1975)
    d. none of the above.
    Answer: b   LO: 5, 6; factual   page: 555

Chapter 16

34. Which of the following is *true* concerning a verdict of "guilty but mentally ill"?
    a. It has been adopted by some states as an alternative to the verdict of not guilty by reason of insanity.
    b. Defendants convicted under this standard serve their entire sentences in a mental institution.
    c. Defendants convicted under this standard serve their sentence in a mental institution until it is determined that they are no longer mentally ill; then they finish their sentence in prison.
    d. Defendants convicted under this standard are given the option of either going to jail or receiving treatment for their "mental illness."
    Answer: a   LO: 8; factual, conceptual   page: 556

35. Which of the following is *true* concerning the verdict "guilty but mentally ill"?
    a. Critics complaint that while it maintains the insanity defense, the defendant does not get the treatment he or she needs to become a fully functioning member of society.
    b. Proponents argue that it recognizes defendants' mental illness while still holding them responsible for their actions.
    c. This verdict ensures that defendants be held accountable for their actions, but also get treated for their mental illness.
    d. It is left to state authorities to determine whether the defendant goes to jail or to a mental institution, but in either case the defendant is required to receive therapy.
    Answer: b   LO: 8; factual, conceptual   page: 556

36. Which of the following is *false* concerning the participation of mental health professionals in the legal system?
    a. Mental health professionals tend to be strong proponents of the notion that psychological disorders can impair people's ability to follow the law.
    b. Mental health professionals tend to be strong proponents of the notion that psychological disorders should be taken into consideration in judging an individual's responsibility for his or her action.
    c. Mental health professionals usually agree on the presence or absence of a defendant's psychological disorder but disagree on the evaluation of the defendant's state of mind at the time of crime was committed.
    d. Mental health professionals are often called upon to provide expert opinions in these cases.
    Answer: c   LO: 9; factual, conceptual   page: 556

Society and Mental Health

37. Which of the following is one of the primary concerns of mental health professionals about the use of rules to determine the acceptability of the insanity defense?
    a. People (normal and abnormal) may not really have as much control as the rules assume we have to choose how to act in a given situation.
    b. Because the rules exist, many people will abuse them and attempt to plead that they were insane, thus literally "getting away with murder."
    c. Despite constant reappraisal and revision, the rules still remain relatively murky and open to too much ambiguity in their interpretation.
    d. Too often people who really need help for their psychological disorders wind up being sent to jail or institutions, but in either case they do not receive the help they need.
    Answer: a   LO: 9; factual, conceptual   page: 556

38. The term for involuntary commitment is:
    a. forced institutionalization.
    b. civil commitment.
    c. civil confinement.
    d. conservatorship.
    Answer: b   LO: 10, 11; factual   page: 557

39. Which of the following is *not* required to commit someone to a psychiatric facility in the United States?
    a. imminent danger to self
    b. imminent danger to others
    c. diagnosis of a mental disorder
    d. need for treatment
    Answer: d   LO: 10; factual   page: 557

40. The standard commonly used for involuntary hospitalization in Great Britain and several other countries around the world is:
    a. need for treatment.
    b. grave disability.
    c. danger to self and others.
    d. inability to care for personal needs.
    Answer: a   LO: 10; factual   page: 557

Chapter 16

41. Which statement is *false* about the shift in criteria for civil commitment in the United States?
    a. It resulted in part from the patients' rights movement in the 1960s.
    b. Opponents of civil commitment argued that people were being incarcerated simply for having "alternative lifestyles" or unpopular political or moral values.
    c. Civil commitment was being misused to institutionalize people who were not mentally ill.
    d. It resulted more from a concern for how mental patients were treated than a concern over their personal freedom.
    Answer: d LO: 10; factual pages: 557-558

42. The criterion that requires that people be so incapacitated by a mental disorder that they cannot care for their basic needs for food, clothing, and shelter is the _____ criterion.
    a. imminent danger to self
    b. self-neglect
    c. grave disability
    d. imminent danger to others
    Answer: c LO: 11; factual page: 558

43. Which of the following is *true* concerning the grave disability criterion?
    a. It requires that persons be so incapacitated by a mental disorder that they cannot care for their basic needs for food, clothing, and shelter.
    b. It is less stringent than the need for treatment criterion because it requires only imminent danger to self.
    c. Because it provides a more clear standard for commitment, it has now been adopted by all but two states.
    d. It has been an effective way to remove the homeless mentally ill from the streets and into institutions.
    Answer: a LO: 11; factual, conceptual page: 558

44. Which of the following cases ruled that, "a State cannot constitutionally confine. . . a nondangerous individual, who is capable of surviving safely in freedom by himself or with the help of willing and responsible family and friends?"
    a. *Durham v. United States* (1954)
    b. *Tarasoff v. Regents of the University of California* (1974)
    c. *Donaldson v. O'Connor* (1975)
    d. *Wyatt v. Stickney* (1972)
    Answer: c LO: 12; factual page: 558

Society and Mental Health

45. In the cases of Kenneth Donaldson, whose father wanted to keep him committed, and Joyce Brown, whom Mayor Koch of New York wanted to be committed, both were able to win release based primarily on the grounds that they were:
    a. being held unfairly against their will.
    b. not mentally ill.
    c. able to take care of themselves and self-administer medication.
    d. not receiving treatment.
    Answer: d   LO: 12; factual   page: 558

46. The criterion of "dangerousness to self" is most often invoked:
    a. when a person is so incapable of caring for his or her personal needs that it may endanger the person's life.
    b. when it is believed that a person is imminently suicidal.
    c. when a mentally ill person refuses to take required medication, which results in the person endangering his or her life.
    d. All of the above are correct.
    Answer: b   LO: 11; factual   page: 559

47. Which of the following statements is *true*?
    a. People with a history of violence are more likely to commit violent acts in the future than people who have not been violent, regardless of psychological history.
    b. People with serious psychological disorders do not have higher rates of violent behaviors than people without disorders.
    c. The majority of mentally ill people engage in violent behavior.
    d. Predictions of mentally ill people's dangerousness to others are more often inaccurate than accurate.
    Answer: a   LO: 13; factual, conceptual   page: 559

48. Which of the following is *not* a useful short-term predictor of violence?
    a. past history of violence
    b. current severe symptoms of psychopathology
    c. substance abuse
    d. criminal record
    Answer: d   LO: 13; factual   page: 560

49. An individual with which of the following diagnoses is the *most likely* to have been violent in the past year?
    a. schizophrenia
    b. bipolar disorder
    c. alcohol abuse
    d. substance abuse
    Answer: d   LO: 13; factual   page: 560

Chapter 16

50. Which of the following persons is *most likely* to exhibit violent behavior?
    a. Victor, a 27-year-old Hispanic male, who has been not taken his medication for bipolar disorder for the past month.
    b. Bruce, a 28-year-old white male, who has been arrested three times--first for driving under the influence of PCP, then for battery, and finally for manslaughter resulting from a barroom fight.
    c. Edward, an 18-year-old black male, who was arrested for selling marijuana.
    d. Edna, a 30-year-old white female, who murdered her husband after 10 years of spousal abuse.
    Answer: b   LO: 13, 17; applied   page: 560

51. Which of the following cases established a patient's right to treatment?
    a. *Durham v. United States* (1954)
    b. *Tarasoff v. Regents of the University of California* (1974)
    c. *Wyatt v. Stickney* (1972)
    d. *Donaldson v. O'Connor* (1975)
    Answer: c   LO: 14; factual   page: 560

52. Which of the following has been adopted or recognized by all states?
    a. the verdict "guilty but mentally ill" (GBMI)
    b. short-term commitment to a treatment facility without a court hearing in an emergency situation
    c. patients' right to refuse treatment
    d. none of the above
    Answer: d   LO: 8, 11, 14; factual   page: 560

53. Which of the following is either not recognized as a right of persons who have been committed or is easily overturned in most states?
    a. the right to treatment
    b. the right to a public hearing
    c. the right to refuse treatment
    d. the right to be placed in the least restrictive treatment setting
    Answer: c   LO: 14; factual   page: 560

54. Which of the following is *not* an instance noted in the text of when a patient's right to refuse treatment can be violated?
    a. when the family has determined that the patient's behavior is bizarre or frightening
    b. when the patient is judged unable to make a reasonable decision about treatment
    c. when it is determined that decisions about a patient's treatment must be made by others.
    d. when the patient is psychotic or manic
    Answer: a   LO: 15; factual   page: 560

Society and Mental Health

55. The notion of informed consent refers to:
    a. providing a patient with a full and understandable explanation of treatment being offered.
    b. allowing a patient to make a decision to accept or refuse treatment based on his or her assessment of the risks and benefits involved.
    c. the patient making a fully informed decision about whether to participate in ongoing research that is carried on in many mental health facilities.
    d. both a and b
    Answer: d   LO: 14; factual   page: 560

56. Which of the following is *true* concerning disputes over a patient's right to refuse treatment?
    a. Most often clinicians and family members pressure patients to accept treatment, so most patients agree to treatment after initially refusing it.
    b. Judges tend to be particularly sympathetic in their rulings to patients' rights to refuse treatment, and particularly their concerns about the risks of treatment.
    c. It is most often the families that want the patient to refuse treatment, but it is the mental health facilities that push for it.
    d. Due to the patients' rights movements, the refusals are generally respected.
    Answer: a   LO: 14; factual   page: 561

57. The term *deinstitutionalization* refers to:
    a. a patient being completely cured, and therefore, the patient is released.
    b. a patient's symptoms being in remission, and therefore, the patient is released.
    c. the move to release patients from mental institutions into the communities.
    d. changing mental health centers into less austere, more caring facilities.
    Answer: c   LO: 16; factual, conceptual   page: 561

58. The original intent of the deinstitutionalization movement was to:
    a. reduce the high costs of treating the mentally ill.
    b. stop the warehousing and dehumanizing of mental patients and reestablish their personal freedoms and legal rights.
    c. put the burden of treating the mentally ill back onto their families, since families are more likely to offer supportive care.
    d. decentralize the governmental intervention in the mental health facilities and treatment concerns.
    Answer: b   LO: 16; factual, conceptual   page: 561

Chapter 16

59. Charles is one of the many homeless mentally ill who wanders the streets of downtown Los Angeles, sleeping in a cardboard box overnight, often not eating, and more often ranting unintelligible or unconventional statements at passersby. Which of the following is probably *not* one of the reasons that Charles is not receiving treatment for his illness?
   a. The deinstitutionalization movement put many mentally ill people on the streets.
   b. Charles is "invisible" to most people, so they are not aware that he needs help.
   c. There are not sufficient facilities in the community to treat people like Charles.
   d. Charles may have chosen to refuse treatment for his psychological problems.
   Answer: b   LO: 16; applied   page: 561

60. Which of the following statements is *false*?
   a. More women than men are found incompetent to stand trial.
   b. The majority of people who are acquitted by reason of insanity are white males.
   c. Mentally ill whites and blacks are equally likely to commit violent acts.
   d. Mentally ill men are more likely than mentally ill women to commit violent acts toward others.
   Answer: d   LO: 17; factual   page: 562

61. Which of the following presents a significant problem in judging mental incompetence for members of ethnic minorities?
   a. Persons from ethnic minorities who commit crimes may be more likely than whites to have severe psychological problems that make them incompetent to stand trial.
   b. Racial stereotypes tend to make evaluators overcompensate and be less likely to determine that a person from an ethnic minority is incompetent.
   c. An evaluator may not speak the same language as the ethnic minority defendant, which may cause misunderstanding between both of them in terms of asking and answering questions.
   d. Because there are relatively standard criteria for making judgments of incompetence, there are no really significant problems in judging mental incompetence for members of ethnic minorities.
   Answer: c   LO: 17; factual, conceptual   pages: 562-563

62. Which of the following is *false* concerning women and their mental competence?
   a. Women are more likely to be judged incompetent than men.
   b. As society has become more aware of spousal abuse, there has been an increase in the number of women who use the insanity defense after killing their abusive partners.
   c. As women become more prevalent in the workplace, they face the stress of working and caring for their families full time, and violence against their infants has increased.
   d. The violence of mentally ill women tends to be underestimated by clinicians, who do not probe for evidence regarding their propensity to violence as much as they would probe a mentally ill man.
   Answer: c   LO: 17; factual   page: 563

Society and Mental Health

63. Which of the following is *false* concerning the incidence of sexual liaisons between therapists and their clients?
    a, They usually involve a male therapist and a female client.
    b. Rates of sexual relationships between therapists and clients have gone from as many as 12% of male therapists and 3% of female therapists having sex with their clients to 1 to 4% of male therapists and fewer than 1% of female therapists having sex with their clients.
    c. The decrease in rates of sexual liaisons between therapists and clients has most likely resulted from increased sensitivity to the effect these liaisons have on clients than any other reason.
    d. The decrease in rates of sexual liaisons between therapists and clients is in part due to the criminalization of such acts and malpractice actions brought by clients.
    Answer: c   LO: 18; factual, conceptual   pages: 563-564

64. The clinician's primary duty is to:
    a. provide competent and appropriate treatment for the client's problem.
    b. ensure that the client will not engage in behavior that is harmful to the client or any other person.
    c. protect the client's confidentiality, even in instances where the clinician believes someone else may be harmed.
    d. avoid multiple relationships with clients, particularly sexual relationships, to avoid any abuse of authority that may jeopardize the client's treatment.
    Answer: a   LO: 18; factual   page: 563

65. Which of the following is *not* a condition under which a client's confidentiality may be breached?
    a. when the therapist believes the client needs to be committed
    b. when the therapist believes the client intends to harm another person
    c. in cases of suspected child abuse or elder abuse
    d. All of these require that confidentiality be breached.
    Answer: d   LO: 19; factual   pages: 564-565

66. Which of the following cases established the clinician's duty to protect people who might be in danger because of their client?
    a. *Durham v. United States* (1954)
    b. *Tarasoff v. Regents of the University of California* (1974)
    c. *Donaldson v. O'Connor* (1975)
    d. *Wyatt v. Stickney* (1972)
    Answer: b   LO: 19; factual   page: 564

Chapter 16

67. Which of the following has *not* been adopted by all states?
    a. the designation of sexual contact between a therapist and client as a felony
    b. a law requiring clinicians to report suspected child abuse or elder abuse, even if it violates their client's confidentiality
    c. a law requiring clinicians to protect persons who might be in danger because of their client
    d. None of the above have been adopted by all states.
    Answer: d LO: 18, 19; factual page: 564

68. Tanya has been seeing Dr. Polk for 3 months. She initially came for what she said was depression brought on by caring for her aging father, who has been deteriorating from Alzheimer's. His behavior has become uncontrollable, and Tanya has been depleting her savings to pay for a visiting nurse to care for her father's medical needs. When Tanya was a child, her father abused her both physically and sexually, and she has always felt a need to have him love her. She now sees that he will never be able to acknowledge that love for her, and she has felt herself become increasingly angry. In fact, Dr. Polk is now suspecting that Tanya has been physically abusing her father. What is Dr. Polk's primary responsibility here?
    a. to breach confidentiality and report the suspect elder abuse
    b. to work with Tanya to get her to stop abusing her father
    c. to ensure that Tanya move her father to a safer environment
    d. to protect Tanya's confidentiality
    Answer: a LO: 19; applied page: 564

69. Jeffrey was referred to Dr. Weiss by the Student Health Services, who felt he needed more intensive treatment than they offered. Jeffrey reported a history of having been in love with a woman, Janna, and after a two-year relationship, she abruptly broke up with him. He is experiencing extreme anxiety and intense anger toward this young woman. At his most recent session, Jeffrey has told Dr. Weiss that he can't stand to see the woman on campus anymore and has begun to plan how to get rid of her. He has already bought a gun and has begun following her. Which of the following cases is most relevant to how Dr. Weiss should proceed?
    a. *Durham v. United States* (1954)
    b. *Tarasoff v. Regents of the University of California* (1974)
    c. *Donaldson v. O'Connor* (1975)
    d. *Wyatt v. Stickney* (1972)
    Answer: b LO: 20; factual page: 564

Society and Mental Health

70. Jeffrey attends college in California. He was referred to Dr. Weiss by the Student Health Services, who felt he needed more intensive treatment than they offered. Jeffrey reported a history of having been in love with a woman, Janna, but after a two-year relationship, she abruptly broke up with him. He is experiencing extreme anxiety and intense anger toward this young woman. At his most recent session, Jeffrey has told Dr. Weiss that he can't stand to see the woman on campus anymore and has begun to plan how to get rid of her. He has already bought a gun and has begun following her. How should Dr. Weiss proceed?
    a. Because of duty of the therapist to protect client confidentiality, Dr. Weiss may do nothing other than help Jeffrey work through his feelings of anger.
    b. It is unethical for Dr. Weiss to breach his duty of confidentiality, however, it is important that he get Jeffrey to turn himself in to the police.
    c. It is unethical for Dr. Weiss to breach his duty of confidentiality, however, it is important that he get Jeffrey to agree to voluntary commitment.
    d. Despite the duty of confidentiality to clients, therapists have a duty to protect persons who may be in danger because of their clients; thus, he must warn Janna.
    Answer: d   LO: 20; applied   page: 564

71. Which of the following is *not* a recent trend discussed in the text with respect to family law in general?
    a. a growing intolerance for child and spousal abuse
    b. an increased commitment to the sanctity of the family
    c. increased rights of individual family members
    d. legal recognition of nontraditional family structures
    Answer: b   LO: 21; factual   page: 565

72. Which of the following is *false* concerning custody arrangements for children of divorce?
    a. At least 25% of the time, parents who are divorcing are unable to agree on the custody arrangements for their children.
    b. By 1995, all 50 states have mandated that unless one parent is shown to be unfit, joint custody of children with access to both parents is best for the children.
    c. Custody decisions can have a tremendous impact not only on the child's life, but on the parents' lives as well.
    d. The standard used by the courts for determining child custody is "in the best interest of the child."
    Answer: a   LO: 22; factual   pages: 566-567

Chapter 16

73. Which of the following statements about judges is *false*?
    a. Judges rarely rule against the recommendations of mental health experts concerning a defendant's competency to stand trial.
    b. Judges typically defer to the judgment of mental health professionals about a person's mental illness and the extent to which he or she meets criteria for civil commitment.
    c. Judges typically accept the arguments of mental health professionals in child custody cases about what is best for the child.
    d. Judges often will waive the statute of limitations to allow someone who recovered memories of sexual abuse in therapy to bring charges against the accused abuser.
    Answer: c   LO: 22; factual   pages: 559,560,566,570

74. Which of the following is an *increasing* trend in child custody and visitation awards?
    a. Mothers are more likely than fathers to be awarded custody of their children.
    b. Grandparents are more often being granted visitation rights.
    c. The awards are reflecting the complexity of child custody cases.
    d. When parents have exhibited high conflict during marriage, courts are less likely to award joint custody.
    Answer: b   LO: 22; factual   page: 566

75. Which of the following has been found from recent studies of the wholesale application of the joint custody mandate in California?
    a. More children suffer from joint custody than benefit from it.
    b. Children whose parents fought during marriage are forced to resolve their conflict.
    c. Children whose parents were embroiled in conflict during marriage learn to negotiate conflict better with joint custody than with single-parent custody.
    d. Many children benefit from exposure to both parents.
    Answer: d   LO: 22; factual   page: 566

76. Which of the following is *not* a part of the American Psychological Association's guidelines for psychologists acting as expert evaluators in child custody proceedings?
    a. The psychologist strives to acknowledge any limitations in the methods or data used.
    b. The psychologist acknowledges and confronts his or her own biases.
    c. The psychologist strives to present his or her client's best possible case.
    d. The psychologist strives to emphasize the child's best interests.
    Answer: c   LO: 22; factual, conceptual   page: 567

77. Which is *not* noted in the text as a possible source of bias in evaluating child custody cases?
    a. education level
    b. gender
    c. race or ethnicity
    d. age
    Answer: a   LO: 23; factual   pages: 566-567

Society and Mental Health

78. Mental health professionals would *not* be involved in which of the following phases of a child maltreatment case?
    a. investigation
    b. evaluation
    c. testimony
    d. A mental health professional may be involved in all of these phases.
    Answer: d   LO: 24; factual   pages: 568-569

79. The most recent and controversial change in the role of mental health professionals in child maltreatment cases is:
    a. investigation by mental health professionals of claims of maltreatment or to determine if maltreatment is likely to occur.
    b. treatment of a child by the mental health worker who is investigating the claim of maltreatment against that child.
    c. testimony by a mental health worker against a parent accused of child maltreatment if the mental health worker has been treating the child.
    d. evaluation of a claim of child maltreatment by a mental health worker who has been working with a child.
    Answer: a   LO: 24; factual, conceptual   pages: 568-569

80. Which of the following is one of the greatest concerns with respect to children being interviewed in child maltreatment cases?
    a. Interviewing children in these cases causes them great trauma by making them relive the experiences.
    b. The mental health professional may ask leading questions in the interviews that contaminate the evidence for trial.
    c. Children are not reliable witnesses because they often cannot differentiate fantasy from fact.
    d. Particularly if the person who is mistreating the child is a parent, the child may be highly traumatized by having to testify against the perpetrator.
    Answer: b   LO: 24; factual, conceptual   page: 569

81. Which is the *least* controversial role that a mental health professional may play as an expert witness in child maltreatment cases?
    a. providing opinions as to whether an accused fits the profile of the typical abuser
    b. providing opinions as to whether the child fits the profile of a typical abused child
    c. providing opinions to explain children's behaviors that may appear to be inconsistent with or contradictory to the children's claims of maltreatment
    d. providing opinions concerning whether the treatment the child experienced was typical of child maltreatment
    Answer: c   LO: 24; factual, conceptual   page: 568

Chapter 16

82. A high-profile case in California that was brought against the owner and teachers of a preschool in which one child first reported strange activities at the preschool, that mushroomed into a courtroom nightmare for everyone involved, was the McMartin Preschool case. Charges alleged that teachers had sexually molested children in their care. The interviewing techniques used with the children led to:
    a. convictions of all of the adults involved on the basis of the volumes of evidence obtained.
    b. convictions only against the owner of the preschool involved on the basis of the volumes of evidence obtained.
    c. dropped charges against the adults because the case took so long the children could no longer remember.
    d. dropped charges against the adults because the evidence was so contaminated that it could not be believed.
    Answer: d   LO: 24; factual, conceptual   page: 568

83. Which of the following is *not* a problem encountered when providing the profile of a "typical" abuser?
    a. There is often contradictory evidence offered concerning what the "typical" abuser looks like; thus, the profile is too ambiguous to be meaningful.
    b. The presence of a similarity between the individual adult and some profile does not necessarily mean the individual is an abuser.
    c. If the adult does not fit the abuser profile, it does not necessarily mean that no abuse took place.
    d. The available data on the characteristics of abusers do not necessarily fit "the pattern."
    Answer: a   LO: 24; factual, conceptual   pages: 568-569

84. Which of the following is *not* an advantage of using mental health professionals in legal proceedings?
    a. They have experience talking with distressed children and adults about sensitive topics.
    b. They are better than other professionals at knowing when a child or adult is lieing.
    c. They may be able to gather more information more objectively than other interviewers.
    d. They are more capable of interviewing children without further traumatizing them.
    Answer: b   LO: 24; factual, conceptual   page: 568

Society and Mental Health

85. One of the greatest controversies in clinical psychology today centers around the debate about:
    a. repressed memories.
    b. recovered memories.
    c. false memories.
    d. All of the above are correct.
    Answer: d   LO: 25; factual   page: 569

86. According to the text, which statement about the repressed memory debate is *true*?
    a. One study found that people can be made to believe that events happened to them that actually did not.
    b. One study found that 49 of 129 women with documented histories of abuse could not remember any abuse incidents at all from their childhood.
    c. One study found that a large number of people who identified themselves as abuse victims could not remember their abuse at some point before their eighteenth birthday, specifically due to repression.
    d. One study found that three-fourths of a group of women with repressed memories of sexual abuse found confirming evidence of their abuse.
    Answer: a   LO: 25; factual, conceptual   page: 570

87. Approximately 1,000 lawsuits have been filed by women who claim to have been sexually abused during their childhood but who had amnesia for the abuse until they had gotten into therapy. Which of the following is *true* concerning these lawsuits?
    a. Generally, the therapists have attempted to dissuade their clients from bringing or pursuing these suits because of the emotional damage they can cause the client and her family.
    b. Therapists are almost equally split in terms of whether they support their clients in these lawsuits or try to discourage them.
    c. Often the suits are encouraged by therapists as a part of the therapy of empowerment.
    d. Generally, it is the therapists who persuade the clients to initiate the law suits as a way of achieving closure and healing.
    Answer: c   LO: 25; factual, conceptual   page: 570

88. According to Elizabeth Loftus (1993), with respect to repressed memories:
    a. women who were sexually abused early in childhood are likely to repress the painful memories until they are triggered by some event later in life.
    b. women who are in therapy are highly vulnerable and seeking answers to their distress, and are easily pressured by their therapists to create memories of abuse.
    c. there is extensive support for the notion of repressed memories, as evidenced by victims of post-traumatic stress disorder.
    d. it is extremely difficult to instill false memories into anyone, whether adult or child.
    Answer: b   LO: 25; conceptual   page: 570

Chapter 16

89. Loftus (1993) and others (e.g., Ceci et al., 1988) state that people can be made to believe that things that never happened to them actually did. On the other hand, Pezdek (e.g., 1997) has conducted research that found it is easy to plant false memories for an event that is consistent with what "might have happened," but not for events that are inconsistent with what "might have happened." This research would offer support for:
    a. repressed memory claims.
    b. those who believe there is no such thing as repression.
    c. those who believe the memories of abuse have been falsely planted.
    d. neither side of this debate.
    Answer: a   LO: 25; conceptual   page: 571

90. When Cathy was about 8 years old, she began to demonstrate symptoms of depression. Noticing the change in her daughter's behavior, Ann took the entire family for counseling. During the sessions, the therapist tried to determine whether Cathy had experienced any form of sexual abuse, but the child denied that this happened. When she was in her mid-20s, Cathy's brother died. At the memorial service, a relative approached Cathy and touched her on the shoulder. The memories of sexual abuse came flooding back and she immediately confronted the man who had touched her. He acknowledged that he had molested her on several occasions when she was a child and said that he had been in prolonged therapy to overcome his deviant behavior. When Ann began to ask Cathy about the process of forgetting, the young woman began to recall that she had remembered it for a while, and then gradually she became completely amnesic for the abuse. This case study would:
    a. support the notion that memories cannot be planted by a therapist.
    b. suggest that we may forget things when they are not important to us.
    c. support the notion that memories can be repressed.
    d. suggest that repression does not exist, although forgetting does.
    Answer: c   LO: 25; applied   pages: 570-572

91. The rules governing the insanity defense suggest that law takes a _____ perspective to psychological disorders.
    a. biological
    b. psychodynamic
    c. cognitive
    d. psychosocial
    Answer: a   LO: 5; factual   page: 572

92. The legal approach tends to legitimize the _____ approach to psychological disorders.
    a. cognitive
    b. behavioral
    c. humanistic
    d. medical
    Answer: d   LO: 5; factual   page: 572

-387-

Society and Mental Health

93. The patients' rights movements focus on the _____ forces that drive people to engage in lawful or unlawful behaviors.
    a. behavioral
    b. psychodynamic
    c. social
    d. biological
    Answer: c   LO: 14; factual   page: 572

94. Which of the following is *not* a guideline set out by the American Psychological Association for providing ethical service to culturally diverse populations?
    a. educating clients to the processes of psychological intervention
    b. educating clients to the values and beliefs of the dominant culture
    c. being aware of relevant research and practice issues relating to the population served
    d. recognizing ethnicity and culture as significant parameters in understanding psychological processes
    Answer: b   LO: 17; factual   page: 575

95. If a therapist is unable to communicate with a client in the language that the client prefers, the therapist should:
    a. learn that language.
    b. encourage the client to try to communicate in the therapist's language.
    c. make an appropriate referral to a therapist who speaks the language.
    d. try to communicate nonverbally.
    Answer: c   LO: 17; factual, conceptual   page: 575

Chapter 16

Essay Questions

96. Discuss the history of the insanity defense and the criteria used to evaluate defendants' pleas that they should be absolved of responsibility for their actions. What are the five criteria that have been used to evaluate these claims? Explain how each criterion broadened or restricted the use of the insanity defense and how it did so. What are some of the difficulties faced when judges and juries attempt to apply these criteria? Which of the five criteria do you think is best, and why?

    A proper answer should identify and discuss the five criteria used to evaluate defendants' pleas that they should not be held accountable for their actions (e.g., the Durham Rule). It should be noted and explained how each criterion affected the insanity defense (e.g., the Durham Rule broadened the criteria for inanity by including any and all mental disorders or defects). Difficulties with these criteria should be discussed as well (e.g., the Durham Rule allows for defendants to be exonerated for any mental illness or defect, even if there is no evidence that the defect caused them to perform the criminal act of which they are accused). Finally, the most favored criterion should be identified and defended (or, if none is adequate, it should be explained what an appropriate alternative might be).

97. Who may be committed to a psychiatric institution? Identify and discuss the criteria and circumstances under which a person may be involuntarily committed for psychiatric treatment. What rights do committed persons have? Do you think that civil commitment is justified? Why or why not?

    A proper answer should identify and discuss the criteria used to justify civil commitment (e.g., dangerousness to others) and the rights of civilly committed people (e.g., the right to treatment). A stance should also be taken on the issue and defended appropriately.

98. The patients' rights movement had the intent of moving the mentally disabled out of mental institutions ("deinstitutionalization") and into community-based facilities. What were the basic "patients' rights" referred to, in connection with both institutionalization and deinstitutionalization? What was the outcome of deinstitutionalization? How might the wrongs that have occurred be corrected?

The student should address the various rights at issue, such as the right to receive treatment, as well as the right to refuse treatment. Deinstitutionalization was aimed at both providing the least restrictive environment possible considering the patient's condition and the focus on placing the mentally ill within the community rather than isolating them or warehousing them in institutions. Unfortunately, the communities by and large did not have the funds to place the patients into group homes, halfway houses, etc., and now many of the mentally ill are wandering the streets, homeless and untreated. The student should present some cogent ideas for resolving this dilemma.

99. Mental health professionals have become familiar faces in the legal system. Describe the many functions that they serve, the roles they play, and the pros and cons of having psychologists involved in these matters.

Mental health professionals now participate in legal proceedings in two important areas: criminal proceedings and proceedings involving children (e.g., custody, child maltreatment, etc.). They serve as investigators, evaluators, and expert witnesses (the student should go in-depth here to describe what they do in each role); their recommendations are given more weight in criminal trials than in proceedings involving children. One of the benefits of involving mental health workers is that witnesses (child or adult) are more comfortable talking to them than to other persons who might interview them; one problem revolves around providing a "typical" profile, since not everyone who commits a crime fits the profile, and many people who fit the profile do not commit the crimes alleged.

Chapter 16

100. Explain the issues involved in the repressed memory debate. What evidence is there to support the existence of repressed memories; what evidence supports claims that memories are "planted" by therapists. How do these memories affect the parties involved (particularly the clients and their families)? Which side of the debate would you support, and why?

Here the student needs to explain repressed memories (events that happened in a person's life for which the person has total amnesia, or the memories appear only in fragmented flashbacks or dreams); recovered memories (memories that had been repressed that surface after some triggering event, such as a woman's child reaching the age when the woman was molested, or a therapist eliciting these memories from a client during treatment); and false memory syndrome (the "planting" by a therapist of memories for events, such as molestation, that never occurred). Among the evidence supporting repressed memories is the fact that in many instances the memories have been corroborated, often by a witness to the event or even by the perpetrator; Loftus' research in planting false or misleading memories suggests the vulnerability of memory to suggestion, however, Pezdek and others have noted that it is much easier to "plant" memories that are consistent with what might have happened than to plant memories that are inconsistent with past possibilities. The student should discuss the issues of empowering clients by working through and confronting these traumatic events, but also the fact that some families have been torn apart by accusations of false memories. Then the student should provide a well-thought-out position for either side and support his or her rationale for that position.

101. Client confidentiality is a critical element of therapy. Without this guarantee, clients may be unwilling to engage in this most intimate of relationships. To what extent does a client justifiably have an expectation of complete confidentiality? When does that guarantee cease to exist? Describe (and name) the case that led to the cessation of complete confidentiality. What do you believe is the consequence of no longer totally protecting this right?

The clinician has a responsibility to the client (to assist the client in overcoming the problems that bring the person to therapy) and to society (to protect anyone, including the client, from harm the client may inflict). Lacking severe harm that may be caused by the client, the client has an expectation of confidentiality, without which she or he would not feel free to express her/his inner most thoughts and feelings--therapy would be jeopardized without this guarantee. The student must address the limits of confidentiality (e.g., intent to inflict harm on others) and the *Tarasoff* case--what happened in the case, and its ramifications concerning the guarantee of confidentiality. The student should then discuss what may occur when the client knows that there is no guarantee of confidentiality in certain instances.